You and your doctor
A NEW ZEALAND GUIDE TO BETTER HEALTH CARE

By the same author:
The General Practitioner in New Zealand (1978)
Primary Health Care and the Community (1981)

You and your doctor

A NEW ZEALAND GUIDE TO BETTER HEALTH CARE

J. G. Richards
MBChB, FRNZCGP, FRACP, FRCP(Ed.)

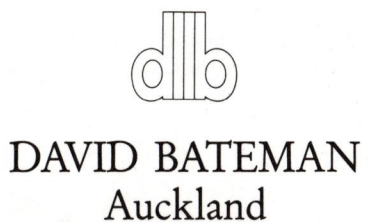

DAVID BATEMAN
Auckland

Copyright © J. G. Richards 1988

First published in 1988 by
David Bateman Ltd
'Golden Heights', 32–34 View Road, Glenfield, Auckland, New Zealand

ISBN 0 908610 85 8

All rights reserved. No part of this publication may be reproduced or transmitted in any form or by any means without the permission of the publishers.

Typeset in Garamond by Typocrafters Ltd
Printed in Hong Kong by Colorcraft
Jacket design — Chris O'Brien
Cartoons — Lincoln Wakefield

Contents

Preface by Dr T. D. S. Seddon, Chairman of Council,
Royal New Zealand College of General Practitioners   9

Introduction   10

Section one — Going to the doctor
1.1	General principles	14
1.2	Telling your story	23
1.3	Taking a child to the doctor	30
1.4	What is a medical emergency?	31
1.5	Why a general practitioner?	32
1.6	The team	36

Section two — Becoming healthy, staying well
2.1	The prevention of illness: the promotion of wellness	42
2.2	Screening for early disease	49
2.3	Commentary on certain screening procedures	66
	(1) Parents at risk of abusing their child	66
	(2) Screening the newborn child	67
	(3) Milestones in the young child's development	68
	(4) Bacteriuria (bacteria in the urine)	69
	(5) Phenylketonuria (PKU)	69
	(6) Congenital dislocation of the hip	70
	(7) Dental caries	70
	(8) Cervical smears (i.e. Papanicolaou or 'Pap' smear)	70
	(9) High blood pressure (hypertension)	71
	(10) Cancer of the breast	72
	(11) Cancer of the lung	75
	(12) Tuberculosis	75
	(13) Cancer of the bowel	75

2.4	The emotions and disease	77
2.5	Diet and health	84
2.6	Special diets	96
2.7	Fitness and exercise	102
2.8	Alcohol and tobacco — threats to health	106

Section three — Some common problems and their causes

3.1	Sore throats	122
3.2	Back problems	124
3.3	Coughs	128
3.4	Abdominal pain	130
3.5	The common cold (coryza)	135
3.6	Headache	137
3.7	Fatigue	140
3.8	Pain in the chest	141
3.9	Fever	143
3.10	Allergic rashes	143
3.11	Problems of face and neck	146
3.12	Vision problems	146
3.13	Weight gain	147
3.14	Vertigo (giddiness)	147
3.15	Earache	149
3.16	High blood pressure	151
3.17	Shortness of breath	152
3.18	Nasal congestion	156
3.19	Non-allergic rashes	158
3.20	Anal and rectal problems	166
3.21	Joint problems	169
3.22	Nervousness	172
3.23	Depression and reactions to loss	173
3.24	Vaginal discharge	174
3.25	Nausea, vomiting and diarrhoea	177
3.26	Pain and irritation of the eye	179
3.27	Menstrual disorders	179
3.28	Acne	182
3.29	Painful urination (dysuria)	183
3.30	Diarrhoea	185
3.31	The menopause	185

Section four — treatment

4.1	Emotional and mental problems	190
4.2	About your medication and reading your prescription	204
4.3	Anti-inflammatory agents	218
4.4	Medicines for the mind and nervous system	225
4.5	The antibacterial medicines ('antibiotics')	235
4.6	Medicines for treating high blood pressure and circulatory disorders	243
4.7	Medicines for the relief of pain	252
4.8	Medicines for the heart	254
4.9	Medicines for the gastro-intestinal system	258
5.	Contraceptives	261
6.	Diabetes	270
7.	AIDS (acquired immune deficiency syndrome)	276
8.	Dementia (including Alzheimer's disease)	279

Appendices

Appendix 1: A brief review of common laboratory tests — 282
Appendix 2: The infectious diseases — a summary — 288
Appendix 3: Cardiopulmonary resuscitation — some questions and answers — 289

Acknowledgements — 291

Reading list — 292

Index — 294

Preface

There is considerable pleasure in supplying a preface for this book as it clearly succeeds in its main aim — to supply information.

This information will be of use not only to patients but also to their carers and relatives, and to everyone else interested in health care.

No general practitioner — and here I speak from 30 years of experience — can serve a population well without working in partnership with the patient and his or her family. The form of this partnership, the variations in the way it works, the healing force that it generates, and the way it builds over time, often being transferred from doctor to doctor, has only recently become more understood. Just how it works, how it can be damaged, how it can be facilitated, are questions being asked, and, as yet, being only partially answered. What is clear so far is that with informed patients, carers and relatives, this healing partnership becomes more effective the more that information is available. This effect is also seen with advice given for preventive health measures.

John Richards has produced a worthwhile book which should cater to a wide spectrum of people. *You and Your Doctor* supplies information on an extensive range of topics and concepts. It is well organised and written in clear language. The effect has been to generally 'de-medicalise' the subject, removing the jargon without patronising the reader. The book sets out to educate and inform. It does it well.

The Council of the Royal New Zealand College of General Practitioners endorses the publication of *You and Your Doctor*.

T. D. S. SEDDON
Chairman of Council
Royal New Zealand College of General Practitioners

Introduction

'The essential unit of medical practice is the occasion when, in the intimacy of the consulting or sick room, a person who is ill or believes himself to be ill, seeks the advice of a doctor whom he trusts. This is a consultation and all else in the practice of medicine derives from it.'
— J. Spence, *The Purpose and Practice of Medicine* (1960)

This book represents a new departure in medical guides. It sets out to place in your hands an easy-to-read book which will help ensure that your family doctor is used to best advantage. In addition, it will give you an indication of what the doctor is likely to ask you, what examinations will be done and what tests you can expect for any of the more common medical ailments. It reviews in detail over 30 problems, outlines possible treatments and describes most of the commonly used medicines prescribed for these and many other complaints.

Section One discusses what you can expect of your general practitioner and offers much good advice on how to prepare yourself or your family for a visit to the doctor. A medical emergency is defined and there is also a short chapter on the doctor's helpers and what they can do for you.

Section Two is concerned with preventive medicine — becoming healthy and staying well. Health maintenance is a topic which has occupied much attention recently and is likely to be of even greater importance in the future. In these pages you will find an account of what orthodox medicine believes is feasible in this area, with listings of the screening procedures which have become established in each age group.

For the first time, the findings of the authoritative Canadian Task Force on the Periodic Health Examination, sponsored by the Department of National Health and Welfare, Ottawa, have been presented in easily understandable form for the interested lay person. Chapters 2.2 and 2.3 are deliberately very full and readers are encouraged to check the sections which relate to themselves, or those for whom they are responsible, to see whether they are receiving all the preventive care that is available and appropriate.

In Section Two further chapters review the place of the emotions in causing disease and discuss diet in relation to general good health and specific medical conditions. There are diets for weight reduction, the prevention of heart disease and the control of allergies. Kilocalorie values are listed for most foods and further tables give useful information about other food content which is difficult to obtain elsewhere. Chapter 2.7 deals with fitness and the value of exercise, includes a warm-up routine suited to a person at any level of fitness and outlines the 'half-as-much' approach for the sedentary and others new to regular strenuous exercise. Section Two concludes with a chapter on the diagnosis and management of alcoholism and tobacco dependence.

Section Three is based on studies of the 30 or so most frequent problems seen by the general practitioner and gives an indication of the most likely causes and the usual diagnostic approach.

Section Four is on treatment. It commences with a chapter on the role of psychological medicine which highlights the fact that not all treatment is drug related. There follows a very practical chapter on how medicines* should be taken and why some preparations get an undeserved reputation for effectiveness. Readers are encouraged to decipher their own prescriptions. Chapters 4.3 to 4.9 present a simplified account of most of the commonly used medicines — how they work and what can be expected of them, together with some indication of possible side-effects. Throughout the text generic names of all medicines are quoted, with the trade names given in parentheses afterwards.

Chapter 5 is about contraception and contains an account of the contraceptive pill, including an outline of how it can be adjusted by the doctor, in consultation with the patient, to minimise unwanted side-effects. Other methods of contraception are also surveyed.

Because diabetes is so common, a chapter on this condition has been included here, together with chapters on AIDS and dementia (including Alzheimer's disease), two further medical problems in which there is currently great interest.

The appendices contain a simple account of the significance of the most frequently used laboratory tests, a summary of the infectious diseases and some practical suggestions on cardiopulmonary resuscitation.

In these pages I have not attempted to discuss 'alternative or ethnic medicine', a field so wide it would need another book to cover it usefully. I would like to emphasise that a great many of the books which are available today espouse unorthodox and often unproven theories of medical treatment. Some of these theories, when put into practice, do more harm than good and delay the receipt of conventional, well-proven therapy. What you read here is, as far as possible, in keeping with what doctors are currently being taught in medical schools. The list on p. 293 contains books on topics discussed which readers may like to study further.

How to use this book

I would suggest that everyone reads Section One, the first two chapters of Section Two and also from Chapter 2.4 through to the end of that section. In Section Three, which deals with common problems and their causes, look for the relevant chapter in the Contents list on p. 5 if you have a medical complaint or have been put on treatment. Similarly, information in Appendix 1 on the common blood and urine tests is likely to be of most interest if you

---

*Note that throughout this text the word 'drug' has been used as little as possible. In fact it is a term which has been used widely for many years for medicines, but latterly much has been heard about 'drug abuse' and the word has been debased, coming to be associated with dependency and illicit activities. To avoid confusion, alternative terms have been used whenever possible in these pages.

have had such tests. Everyone should read Chapter 4.2, 'About your medication and reading your prescription.'

Concerning Section Four, where generic and trade names of medicines are quoted, I must confess that it has not been possible to list all the brands of all the medications on the market. If you seek information about a medicine which you are taking, look for it first in the index. If it is not listed there, try to find out what its official (generic) name is and check for that in the index. If you are still not successful, it may be possible to determine which major family of medicines it belongs to and so get information about the whole group.

Some doctors who have read this book, while applauding its purpose, have considered that it is too full. I believe, however, that as a profession we tend to underestimate the ability of the public to understand medical matters and assimilate health-promoting advice. I am convinced that an informed patient is the doctor's best ally. Studies clearly indicate that patients who understand the nature of their condition, and the significance of what the doctor says and does, are much more likely to persevere with treatment or preventive measures, and so have a greater chance of keeping healthy. It is my hope that *You and your doctor* will help towards the achievement of that end.

SECTION ONE
Going to the doctor

1.1 General principles

'The more complex medicine becomes, the stronger the reasons why everyone should have a personal doctor who will take continuous responsibility for him and, knowing how he lives, will keep things in proportion, protecting him if need be from the zealous specialist.'
— T. F. Fox, 'The Personal Doctor', *Lancet*, 1960

It should be a basic premise in health care that all should have the right — and it should not be regarded as a luxury — to have a medical advisor who is familiar with their background, both medical and social; someone with whom they feel comfortable and not in any way threatened; someone to whom they can confide their concerns about health, both physical and emotional, and with whom they can discuss their health needs in the present and in the future; someone who is capable of managing the majority of their ailments, can advise about other levels of care, and who can provide continuity and examine problems in the context of the family and the community.

What can you expect of your general practitioner?
(a) A well trained professional who has completed an accredited university course and obtained at least a basic medical degree.
(b) A doctor who has specific postgraduate training or experience directed to the needs of general practice. This training will usually require at least three years of in-service supervised experience prior to independent practice.
(c) A doctor who will listen with care and concern to the description of your problems and who is prepared to give you adequate time.
(d) A doctor who as far as possible will give your problem his or her full attention throughout the time you are present in the consulting room. (Telephones and other interruptions are sometimes unavoidable.)
(e) A doctor who will bring to bear on your problems the full benefits of his or her experience and who makes a point of keeping abreast of medical advances.
(f) A doctor who will tell you what is thought to be the problem, what treatment is available, and the likely outcome of the treatment if you accept it.

(g) A doctor who will keep strictly confidential the information supplied by you. If it is important that other people be informed, your permission will be sought before this is done.
(h) A doctor who will not make unjustified assumptions about you or jump to conclusions, and is not judgemental.
(i) A doctor who will allow you to ask questions about any aspect of the disorder or its management.
(j) A doctor who will encourage you to take part in the decision-making process so that you have the opportunity to refuse the treatment or course of action suggested, if you think it seems undesirable.
(k) A doctor who will maintain a continuing interest in your welfare and will also provide emergency care, personally or by deputy, should you require this at any time.
(l) A doctor who will take an interest in disease prevention and who if you are already ill will advise you how to avoid recurrences and/or minimise complications.
(m) A doctor who will be reasonably accessible so that you can seek advice without undue delay.
(n) A doctor who will provide an equal standard of care to all patients regardless of age, race, religion, sex or other considerations.
(o) A doctor who will be prepared to attend you in your own home should that be necessary.
(p) A doctor who will keep adequate records of your medical history and treatment and of risk factors in your constitution and background.
(q) A doctor who will look upon you as a person, and not merely as the bearer of a disordered organ. This will include taking an interest in you as a family and community member.

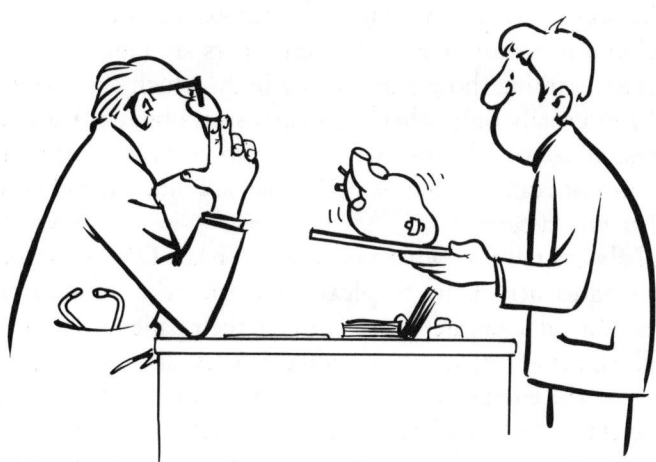

(r) A doctor who will provide adequate facilities to enable the provision of high quality care.
(s) A doctor who knows his or her own limitations and who will be prepared to refer you on to specialist services where appropriate.

(t) A doctor who maintains good physical and mental health so that he or she can provide the highest possible standards of patient care.
(u) A doctor who is not embarrassed or upset if you ask for a second opinion.

What you should *not* expect of your general practitioner

(a) A prescription for medicine at every consultation.

(b) A definite diagnosis for every symptom. Studies have shown that in any one month approximately 75 per cent of the population experiences some abnormal symptom or sign. Most of these complaints are fleeting and of no serious consequence to patient or doctor and will resolve without treatment. General practitioners are taught to be adept at sorting the wheat from the chaff, and usually they can at least be quite certain whether a condition is going to require urgent attention or whether a delay is acceptable. Often it is prudent for the doctor not to venture a diagnosis in ill-defined conditions as this may well create unnecessary anxiety in the mind of the patient. If symptoms or signs persist, it may later become important to isolate the exact cause of the problem if that is possible.

Sometimes because patients seem to expect it, doctors may give vague labels to a collection of symptoms which do not fit any recognisable disease pattern. A favourite one is 'the menopause'. Many women with an unexplained symptom have in the past been told that their problem is part of the 'change of life' or 'menopause'. Some women become even more apprehensive, especially if they have friends or relatives who are quick to embellish their existing ideas with alarming stories about the problems they may encounter. Many women do get problems at this time in their life, but a great many things are attributed to the 'change' which have little or nothing to do with it.

(c) A complete examination at every consultation. A full examination, which is always very time consuming, is seldom necessary. General practitioners are taught to review a patient's medical history and then examine those parts of the body which are essential to the formulation of a diagnosis. It is usually only when the diagnosis is obscure that a full examination is desirable. Sometimes, of course, doctors are lazy or so pressed for time that even those parts of the examination that really should be performed are omitted and you do not receive the quality of care that you deserve.

(d) A doctor who will always tell you what you want to hear. Doctors want to be liked by their patients and have an earnest desire to please. Sometimes it is important that patients be told unpleasant facts. Some doctors are reluctant to tell their patients that they are alcoholics, for example. They will tell patients that they should drink less alcohol and give other relevant information, but never say the fateful words. There are two reasons for this. Firstly, it is often hard to be absolutely certain of physical or emotional dependence on alcohol, and secondly, the doctor's concern that making such a diagnosis is being judgemental and that the patient will seek medical attention elsewhere.

Many true alcoholics will not take significant steps to tackle the problem until someone has the courage to put the label 'alcoholic' on them. As a result there are often serious delays before appropriate treatment is obtained.

(e) A doctor who can afford to give you unlimited time without extra charge. If you take up a lot of the doctor's time and the fee is not increased to allow for this (assuming that the doctor is working on a fee-for-service basis), it is reasonable to assume that the doctor will be out of pocket. The expenses of the practice, which usually amount to about 50 per cent of the fee, continue at all times regardless of what the doctor is doing.

(f) A doctor who is always 'sweetness and light'. Doctors are human too, and everybody has their 'off' days when they are not at their best and we all have our personal worries and upheavals. Inevitably the quality of work performed will reflect this from time to time. Tiredness can also be a factor. If your doctor is regularly below par and not performing adequately, it may be time to seek a change.

A special relationship

The relationship between you and your doctor should be a very special one, as will be emphasised at various times in this book. It is a mistake for you to regard a visit to the doctor in the same light as say a visit to the grocer or even a visit to a pharmacist. This is not to belittle the role that such people play in our everyday lives and in meeting certain physical needs, but a good medical practitioner should be particularly sensitive to your feelings, and be aware of, and take into account, a multitude of psychological forces, especially in the presence of sickness.

Life and death decisions

The choice of doctor is a very personal and important decision and in some instances may ultimately make the difference between life and death or between sickness and health.

It is not every day that a general practitioner is called upon to make decisions that can make the difference between life and death, but it does happen more often than most people realise. The most obvious situation is that of a medical emergency such as an acute asthma attack or an epileptic fit. Under these circumstances it may be crucial that you receive the right medication, in the right dosage, at the right time. Less obvious situations may be the choice of medicines in a chronic condition or the combination of two or more medications.

Another very difficult decision may be whether to hospitalise or not. If every general practitioner hospitalised all the patients who caused any anxiety, the hospitals would not be able to cope, and patients with conditions which can only be dealt with in hospital would not be able to get the help they need. So the general practitioner has to weigh up who can safely be cared for at home and who needs hospital admission. A hospital admission has intrinsic hazards and sometimes you may be better served by remaining at home when this is feasible. A lot of people, particularly the elderly and young children, will pick up infections in hospital which they would be unlikely to catch if they were nursed at home. Similarly, some elderly folk are perfectly well able to find their way around their own home, but as soon as they are moved to another environment they become confused and disorientated.

Limitations

Good doctors are aware of their own limitations and will refer you to a more experienced or knowledgeable colleague when appropriate. Remember, however, that such a recourse to authority is not always immediately available and general practitioners may also have to make a decision on how long you can reasonably wait for a second opinion without detriment to your health.

Where the delay seems unreasonable, the general practitioner can sometimes bring influence to bear to ensure that the consultation with a specialist or respected colleague occurs earlier than it otherwise would. General practitioners will keep a check on the work of specialist colleagues, learning who does what, does it best, gets on well with certain personalities and so on. In this way a general practitioner may help you to choose the best person to meet your specific needs. Often, general practitioners will ask you if you have any special wishes concerning the choice of specialist, and usually these are granted. Sometimes the general practitioner knows that a specialist suggested by you has limitations in some particular area, and may gently attempt to dissuade you from seeing that person.

One has to remember that no one person can be an expert at everything and this applies to the specialties no less than to general practice. Most general practitioners have a wide range of expertise but obviously have to refer some problems, but only about 3 per cent on average. This percentage will vary a little from place to place and from person to person. Newly qualified doctors may refer because they are aware of their lack of experience or they may not refer because they know they are up-to-date with recent advances. Older practitioners may or may not refer, for exactly the opposite reasons.

Confidence

Some patients may lack confidence in a young doctor who appears inexperienced and often an aware doctor will sense this early and offer a referral before being asked for it. This may save you from what is often perceived as an embarrassing situation — asking a doctor for a second opinion.

Unfortunately not every specialist recognises such consultations for what they are; that is, not so much a request for a diagnosis or assistance with management, as a call for help in reinforcing patient confidence in their own doctor. Nevertheless, if you are not satisfied with a diagnosis or treatment, you should not be shy about requesting a specialist opinion. In medical matters, peace of mind is very important.

Consumer studies

A number of studies have been done in an effort to determine what sort of doctor patients want. I did such a study some years ago in New Zealand using a questionnaire modified from one used by Anne Cartwright in Britain. The results which she obtained and mine were very similar.

The qualities most valued in a general practitioner were a good manner and approachability. Knowledge, capability and thoroughness came a distant second. The qualities most often deemed to be absent in general practitioners were good communication and satisfactory interpersonal relationships.

Changing doctors

Many people express concern about the idea of changing their doctor, believing that it contravenes 'medical ethics'. They do not realise that medical ethics relate to the doctor's behaviour towards patients and colleagues. You, the patient are not bound by any code of ethics other than the normal rules of human behaviour established in any civilised community. There is no ethical objection to you changing doctors at any time. Sometimes, of course, there are good practical reasons why this may be undesirable. If you, the patient, have had good caring service from a doctor for many years and the doctor has come to know you well, it is probably unhelpful to interfere with that relationship. Usually a doctor who is thoroughly familiar with your past history and social circumstances will be much more effective than one who has only limited and recent knowledge, although this of course will depend greatly on the nature of the complaint.

There is also the problem of having to explain an often complicated past history to a new doctor and perhaps having to resurrect embarrassing matters, now half forgotten.

On the other hand, some doctor-patient relationships over a long period of time slip into a casual familiarity which becomes counter-productive. A doctor who is seeing a patient very frequently for some complaint such as high blood pressure may fail to detect relatively insidious changes such as those caused by deteriorating thyroid function (i.e. hypothyroidism). A new doctor may identify such an abnormality at first glance. There are probably few doctors who have worked as locum tenens who have not had the satisfaction of diagnosing such a condition which has been overlooked by the usually more experienced doctor that they are relieving.

Dissatisfaction Where there is dissatisfaction with a doctor, it is much better to change to another than to persevere with an unproductive relationship. Unfortunately this is not always possible and in some countries there are bureaucratic barriers to the easy transfer from one doctor to another.

Use this privilege to select the best doctor for you, remembering that the best doctor is not necessarily the one who treats you exactly the way you think you should be treated. For example, some people expect their doctor to prescribe antibiotics for every trivial infection rather than use judgement and experience.

More than one doctor

Some people elect to be attended by more than one doctor. This often happens in large cities. When you are at work, it is possibly more convenient to attend a doctor whose office is adjacent to your workplace. This saves taking time off work in order to see your usual doctor who probably consults in a suburban practice close to your home. This can be satisfactory providing there is first-class communication between the two doctors. If there is not, as is usually the case, neither knows what is going on and sometimes the two will work at cross purposes. Furthermore, neither will know who has primary responsibility for you. A system of patient registration with a single nominated doctor, as in Britain, does away with this difficulty.

Doctors are not supposed to tout for work, but with the new emphasis on preventive medicine there is often a need to recall patients for inoculations or for special checkups. Any doctor who writes to you suggesting that it is time for a preventive inoculation (for example against german measles (rubella)) is in danger of criticism from other practitioners, if another doctor is treating you also. This can be perceived as 'stealing' patients and for this reason some doctors are reluctant to institute such services for anyone other than those who they feel confident obtain *all* their medical attention from them.

What is perhaps more common is for a patient to live in an outer suburb but regularly attend only a central city practitioner. Such city practitioners are seldom able to provide night or weekend services for their far-flung patients and so when an emergency occurs at home, the patient has no one to turn to.

Out-of-hours calls to an unknown practitioner If you are lucky, a phone call to a local practitioner will produce a sympathetic response and usually in a real emergency some help can be obtained. Sometimes, however, the local practitioner takes the view that he or she can only be responsible for a defined group of patients and cannot be available to the whole city and advises you to call your own doctor. If you are left stranded you really have little other than your own lack of forethought to blame for the situation. For this reason it is best when seeking a doctor to try to find what arrangements are made for out-of-hours services. If these are unsatisfactory, then you should look for another doctor who can provide adequate out-of-hours care.

Problems in rural districts

In rural districts the problems can be more difficult. Frequently there is only one doctor and change is impossible without much travel and the prospect of long delays or lack of attention in emergencies. In many circumstances it is best then for you to discuss with the doctor any dissatisfactions you may have with the quality of care that is provided. This takes a lot of courage, but at least it gives the doctor an opportunity to explain the reasons for his or her actions and to make changes where these are appropriate. It may be that your expectations are unreasonable and sometimes an effort should be made to see the doctor's point of view.

Such an approach often clears the air and lays the way to the development of a really good working relationship. If, however, it seems that differences are irreconcilable, then it is usually wise to make a clean break, if that is possible. You should then decide who is going to be your new doctor so that your former practitioner can forward your records to the new choice.

Sometimes, after they have attended a new doctor a few times, patients realise that they were getting better attention from their former doctor. This should not happen too often, because before changing, it is sensible to make judicious inquiries about any proposed new practitioner from friends and acquaintances who attend that doctor. Remember, however, that we are all different and a doctor who suits one personality may not suit another.

Some suggestions

The following suggestions may be useful in helping you to get the best value from your general practitioner.

1. Make sure that you have a general practitioner who accepts responsibility for your medical care, i.e. regards you as his or her patient. Before you decide on a particular doctor, find out from the receptionist what consulting hours are kept and what out-of-hours services are provided.

2. Find out the best time to ask for house calls, should these be necessary, and how long ahead you need to book for non-urgent appointments. Do not wait until you are down to your last tablet before seeking an appointment.

3. Sometimes doctors are fully booked and when asked for a consultation the receptionist may offer an appointment several days ahead. If you feel sure that a consultation is needed as soon as possible, explain fully what is wrong, and if necessary ask to speak to the doctor. (See section on 'The team', p. 36.) Try to ring for an appointment early in the day rather than waiting until the last possible minute in the evening, in the hope that the condition will improve. Most doctors would prefer to see an occasional patient, perhaps unnecessarily, early in the day, rather than have a long list of patients to see when tired at the end of a busy day.

4. Have a clear idea of what you want the doctor to do for you in the time available. Before you see the doctor, think over carefully how you are going to describe your symptoms briefly but fully, ignoring irrelevancies. (See section on 'Telling your story', p. 24.) If you have several problems, tell the doctor about them all at the beginning of the interview so that the time can be divided up profitably. From the doctor's point of view there are few things worse than a patient who mentions a major problem for the first time just as the interview is drawing to a close.

5. Do not leave out, or make light of, important symptoms with the idea that the doctor is so clever that they need not be mentioned.

6. If you have a major problem to discuss or several family members to be seen, ask the receptionist to give you extra time and be prepared to pay for it if necessary. Many doctors like a double appointment for a first maternity visit also.

7. Always remember that time is very important to the doctor, just as it is, of course, to most patients. If possible, do not cancel an appointment at short notice. Your doctor may not be able to fill the appointment in the time available, possibly losing money as a consequence. It also means that other people may be denied access.

8. It is preferable to have all the family in the care of one doctor. A doctor can usually serve you best when having a knowledge of the whole family. Similarly, if possible, try to get all your medical advice through the same doctor. If you do have to get advice elsewhere, see that your usual general practitioner knows about this, so that a complete record of your medical history may be maintained.

9. Do not be afraid to ask any question of your doctor. Part of the doctor's task is to help you understand your complaint and how best to deal with it. This is much better than saying 'the doctor did not tell me anything'. Maybe you gave the impression that you did not want to know.

10. Make sure that you wear clothes which will come off easily and quickly so that time will not be wasted while you struggle with tight clothes when the doctor decides to examine you. Similarly, never assume that the doctor will not require to do an examination, however trivial the complaint may appear to you.

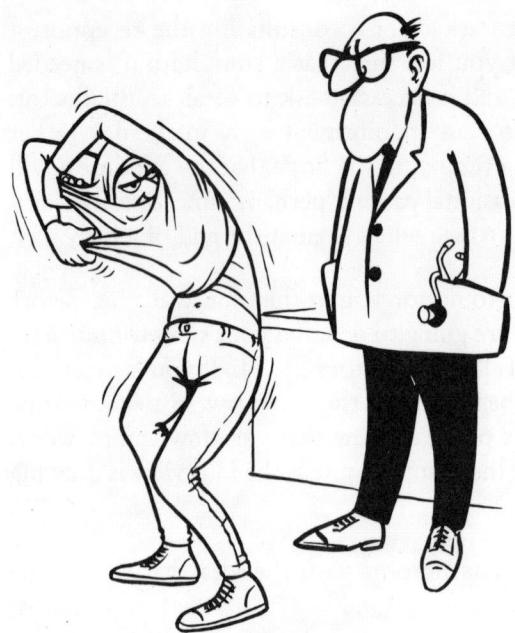

11. If you want to transfer to another general practitioner, it is both courteous to the doctor who has been looking after you and, of course, to your advantage to discuss the move, or at least notify your doctor so that your records can be transferred.

12. It is always in order to ask your doctor to arrange a second opinion, if you feel you need one.

13. It is often important for doctors to have details of very confidential matters. For this reason people often prefer to have as their doctor someone who is not a close personal friend or relative. Thus, if you are a close relative of a doctor or see a doctor socially quite frequently, it may be very difficult to tell that doctor about some sexual indiscretion, a misdemeanour of which you are not very proud, or even intimate details of a perfectly ordinary marriage.

Most people on such occasions prefer a doctor who is not a personal friend, nor someone who is met up with regularly on a social basis.

14. In a similar way, most doctors prefer not to take responsibility for the medical care of their own families. Close involvement and excessive concern can lead to a lack of objectivity on the part of the doctor so that judgment is clouded and mistakes are easily made. Many doctors' families have difficulty in understanding this reluctance and they try to pressure their spouse or parent into giving them treatment. If treatment is unsuccessful, confidence is seriously undermined.

15. In each district there is a complaints officer who can be contacted, if you have a complaint against a doctor. This is a service sponsored by the Medical Association.

1.2 Telling your story

'Hannah More wondered why people should be so fond of the company of their physician till she recollected that he was the only person with whom one dared to talk continually of oneself, without interruption, contradiction or censure.'
— Sir Robert Hutchinson, *British Medical Journal*, 1934

It is often a good idea to spend some time before you visit the doctor considering just how you will explain your problem. If it is a first visit, the doctor or the nurse may want a lot of background information. Here are some of the things that may be required for your record, which is often referred to as your *medical history*.

Basic information
Full name, address, phone number (home and work), next of kin, insurer (if insured), date of birth, country of birth, marital status, religion, occupation. Past illnesses. Immunisations, with dates. Illnesses suffered by your parents, brothers and/or sisters or other close relatives, including mental illness.
Any illnesses that you are known to be predisposed to.
Any hospital admissions, with dates.
Any problems such as allergies, particularly to previously administered medicines.
Any special dietary regime that you have adopted.
Whether you smoke or drink and the amount. (Be honest.)
Any medicines that you are taking. Remember to mention the contraceptive pill and any proprietary medicines or vitamins that you are buying from the chemist.
Any exposure to chemicals or other hazards at work.
It may also be very important for the doctor to be aware of any major problems in your life, e.g. anxiety about examinations, or disagreements with parents, or tension between a married couple.

The reason for the visit
It is useful at the commencement of the consultation to make known to the doctor what you believe to be the main reason for your visit. Thus it could be that the real reason for

seeing the doctor is that you are afraid that something you have noticed could be due to cancer. There is nothing to be ashamed about in saying this; it is a very natural and almost universal fear. Alternatively it could be that all you want is the doctor to confirm that you are unwell and unable to work and provide you with a note for your employer.

Rather than indicating what they want from the doctor, many people start by describing the symptoms and the doctor sometimes prescribes medicines which are not really wanted or needed because the patient has failed to make it clear that they are there only because their employer demands a note. Just because a patient is sufficiently unwell to warrant time off, does not mean that they are going to need medication.

Telling your story

It is probably now time to describe the symptoms or signs which have led you to seek medical attention. Try and recall exactly when they started and what was the very first thing you noticed. Then describe in as much detail as you can, with times, the development of the problem.

Thus you might start by saying: 'On Tuesday evening four days ago, I first noticed that my throat was sore. By next morning it was considerably worse and I had developed an irritable cough and a congested nose. At the same time I noticed that I felt feverish, and that night I had a sweat. Two days after the onset, the cough had started to become productive and the material I produced was thick and had a grey-green colour. I also noticed about this time that there was a discharge from the back of my nose into the throat. Yesterday my left ear had a sharp throbbing pain which was only eased by aspirin and it remains very sore today. I notice that I seem to hear less well from that ear. I am feeling really wretched and have not had much interest in food for three days. I also have a dull headache which seems to be there particularly when I feel feverish. The whole of the head is involved but it is relieved a little when I lie flat in bed.'

Providing such a clear history can save an amazing amount of time and means that the doctor has a really good idea of how you have been affected. Sometimes it is worth adding something such as, 'The pain in the ear is the thing that bothers me most and I wonder if my hearing is going to be permanently damaged.'

Many people give their history in such a jumbled, piecemeal way that it is like putting together a jigsaw puzzle. Most doctors are good at this, but it can be very time consuming and the main message can be missed.

Describing symptoms It is also helpful to give as much information about individual symptoms as you can.

Pains are particularly hard to describe. Try to sort out the characteristics of the pain first in terms of the type of pain. Thus, is it a sharp pain or a dull pain; a tearing pain or a stabbing pain; a constant pain or an intermittent one? How severe is it?

Does the pain rise slowly to a crescendo and then fade away, perhaps disappearing altogether for a time? What are the time characteristics of the pain? Where is the pain? Is it always in the same spot and does it seem to radiate anywhere?

What things (such as movement) make the pain worse and what things (such as local heat or rest) make the pain easier? Are there any other symptoms which occur at the same time as the pain, such as sweating or nausea? The doctor will probably also want to know whether you have ever suffered such a pain before.

If your description is complete, it may in itself be enough to give the doctor a clear indication of the most likely diagnosis.

Body systems

There are a variety of questions a doctor may ask relating to particular body systems. Thus, for the **digestive system** the following questions might be asked:
Have you a good appetite?
Are you on a diet?
What is your weight doing?
Do you eat between meals?
Do you have difficulty swallowing food?
Does the food seem to stick on the way down?
Do you get a sensation of sour/acid material coming up to the back of your throat?
Do you get any sensation of burning or other discomfort behind the breastbone (sternum)?
Do you suffer from 'indigestion'. How does it affect you? What seems to bring it on?
Do you get pain in the abdomen?
Is the pain always in the same place?
Have you had any vomiting or diarrhoea?
Do you bring up much wind? Do you pass much wind from the back passage (flatus)?
Are your bowels regular? Do you have more than one motion daily? Are the bowel motions (faeces) properly formed? Are they discoloured — either very pale or very dark?
Is there ever blood with the motions?
Is there mucus with the motions? (Mucus is white or colourless, usually slightly oily, material.)
Do you suffer from haemorrhoids (piles)?

For the **genito-urinary system** the doctor might pose the following questions:
Do you have pain on passing water?
Do you have to rush to get to the toilet (i.e. urgency)?
Do you pass water very frequently?
Do you have to get up at night to pass water (If 'yes' — how often?)
Is your water discoloured? Have you ever passed blood?
Do you get abnormally thirsty?
Have you had a rash or irritation around the water passage?
Do you have trouble starting to pass urine?
Does your water come away when you do not wish it?
Does sneezing, coughing, lifting or reaching up cause you to pass a little water?
Do you wet the bed at night?

For women:
Are your periods regular?
Are you using contraceptives?
Is the amount of the loss greater than usual?
How many pads do you use for each period?
Is there any blood loss between periods?
Is there any discharge between periods?
Do you suffer any irritation in the genital area?
Is there any pain on intercourse?
Is there pain with the periods?
Is there pain between periods?
Are you able to achieve orgasm?

For men:
Is there any discharge from the penis (i.e male organ)?
Have you had any sores on the penis?
Is there irritation of the penis?
Is there difficulty in retracting the foreskin?
Has there been any swelling or pain in or around the testicles?
Do you have a good stream?
Do you tend to dribble after you have passed water?
Are you able to achieve orgasm?

For the **musculo-skeletal system** questions might include:
Do you have any joint problems? Are they worse at any particular time of the day or night?
Do you have any joint stiffness?
Do you suffer from backache or neck problems?
Have you ever had sciatica or 'lumbago'?
Have you any aching muscles?
Have you ever experienced any injuries to your joints or back?

For **the skin**:
Have you any skin blemishes?
On what part of your body are your skin problems? How do they affect you?
Do the areas weep? Do they itch?
Have you had similar problems before?
Have you noticed things which make the problem worse?

For the **nervous system**:
How is your eyesight?
Do you ever see lights or spots before your eyes?
Do you have difficulty focusing your eyes?

Do you ever see double? Does the double vision go if you cover one eye?
Do you ever see haloes around objects?
Do you ever experience a sensation that things are moving around you or that you are moving while everything else is static?
Do you experience noises in your ears?
How is your hearing?
Do you suffer from headaches? Which part of the head?
Do you get 'pins and needles' in any part of the body, which does not go away rapidly, as when a limb 'goes to sleep'?
Have you any part of the body where the feeling has been lost?
Is your coordination satisfactory?
Do you suffer from unwanted movements of your head or limbs?
Is there any weakness in your limbs or other part of the body?
Have you got complete control of your bowels and bladder?
Is your balance satisfactory?
Do you suffer from fits or blackouts?

Endocrine and metabolic systems:
Does the hot or cold weather affect you unduly?
Have you experienced unexplained tiredness? Do you feel that you are slowing up?
Do you have swollen hands or ankles?
Is your hair falling out? (*For women* — Will your hair take a 'perm'?)
Do you perspire? (Not at all, a little or a lot?)
Do your hands and feet get excessively hot?
Do you suffer from palpitations (regular or irregular thumping of the heart when at rest, or irregular beats on exertion)?
Have your hands developed a tendency to fine trembling?
Do you feel nervous?

Heart and respiration:
Do you get chest pains?
What sort of pains, and when do they occur?
Do the pains radiate to any other part of the body?
In what part of the chest do they occur?
Do you have any other symptoms when the pain is present?
Are you a smoker?
Have you a cough?
What sort of material do you bring up when you cough?
Is it ever bloodstained?
Has it changed in character recently?
Do you get short of breath easily?
Do you get wheezy?

Heart and respiration (cont.)
Can you lie flat in bed or do you have to sit up?
Is the breathlessness worse at any particular time of the day or night?
Do you ever faint or feel light-headed?

Psychiatric:
Do you feel tense and nervous?
Have you ever had a 'nervous breakdown'?
Are you subject to depression?
Do you sleep well at night?
Are you lonely?
Do you have good support from family and friends?
Do you feel that everybody is against you?
Do you feel angry that fate has been so hard on you?
Do you have feelings of worthlessness?
Have you ever seriously contemplated suicide?
Do you feel that you are being persecuted?
Do you find your sex life satisfying?

This is by no means a complete list of questions commonly requiring answers. Individual symptoms will sometimes require special elucidation. Some questions are important in several body systems and some disease processes will involve numerous body systems.

The general practitioner will want information according to which body system is thought to be involved.

Your own words
Doctors prefer you to tell your story in your own words rather than having to ask questions presented in the form indicated above. In this way they feel they are not putting ideas into your head and influencing unduly the way the story is told. It is important that it be told 'like it is' rather than trying to fit the story into some preconceived idea of the disease process. These days doctors are taught to use 'open-ended' questions which often start with the words 'Tell me'. Thus a doctor may say, 'Tell me about the pain in your chest'. It is then up to you to explain in as much detail as possible the exact character of the pain. Usually at the end of this the doctor will ask some specific questions designed to clarify further the description of symptoms, but the more information that comes in your own words without prompting, the better.

Sometimes it is worthwhile for you to jot down on a piece of paper before the interview all the points which you wish to make known to the doctor.

Most doctors are happy for you to refer to such notes, but do not much appreciate having the notes thrust under their noses. They much prefer to hear the story from your own lips. In this way they are better able to identify the way you feel about the problem. Otherwise there is a lot of non-verbal communication which goes unexpressed.

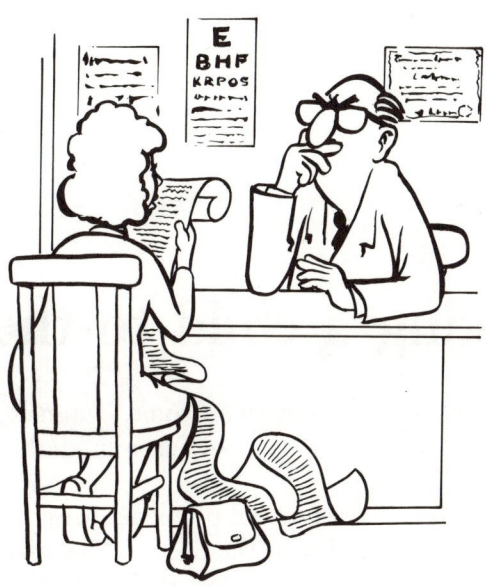

A note about time Any medical consultation should be thought of as a meeting between friends and it is appropriate that at the beginning some pleasantries should be exchanged. It may be important that you and the doctor get to know each other better and feel at ease and it can be an opportunity to obtain information about the wellbeing of your family or aspects of your lifestyle. However, too much discussion about the weather or holidays and the like can be time-consuming and unproductive. As there is a limit to the number of patients that a doctor can reasonably see on any one day, there has to be a limit to the time that is available to any one patient. If you take up more time than is allotted to you — and this is sometimes unavoidable — it will usually mean that someone else gets reduced time or that your doctor will have less time for family life and relaxation at the end of a busy day. Most doctors try to give each patient at least 15 minutes although in some big practices only ten minutes is possible. Occasionally a useful consultation can be briefer than this, but if you are to be adequately examined, advised, a prescription written and questions answered, anything less than ten minutes passes very rapidly and is likely to lead to omissions.

Some doctors regularly work much longer hours than is desirable, often giving a great deal of themselves in the process. If such doctors do not get frequent holidays or other breaks from routine, they are in serious danger of 'burnout' — a phenomenon well known amongst the helping professions. This can lead to an abandonment of general practice or else to a much less dedicated, rather disinterested type of practice and may make them the subject of considerable public criticism. Often they become the malcontents of medicine.

1.3 Taking a child to the doctor

'Infants do not cry without some legitimate cause.'
— Ferrarius, 16th century

Taking a child to the doctor has some special problems. Most youngsters appear to be very apprehensive on the occasion of a visit to the doctor. This may be just a natural fear of a new and unknown environment or it may be that they have sensed your anxiety. Sometimes it is because they feel sick and miserable.

Most doctors acquire some skill at gaining the confidence of their younger patients but this will be aided by a relaxed parental attitude. Even offering rewards in advance for good behaviour while at the doctor may suggest to the child that the encounter is likely to be an ordeal. Honesty with the child is very important. I often hear parents telling their children not to worry, that an injection won't be felt or that it won't hurt, whereas we all know that usually it does.

I am also unhappy with the parent, trying to control a child, who declares, 'If you don't behave, the doctor will give you a hiding'. This immediately creates a fear of the doctor and is similar to the parents who constantly threaten a visit from a policeman.

As far as possible, you should try and control your children while in the doctor's office. Some children are remarkably active and inquisitive and sometimes almost every item of equipment in the room is disturbed in the course of a consultation. As many of these items are delicate and expensive, the doctor may have difficulty giving full concentration to the matter at hand while trying to keep an eye on a restless child. On the other hand, perfect behaviour is not expected and some parents scold a child for almost the slightest movement. This too can make the interview an ordeal.

Some doctors elect to reward good behaviour with sweets. This form of bribery is often effective but I think other rewards are more appropriate. Such actions make a number of non-verbal and incorrect statements to both parents and child, i.e. 1) sweets are a suitable reward for good behaviour, 2) sweets are acceptable food for children.

Usually children are just as pleased to have a picture of an animal or a vehicle stamped or drawn on the back of their hand as a reward.

There are now available some very good children's books which describe a visit to the doctor. These can be read to children and are an excellent way to prepare a youngster for this new experience.

1.4 What is a medical emergency?

What should be regarded as an emergency? This is one of the biggest worries in many households, and it is very hard to provide all-encompassing guidelines. Perhaps the best thing one can say is that when in doubt it is better to call a doctor and be on the safe side. No one should gamble with health.

Many mothers tend to wait until the father comes home before making a decision about their children. I have already commented that it is better to call early in the day if possible, rather than waiting until the evening when probably the doctor is looking forward to a well-earned rest. The condition of children fluctuates so rapidly that often even experienced professionals have difficulty in making this decision in youngsters.

In general, one can say that for all ages:
(**a**) Anyone who is drowsy and lethargic or is experiencing periods of unconsciousness or semi-consciousness without obvious reason probably needs medical assessment. Unconsciousness due to a head injury requires medical attention, as does unexplained neck or back stiffness.
(**b**) Anyone with severe unexplained pain — particularly chest or abdominal pain — should see a doctor promptly.
(**c**) High fever (over 40°C), particularly when the cause is uncertain, or when it is associated with convulsions (fits), clearly needs attention.
(**d**) Extensive loss of blood or other fluids from the body, a rapid, thready pulse, cold sweat, faintness and pallor, either in combination or singly, suggest a need for urgent attention. This includes severe vomiting or diarrhoea.
(**e**) Weakness or numbness of limbs or other parts of the body may be a danger signal if it has not been observed before, as may slurring of speech, confusion or giddiness.

Other urgent situations include:
(**f**) Earache, particularly if it is associated with a temperature and a stuffy nose.
(**g**) Injuries, particularly of the head, but if severe in any site. Any injury where a fracture is a possibility.
(**h**) Shortness of breath or wheeziness, noisy breathing, unless the condition has been well diagnosed and you believe you have the means at hand to control it.
(**i**) Any changes in vision that are of sudden onset.
(**j**) Anyone experiencing a strong desire for suicide.

1.5 Why a general practitioner?

'The essential and inescapable fact is that a specialist is expert for one purpose. . . . Disease is no specialist. Patients do not consult us because certain organs are affected but because they feel ill. They come with symptoms and the earlier and therefore the more curable their malady is, the more vague will those symptoms be, the more difficult the elucidation of the cause, the greater the need in the first place, of a general investigation by one whose daily practice covers the whole of disease.'
— Sir Heneage Ogilvie, *Lancet*, 1948

In most communities the general practitioner (known in the USA as the family physician or family practitioner) represents the first point of medical contact.

Some people attempt to by-pass the general practitioner and deal directly with the specialist. Often they believe that the day of the general practitioner is past and take the view that medicine is so complex that any doctor who is a 'jack of all trades' cannot possibly be competent at anything. What is sometimes not recognised is that the well-trained family doctor of today is capable of coping very well with the vast majority of medical complaints.

Economy

Where there is such a system of first-contact medical care (or 'primary care' as it is often known), it is a very economical way of providing medical services both from the point of view of the individual, who may be required to pay personally, and the state, which usually accepts partial responsibility for the cost of the provision of health care.

In contrast, if everyone was to seek specialist care in the first instance, the cost of care would be greatly increased and the specialist services would be inundated with problems which could be dealt with by medical professionals with much less expensive and sophisticated training. One effect of this is a dilution of specialist experience so that the specialist sees fewer of the really complex cases and so develops less facility in managing them.

Thus in some parts of the world, paediatric specialists who provide first-contact care also provide much well-baby supervision. As a consequence they have much less time available to deal with more complicated problems referred from other practitioners. This contrasts with some other countries where the paediatrician's activities are confined almost entirely to dealing with unusual and obscure problems so that they become very adept in managing such rarities. In fact it would appear that in the USA many paediatricians and internists (specialists in general medicine) provide care that is little different, although usually more expensive, from that which general practitioners provide in other countries. The major difference would appear to be the age groups attended, the paediatrician dealing with young babies, children and adolescents, the internist managing adult medical problems. The general/family practitioner tries to bridge all age groups and this would appear to have numerous advantages.

What is a general practitioner?

Over recent years many definitions have been proposed. Here is a selection. The first is my own.

'The general practitioner is a doctor who provides personal, family and community orientated comprehensive care on a first-contact and continuing basis.'

The Australian College of General Practitioners defines the general practitioner as *'one who provides primary, comprehensive and continuing total patient care to individuals, families and those with whom they interact.'*

The definition by the British College of General Practitioners really sounds more like a job description: *'The general practitioner is a doctor who provides personal, primary and continuing medical care to individuals and families. The general practitioner attends patients in their homes, in the consulting room and sometimes in hospital. The general practitioner accepts responsibility for making an initial decision on every problem patients present, consulting with specialists when it is thought appropriate to do so. The general practitioner will usually work in a group with other general practitioners, from premises that are built and modified for the purpose, with the help of paramedical colleagues, adequate secretarial staff and all the equipment which is necessary. Even in a single-handed practice the general practitioner will work in a team and delegate when necessary. Diagnoses will be composed in physical, psychological and social terms. The general practitioner will intervene educationally, preventively and therapeutically to promote the patient's health.'*

Finally, the Academy of Family Practice in the USA states: *'Family practice is comprehensive medical care with particular emphasis on the family unit, in which the physician's continuing responsibility for health care is not limited by the patient's age or sex, nor by a particular organ system or disease entity.*

Family practice is the specialty in breadth which integrates biomedical, behavioural and social sciences. The core of knowledge of procedural skills encompassed by the discipline of family medicine prepares the family physician for a unique role in patient care, including the use of cognitive and procedural skills in diagnosis and management and as a personal physician who provides and coordinates health care delivery.'

The American Academy as a corollary goes on to define 'family' as *'a group of individuals with a continuing legal, genetic and/or emotional relationship. Society relies on the family group to provide for the economic and protective needs of individuals, especially children and the elderly.'*

What then do these brave words mean?

(a) Personal care
This is largely self evident and refers to the one-to-one relationship that ideally should develop

between you and your doctor. It is an intimate, confidential situation which should encourage both you and your doctor to be frank and open with each other, facilitating the best possible two-way communication.

This situation is promoted by —

(b) Continuing care

Where the one-to-one care is a continuing process, personal care tends to flourish. The better you and your doctor come to know each other, the better able the doctor is to understand the various influences under which you operate. By seeing you on a number of occasions the doctor usually gains a very useful idea of your inherent characteristics, past medical history and misadventures. Such information may have a profound influence on the way your problems are subsequently sorted out. Additionally you come to understand the doctor better and feel more comfortable in the doctor's presence.

This is a particular advantage that the general/family practitioner has over the specialist, whose services are much more likely to be given on a 'one-off' or episodic basis.

Continuing care also facilitates —

(c) Comprehensive care

The popular term for this is 'whole person care' or 'holistic care'; sometimes it is spoken of as 'total patient care'. The implication is that your problems should not be seen in isolation but in the context of the whole person — body, mind and spirit — recognising that none of these aspects of your personality should be considered distinct and independent. The term 'comprehensive care' can refer also to your environment or to the recognition that many people do not suffer from only one medical disorder but several, and that each may have an influence on the others.

(d) Family and community-orientated care

This is also an allusion to the environment. 'No man is an island' wrote Donne. Your problems must be seen in the light of their effect on the family and also the effect of the family and the community on you.

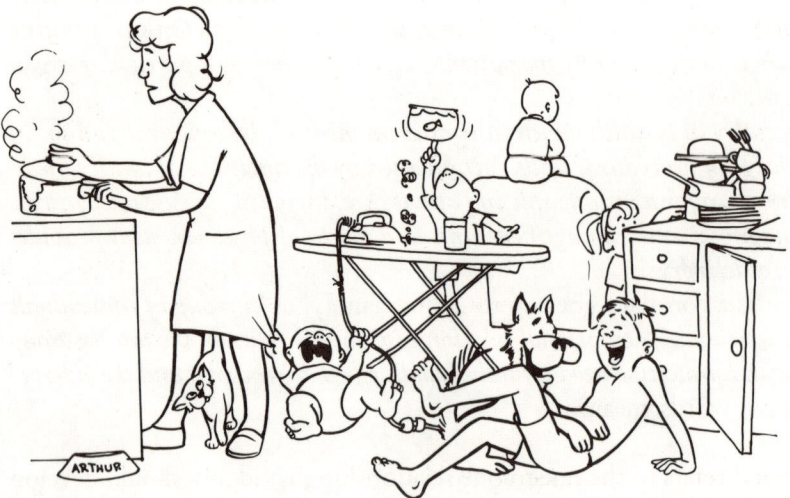

The most dangerous workplace, from the point of view of injury, is in the home.

Work-related disorders are included in this category. Doctors should never ignore the possibility that a disorder is related to a patient's occupation. Not only are many complaints the result of occupational exposure, but many illnesses have an important influence on a patient's ability to cope with work. It must be remembered also that the most dangerous workplace, from the point of view of injury, is the home.

(e) First-contact care

This relates to the general practitioner's role as the first port-of-call for most problems. It is also the reason why the work of the general practitioner is often referred to as 'primary care'. Hospital treatment and specialist care is sometimes referred to as 'secondary care', and rehabilitation may be spoken of as 'tertiary care'.

General practitioners are often called upon to make the very important decision on whether to take personal overall responsibility for a problem presented, or whether to refer a patient elsewhere. Emergency services come into this category and in general it can be said that the community expects general practitioners to provide emergency services for those patients under their care.

As nobody can be expected to be available 24 hours a day, seven days a week, general practitioners often have to delegate their responsibility. In some situations this care is provided by organisations specially set up for the purpose and paid for in part by the doctors using the service and in part by the patients receiving the care. These organisations are often known as 'deputising services' and usually they do the work well. The disadvantage is that such a service is less personal and usually the general practitioner who uses the service has little or no control over who is employed to provide it. In my view the optimal out-of-hours service is provided by small groups of general practitioners who know and respect each other's work and who if necessary have access to each other's records, rostering themselves for such duties.

In conclusion, I quote from a 1948 British Medical Association report on 'The Training of a Doctor':

'An enumeration of the desirable qualities of the ideal general practitioner reveals that only a superman could possess them all. He should have inexhaustible tact, wisdom, patience, discretion, and that "imperturbability" which Osler placed in the forefront of the qualities of a physician or surgeon. He needs to be gentle, yet firm in speech and action, and his manner must inspire confidence and trust. He should have a kindly humane approach to his patients and, however pressed he may be for time, each patient should be made to feel that his illness is of real concern to the doctor. The general practitioner needs a deeply imaginative sympathy which enables him to understand his patient's fears, anxieties, pain and discomfort. . . . He must be able to put himself in the patient's place. . . . The general practitioner is guide, philosopher and friend to patients of all classes and shows himself equally at ease with the duke and the dustman, the bishop and the boilermaker. Such "bedside" qualities must be supplemented by sound medical knowledge and efficient practical work and the practitioner's art must be applied through scientific methods — observation, discrimination, solution, diagnosis and decision. His general conduct in professional and private life should be guided by high moral principles, and in his practice he should adhere steadfastly to the spirit of the Hippocratic Oath.'

1.6 The team

'The lone hand has advantages as well as the much advertised team work, but each in its own place.'
— Sir Alexander Fleming (1881-1955), discoverer of penicillin

The practice nurse
For many years doctors have employed nurses to assist with medical tasks in the practice. Smaller practices sometimes try to combine the roles of nurse and receptionist, but usually their functions are quite distinct.

Traditionally nurses have been responsible for doing dressings and giving injections, but latterly their area of involvement has been greatly expanded in many practices.

As a patient, you may find it easier to talk to a practice nurse than to the general practitioner, perhaps because you share the same ethnic background, sex, or socio-economic status. If you feel this way, you should have this opportunity, even if the doctor has to be included in the consultation later, because of his or her more specialised knowledge.

If you feel that you would like to speak to a practice nurse, before, after or instead of the general practititioner, you should never be afraid to ask for this.

Complementary roles
The truth is, doctors cannot be all things to all men (or women) and every effort should be made to make the roles of practice nurse and general practitioner complementary. This can work in many ways. Thus a male doctor may have difficulty in seeing the female point of view. The practice nurse, if female, may in certain circumstances help to meet this need. This, incidentally, would suggest that there might be a place for male practice nurses in the offices of female practitioners. Similarly, some doctors may not be good at providing health education or explaining to patients how their medicines should be taken. Such doctors should endeavour to employ practice nurses who have competence in these areas.

Practice nurses can also play a part in screening procedures and in special clinics such as those for the overweight, antenatal care, diabetes and so forth.

Of course, if you do not wish to be involved in any way with a third person — usually a practice nurse — that is your privilege, and you should make this known to the receptionist at the time of making an appointment. Sometimes there are matters which are so confidential that it is very embarrassing to involve others.

The social worker

A few practices are large enough to justify the employment of a fulltime social worker. The social work role in medicine is usually centred around the placement of people in appropriate rest-home or hospital care, the provision of community services such as meals-on-wheels, assistance in obtaining social welfare benefits and the like. The social worker is a very significant community resource and since alert general practitioners are often the first to perceive problems in the community, they are an important source of referral.

Some social workers also accept a role as counsellors. A few general practitioners have neither the time, the experience, nor the interest to involve themselves deeply in counselling. In such cases this is usually undertaken by a person with a training in psychology, or by social workers. Some people also get counselling through the Church, although this is much less used than in the past when many more people sought emotional and spiritual support from their religious advisors. In a sense the doctor and the counsellor appear to have assumed the mantle of the cleric.

The receptionist

The receptionist is usually responsible for making appointments. In a way the receptionist is the doctor's 'shop window' and a good receptionist can make a great difference to the success of a practice. The best receptionists have a warm, welcoming manner towards patients and will do their best to ensure that you get attention at a time which is convenient to you. With experience, some can even judge how long individual patients will require with the doctor.

Difficulties can sometimes happen when the appointment book is full and there arises a problem which could be urgent. Should the patient be squeezed on to the already full list or is it reasonable to ask him or her to wait a day or even longer? This is where a clear explanation from you can be so helpful. If the condition is such that you really feel you should be seen immediately, or even sometime later the same day, it is best to make this quite clear to the receptionist. In fairness to other patients, you should not be unreasonable in these demands but usually you have a fairly good idea of the seriousness of the condition. (See section on what to regard as an emergency, p. 31.)

If you still feel sure that you are not being afforded attention as promptly as desirable, it is best to ask the receptionist to let you speak to the practice nurse, or the doctor. Sometimes it is all too easy to be put off by a reassuring receptionist trying to protect a doctor who is already quite probably overworked. Good communication is essential at this point and the role of the receptionist can be a vital one.

If you are known to the practice, the doctor will recognise a responsibility to you, and will always want to see you promptly should a real emergency arise. This situation highlights the importance of having a personal doctor who recognises you as his or her patient. Once you are accepted by a practitioner as a patient, that practice has a moral, and in some countries a legal, responsibility to provide medical care if called upon to do so in an emergency.

If you have no formal association with a practice, it can sometimes be difficult to find a doctor who will accept responsibility for you at short notice, although few will refuse a request for help if there is no other source of medical care available.

Apart from making appointments and greeting you on arrival at the doctor's office, receptionists usually accept some responsibility for the administration of the practice.

Other team members
Yet other members of the team are the *district nurses*, who visit homes and provide a variety of nursing services to people disabled by illness. *Occupational therapists* can be called upon to advise on how hazards in the home can be minimised, and dietitians assist in matters relating to diet. *Physiotherapists* ('physical therapists') give treatment to muscles, ligaments and other structures which are causing pain or require strengthening. They will also advise about posture.

All of these assist in the process of rehabilitation, which is really another way of describing the restoration of patients as far as possible to their normal activities at home and/or the workplace. The term relates to both physical and mental functioning. Wherever possible, patients are kept in their own homes, but clearly there are times when institutional care is unavoidable. Sometimes general practitioners continue to care for their patients in these circumstances, but often the care is relegated to hospital doctors who specialise in particular problems.

Medical students
Today medical students spend some weeks gaining experience in general practice. This is comparable to their other practical experience which in the past has been confined almost entirely to hospital. Medical educators have at long last realised that they are educating doctors for practice in the community as well as in hospital. The work in each situation is really quite different and one is no less important than the other. Who would even dream of trying to train a carpenter in an engineering workshop? Clearly the best place to teach future doctors about the way things are done in general practice, is in general practice. As a result, you can expect to encounter students in general practices, just as you may in hospital.

In many ways, if you are seen by students you are specially privileged. Usually the student has fewer time constraints than the doctor, and you get the benefit of the student's knowledge and interest as well as the subsequent consultation with the supervising doctor. As in so many situations, 'two heads are better than one'. Hopefully you will welcome the opportunity to see a student, but always you have the right to refuse. Occasional embarrassment is perfectly understandable and it would be a foolish doctor who did not make allowances for this.

Fragmentation of care
In the area of teamwork the art is to achieve coordination and cooperation without significantly interfering with personal care and continuity. It is a source of concern to many general practitioners that there now seems to be a trend to fragmentation of care. Clinics are set up to serve specific purposes — usually purposes which are well within the province of the general practitioner, e.g. for well-baby care, family planning, cervical smears, occupational health and so on.

There is a place for some of these as a few general practitioners do not wish to provide such services, and sometimes patients are reluctant to ask their own doctor for them. Unfortunately these special clinics have a tendency to proliferate and the range of services provided broadens. As a result, general practitioners who are attempting to provide whole-person care may find that they seldom meet some of their patients and consequently their understanding of those patients' problems may be restricted.

Some people today say they do not get the personal attention that they remember receiving from family doctors in the past. In fact, there are many doctors who are very willing to give just as good and caring service as did the horse and buggy doctor of such revered memory, but it is very difficult to provide a truly personal service to anyone who is receiving medical advice from a wide variety of sources.

The patient

There is, of course, one other member of the team who should not be overlooked and that is you, the patient — the most important member of all.

You can and should make an important contribution to decision-making in matters relating to the management of your own illness. This is best achieved when you have a thorough understanding of what is available by way of treatment and the consequences of withholding treatment. Usually family doctors will provide this information. This book is an attempt to supplement and reinforce the information which is given you, so that you may be an even more effective team member.

SECTION TWO

Becoming healthy, staying well

2.1 The prevention of illness: the promotion of wellness

'To administer medicines to diseases which have already developed . . . is comparable to the behaviour of those persons who begin to dig a well after they are thirsty, and of those who begin to cast weapons after they have already engaged in battle.'

— Huang Ti, The Yellow Emperor (2697–2597 BC)

Much is heard these days about preventive medicine and there is no doubt that both doctors and the public earnestly desire to see more done in this field. Unfortunately the payment systems for most doctors have not been designed to promote health. Most countries have a sickness-orientated system which rewards doctors for alleviating ill health but does little to encourage them to keep people well.

However, many doctors have come to realise that they should accept a responsibility to promote positive health. They are taking to heart the old saying, 'It is better to have a fence at the top of a cliff than an ambulance at the bottom.'

The World Health Organisation (WHO) has defined health as *'a state of complete physical, mental and social wellbeing — not merely the absence of disease or infirmity'* — which is probably an impossible ideal. I rather prefer a definition which says health is *'a satisfactory adaptation of the individual to his or her total environment — physical, psychological and socio-cultural'*. Somehow the term 'satisfactory' seems more attainable and less all-embracing than the WHO use of the term 'complete'. There are very few absolutes in this world. Katherine Mansfield put it very well when she wrote, *'By health I mean the power to live a full, adult living breathing life in close contact with what I love . . . I want to lose all that is superficial and acquired in me and to become a conscious direct human being. I want by understanding myself, to understand others. I want to be all that I am capable of becoming so that I may be a child in the sun. Warm, eager, living life — to be rooted in life — to learn to desire to know, to feel to think to act. That is what I want.'*

Preventive medicine attempts to achieve just this.

Primary and secondary prevention

It is customary to describe preventive procedures as being either *primary* or *secondary*. 'Primary prevention' is doing those things which prevent disease occurring in the first place; 'secondary prevention' is preventing the complications of an existing disease process. Into the primary category come all the public-health measures which have evolved over the years such as the provision of clean drinking water, washing hands after visiting the toilet and before handling food, keeping food uncontaminated and away from flies and bacteria, washing dishes after use, the avoidance of shared eating and drinking utensils, etc.

Primary prevention also includes the various *preventive injections (inoculations)* which are recommended. Here is a list of current recommendations. (The timing varies a little from one country to another.)

TRIVAC (for diphtheria, pertussis (whooping cough) and tetanus) — 6 weeks of age
TRIVAC+polio — 3 months
TRIVAC+polio — 5–6 months
Morbilli (measles) — 12–15 months
DIVAC (for diphtheria and tetanus)+polio — 18 months
Polio — 5 years
Rubella (German measles) — girls 12 or 13 years of age
Tetanus booster — 15 years and then every 20 years

Where hepatitis B inoculation is recommended, this should ideally be given first within 12 hours of birth, again at six weeks of age and finally at five months of age.

These inoculations represent possibly the most effective primary prevention that we have. Diet (see p. 84) can be either primary or secondary prevention.

Unfortunately, progress in most areas of primary prevention is painfully slow. We still have much to learn about the causation of disease and particularly the influence of lifestyle on the development of ill health. One difficulty is that there is seldom a clearcut association between environmental factors and most of the common diseases. Doctors are reluctant to recommend widespread environmental and lifestyle changes in the absence of definite scientific evidence of their benefit.

Below is listed the best known of the factors recognised as detrimental to health:

(a) smoking
(b) alcohol
(c) inactivity
(d) motor vehicle accidents
(e) drugs
(f) stress
(g) unsatisfactory diet

Smoking

There are many health problems which clearly appear to be a result of smoking and one can only applaud the efforts of organisations such as ASH which have been set up to try and dissuade people from this habit. These health problems are discussed in Chapter 2.8 on alcohol and tobacco (pp. 106–19).

Alcohol

Alcohol is a problem for several reasons. Not only can it have damaging effects on the body, but it also loosens the inhibitions so that people may behave in ways which are potentially damaging to others. Thus many motor-vehicle accidents and much domestic strife can be attributed to alcohol. In fact, from time to time when there have been brewery strikes or other causes of failure of alcohol supplies, it has been notable how significantly the crime and accident rate has fallen on such occasions.

Alcohol is interesting, however, in that it causes a dilatation of the blood vessels and as a result is considered helpful in improving impaired circulation of the blood. There is also some evidence that a small intake of alcohol taken on a fairly regular basis provides some protection from coronary artery disease and subsequent heart attacks. Such information is inclined to give encouragement to those who seek an excuse for regular drinking and has the potential to do more harm than good.

Many believe that the physical damage from alcohol is particularly likely to occur if a heavy drinker also takes an inadequate diet, as is often the case. (The problems of alcohol are further discussed on pp. 108–14.)

Inactivity

The importance of exercise remains uncertain. It seems generally agreed that inactivity is harmful. What is in doubt is how much exercise is optimal. There seems to be a tendency for any part of the body which is not used regularly to become less efficient and this may well apply to the heart as much as to other organs. Heart disease is one of the two major killers of our modern civilisation and we are only slowly coming to learn about its causes.

Most people who undertake regular and very vigorous exercise do so in the belief that this will help to forestall heart disease caused by blockage of the arteries to the heart (i.e. coronary arteries). They may be right, but some recent evidence from research in Framingham would seem to show that much less exercise is just as useful from the point of view of preventing coronary heart disease.

There can be no denying that those who jog, for example, get a great deal of satisfaction from it, and this may be psychologically beneficial, and many also derive a feeling of wellbeing which some have considered addictive. The detractors of jogging point to the number of people who die during or after their jog and the incidence of arthritis in weight-bearing joints that occurs in joggers, not to mention the repetitive strain injuries that can develop. These detractors claim that the dangers outweigh the advantages. The truth is that we still do not know, and the best that your medical advisor can do is to suggest a middle course involving a reasonable amount of activity without becoming obsessional about it. (Exercise is further considered in the section on pp. 102–5.)

Motor vehicles

Motor vehicle accidents are a very prominent cause of death and disability, particularly amongst the young. If the annual mortality from accidents on the roads were caused by bacteria or viruses, we would be horrified at the severity of the epidemic. The problem is an interesting one because we know its causes and to a large extent we know how to prevent road accidents — obvious ones would be to restrict motor vehicles to a very low speed and to prohibit alcohol drinking before driving, absolutely. However, as a society we love our cars and the convenience they afford us and we have accepted that, for us, the advantages of this form of transport outweigh the costs, both in human and monetary terms. Measures such as seat belts and crash bars are important ways by which lives can be saved.

Drugs

Another item in the list of things harmful to health is drugs, and in a sense *alcohol* is the most dangerous of the drugs at present in common use.

Most people when they speak of drugs are referring to 'drugs of addiction' and they are thinking at such times of morphine, pethidine, heroin, cocaine, LSD, amphetamines and the like. Doctors often use the term 'drugs' when speaking of the many medicines which are now available for the treatment of disease processes and the alleviation of pain, both physical and mental. The majority of the medicines which doctors use are not habit forming and patients can take them without any fear of 'drug addiction'. Perhaps a better term is 'pharmaceuticals' or 'medication'. The whole question of the use of pharmaceuticals is looked at in Chapters 4.1–4.9 and Chapters 5, 6, 7 and 8.

The dangers of so-called 'recreational' drug use are so well known that with the exception of alcohol and tobacco, they will not be discussed further in this book.

Stress

A further sometimes injurious factor in the lifestyle of most people is *stress*. None of us can avoid stress entirely, and life would be dull indeed if we did. Some tolerate stress extremely well, while others merely appear to do so; many tolerate it very poorly. There is evidence that moderate degrees of stress are good for us, but when the stress is severe, it can have a deleterious effect. Many people respond with obvious physical symptoms which may take the form of headaches, sweating, a desire to pass urine frequently, diarrhoea, etc.

W. B. Cannon, a physiologist, in 1915 described the 'fight or flight' symptoms which he demonstrated were largely caused by the production of a substance called adrenalin (i.e. epinephrine) in the body. Many of the typical symptoms of severe anxiety can be reproduced by an injection of adrenalin. Cannon believed that the adrenalin was produced to give the body temporary extra strength and vigour to either stop and fight with an enemy, or else to flee. In 1956 his message was taken up and popularised by Hans Selye in his book *The Stress of Life*.

The theory has been further extended to suggest that if the adrenalin is not utilised by the body for its intended purpose, it will be destroyed in some way, and that the process is capable of leading indirectly to blood vessel damage and perhaps over a long period of time, the development of blockages in the coronary or other arteries. The suggestion has been made that because of this, if one becomes very tense or angry and this is bottled up, as it often must be in a civilised community, it is wise to utilise the adrenalin by going for a run or undertaking some other energetic pursuit.

General practitioners early in their careers become very much aware of the part that our state of mind plays in health and illness. People who have a lot of worry or anxiety, or who become depressed, seem to have a much lower resistance to many disease processes. This will be discussed further in Chapter 2.4 on the emotions and disease, where it is shown how it is possible to predict roughly who is at risk of illness as a result of life's vagaries. (See p. 78.)

Diet

Faulty diet is the last of the remediable factors with which we need to concern ourselves in the maintenance of good health. This will be discussed in Chapter 2.5 on pp. 84–95.

Preventing coronary heart disease

Easily the greatest killer in the western world is coronary heart disease. Much research has gone into trying to discover the principal factors in its cause. Very slowly and after extensive debate, the facts are beginning to emerge, but there is still a need for further study. Most of the lifestyle factors already mentioned seem to be involved.

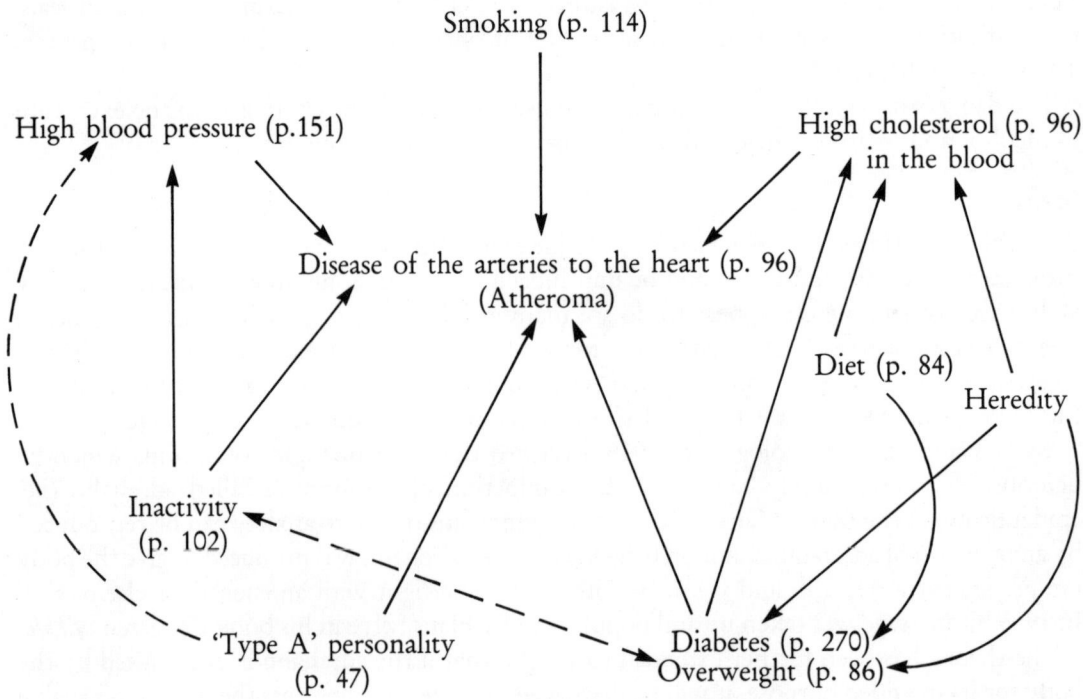

Certain people inherit a tendency to high cholesterol in the blood either on its own or in association with diabetes, and their risk of disease of the arteries to the heart (i.e. coronary arteries) is increased. A few people with very high levels of cholesterol (known as hypercholesterolaemia) are apparently subject to consequent heart attacks at a very early age. There are now a number of medicines which are effective in bringing the cholesterol level down, and this seems to reduce the chance of heart attacks. A strict diet can also help. (See pp. 96–102.)

Diabetes is a risk factor but it remains unclear whether this is primarily related to the diabetes per se, the elevated blood sugars or the high cholesterol.

The role of exercise, or the lack of it, seems the least understood, but as stated, most authorities take the view that inactivity increases the risk.

Both smoking and high blood pressure are very significant causative factors. The dangers of heart attacks from smoking greatly outweigh the better recognised danger of lung cancer.

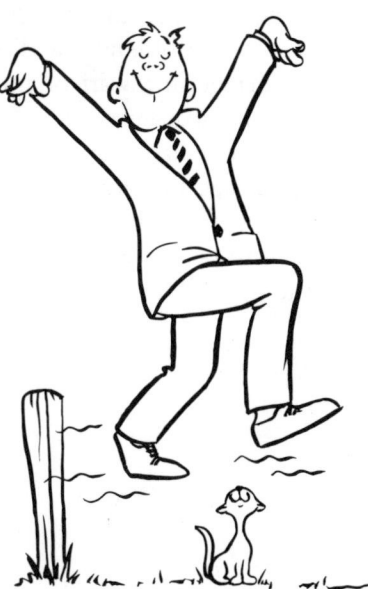

'Type A' personality

Finally there is the 'Type A' personality. Some workers have broadly classified people into two categories: those with Type A personalities are hard driving, aggressive, impatient, restless people, always conscious of the passage of time, always dynamic and forceful. The others, considered to be 'Type B', are much more placid, relaxed and contented; they are usually relatively unambitious and much more passive. The former are likely to be under constant stress and studies suggest they are more prone to coronary artery disease and heart attacks. Sometimes, by changing their attitudes and learning relaxation techniques, such people can reduce their risks. Clearly these two personality types represent opposite poles of what must be a spectrum and most people would see themselves as somewhere between the two. The classification is too crude, but does help to highlight the fact that stress can play a part here, as in so many other disorders.

Secondary prevention

Much of what is done by the doctor comes into the category of *secondary prevention*. As a profession we have more skills at this and also more success. It involves the recognition of disease processes at their very earliest stages with a view to either curing the disease or else alleviating or preventing the complications.

Most patients seek the doctor when they become aware of an abnormality in their health and in many conditions, the earlier a visit is made to the doctor, the better. Doctors are trained to sort out those conditions which require urgent attention from those which do not.

Often patients are advised of danger signals, by advertisements. Among the best known must be those promulgated by cancer societies concerning the danger signs for cancer. Here is the usual list:
1. Any sore which does not heal.
2. A lump or thickening in the breast or elsewhere.
3. Any unusual bleeding or discharge.
4. Any change in a wart or mole.
5. Persistent hoarseness or cough.
6. Persistent indigestion or difficulty with swallowing.
7. Any change in normal bowel habits.

Today doctors sometimes make efforts to identify disease before people develop symptoms sufficient to bring them spontaneously to the office. This is the process known as *screening* and the possibilities in this area are discussed in detail in the next chapter.

2.2 Screening for early disease

> 'Then gently scan your brother man
> Still gentler, sister woman.'
> — Robert Burns (1759–96)

One approach to preventive medicine is for the doctor or other health worker to organise screening campaigns. These are based on the belief that if a simple, reliable and inexpensive diagnostic test can be found, it may be useful to apply that test to whole populations in the hope that by finding a disease early, some intervention will be possible that will influence the course of the condition to the benefit of the patient. No good purpose is served if a disease is diagnosed and doctors are unable to do anything about it; the patient would usually have been better left without this knowledge.

Wholesale screening of this sort tends to be very expensive and can only be justified if the benefits to the community outweigh the cost. This requires a good yield of treatable disease. It is also very important that the diagnosis be accurate. Some tests tend to over-diagnose so that people, initially at least, are led to believe that they have something wrong with them, when in fact further testing shows that they are well. Such 'false positive' tests, as they are called, create a lot of unnecessary anxiety and may do more harm than good. Alternatively, the tests may not be sufficiently sensitive and people suffering from a disease may be told that they are well. These are called 'false negatives', and they too can be harmful, for patients may be wrongly reassured.

The success of tests such as these depends on many factors. Frequently they are more rewarding in ill-educated communities because better educated people tend to take themselves promptly to the doctor if they notice an abnormality, while less knowledgeable people tend to ignore important symptoms or take a stoical attitude towards them. Thus some people will ignore discharging ears and treat them with as little concern as they would a runny nose.

Young children are an important target for health workers interested in screening, because children usually do not realise that they have an abnormality. For example, a child who has deficient hearing will be unlikely to complain because it has never known what it is to have good hearing. Elderly people can be yet another worthwhile target group because they may ignore treatable disease, attributing it to the fact that they are getting old.

A further source of successful screening is symptomless disease, and high blood pressure would be the best example. High blood pressure can be very severe without the patient being aware of it. Some other conditions such as cancer of the neck of the womb (i.e. cervix) and cancer of the breast may also have few symptoms in the very early stages.

For a screening programme to be successful, cooperation is essential, and most attempts at screening have discovered that the people who are at greatest risk of disease are often the very ones who refuse to cooperate with the testing, or who when an abnormality is discovered, fail to take steps to have it treated.

Screening criteria

At the risk of repetition, here is a list of criteria which the World Health Organisation has recommended should be satisfied in order to make a screening programme worthwhile:

1. The condition must be an important one — something which, if left untreated, would lead to disability and/or death. The long-term benefits of treatment must exceed the detrimental effects of the treatment.
2. There should be a recognised latent or early symptomatic stage, i.e. a stage before the patients are sufficiently aware of the problem to take themselves to the doctor.
3. There should be a reliable test or examination with a low incidence of false positives and false negatives (unless false positives are easily eliminated).
4. The test or examination should be acceptable to patients, and safe.
5. Facilities for full work-up of any disease discovered should be available.
6. The cost of finding cases should be economically balanced in relation to the total national health spending, i.e. it must be cost effective.
7. As far as possible the task of finding disease should be a continuing (or repetitive) process and not a once-and-for-all project.
8. The natural history of the condition from latent to declared disease should be understood and also its subsequent course if left untreated.
9. There should be an agreed policy amongst doctors as to which cases discovered are appropriate for treatment.
10. There should be a known, effective treatment such that the quality of life of the patient is improved, not merely advancing the time for which the patient experiences disease.
11. Treatment should be available and acceptable to patients, and the majority of the patients must be prepared to comply with the treatment recommended.

In most screening programmes only one test is done, but in some parts of the world organisations have been established to provide a whole battery of screening tests at the one time. Obviously there is the possibility of economies of time and money being achieved in this way. Nevertheless, such batteries of tests, because of their number, are often expensive, and current evidence would suggest that they are seldom justified. This type of screening has been called 'multiphasic screening' and it is usually preferable and cheaper to visit a general practitioner who is willing to take a full history, examine relevant parts of the body, and then arrange for blood tests and X-rays if the evidence suggests they are warranted. With the exceptions of hypertension and cancer of the cervix mentioned above, surprisingly little disease is found in patients who are free of symptoms and signs, and most of the really useful screening procedures can be done readily in the general practitioner's office without the use of high technology.

ANTENATAL SCREENING

Remember too, that some procedures are themselves hazardous and one should particularly try to minimise, if possible, the radiation that is inevitable from X-rays.

'Case finding'

Another form of screening, which is more economical, is called *case finding*. This is the situation in which a doctor takes the blood pressure of a patient who comes about say, a sore throat. There is no medical association between sore throats and blood pressure, but the visit provides a good opportunity to check for a common and usually symptomless disease. In a similar way many doctors will do cervical smears from time to time on patients attending for repeat prescriptions for the contraceptive pill. This is not to imply that there is an association between taking the pill and cancer of the cervix, but simply because it is a convenient opportunity.

Interestingly, the yield of positive findings is proportionately greater in case finding than in screening random groups of people and this is because of the known tendency for disease processes to cluster. Thus it can be said that if a person suffers from one disease process there is a greater than average chance of that person suffering from yet another disease process. The reason for this is seldom clear except when the diseases are related to poor hygiene or poor diet. Sometimes it seems to be associated with the diminished resistance that occurs in people who are under stress.

The other area that has proved fruitful for screening, not unexpectedly, is the 'at risk' patient. These are patients who for one reason or another are known to be at greater risk than usual of developing a particular disease. As we go through life, our risks for certain conditions change. This is borne out by the causes of death in different age groups. Thus motor-vehicle accidents are a much commoner cause of death in the young than in the elderly. On the other hand, cancer is relatively rare in young people but quite common in older age groups.

The rest of this section will be devoted to looking at what disorders may warrant screening procedures in the various age groups, starting with the unborn baby and mother. The tables are based on the findings of the Canadian Task Force on screening. You should look through these tables for the one which relates to the age bracket you are interested in. Following the tables there is a commentary on certain screening recommendations.

Patients seeking to have screening tests done by their general practitioner should make a special appointment for this purpose. In many cases a double appointment will be required in order to ensure sufficient time is available.

(1) Antenatal (prenatal) screening

Things doctor will look for or try to prevent	Time of search and action doctor will follow	Factors for consideration
1. Factors possibly leading to deficient oxygen supply during and after birth	First visit and follow-up visits	Toxaemia, kidney and heart complaints. Diabetes. Previous problems in childbirth. Abnormalities of birth passage.

Antenatal screening (cont.)

Things doctor will look for or try to prevent	Time of search and action doctor will follow	Factors for consideration
2. Abnormalities of spinal canal	4–5 months pregnancy	A blood test is available but only warranted if the parents are prepared to accept termination of pregnancy if further tests show spina bifida (a birth defect of the spinal canal) present.
3. Down's Syndrome ('Mongolism')	First visit	Previous Down's Syndrome child in the family. Mother over 35 years. Evidence mother has characteristic abnormality of genes.
4. Rubella (German measles)	First visit	No history of the disease. No history of immunisation.
5. Gonorrhoea	First visit	Known history of casual sex, by either partner, prostitution, etc.
6. Syphilis	First visit	Known history of casual sex, by either partner, prostitution, etc.
7. Inadequate diet and underweight baby*	First visit and follow-up visits	If diet thought to be inadequate.
7a. Iron deficiency	Check blood at first visit and repeat at approx. 28th week	
8. Parenting problems*	First visit and follow-up visits	Particularly unplanned children, problem families, etc.
9. Alcohol	First visit and follow-up visits	Complete avoidance should be recommended during pregnancy.
10. High blood pressure*	Check at all visits	Check for abnormal protein in urine.
11. Diabetes mellitus	First visit and follow-up visits	Previous large babies. Previous babies born dead. Recurrent abortion. Development abnormalities in previous child. Family history of diabetes. Overweight.
12. Mother and baby's blood groups not compatible — ABO abnormalities (Rh status)	First visit	

*See notes following.

Antenatal screening (cont.

Things doctor will look for or try to prevent	Time of search and action doctor will follow	Factors for consideration
If Rh negative	Check blood again at 20 weeks, every month to 28 weeks, and after that every 2 weeks.	
If Rh positive	Check blood between 32 weeks and 36 weeks	
13. Early labour	First visit	Previous history. Surgery to uterus (womb)
14. Recurrent abortion	First visit	Possible genetic abnormalities, disorders of the endocrine glands, disorders of uterus.
15. Bacteria in the urine*	At 12 weeks and every 12 weeks thereafter	History of infections in the urine (cystitis).
16. Breast feeding	Discuss at various visits	
17. Post-birth depression	Check for this at post-natal visits	Previous history of depression

Other things which may be considered at this time are the possibility of the mother having toxoplasmosis — an infection which can affect the unborn child; the question of whether the mother smokes and its possible effect on the infant's birth weight; any medicines that are being taken, with a view to identifying any known to be harmful to the baby; the possibility of the mother being dependent on drugs; the state of the mother's teeth with a view to preventing deterioration. The doctor will, of course, also check that there is only one baby and not twins or triplets. The position of the baby will also be noted to ensure that the head is coming first and not the feet or arms.

(2) Infants at birth and first week of life

Things doctor will look for or try to prevent	Doctor will do	Factors for consideration
Deficient oxygen supply	Physical examination	Abnormalities of heart, overwhelming infection, fits, etc.
Bleeding disorders	Give Vitamin K_1	Baby due

*See notes following

Infants at birth and first week of life (cont.)

Things doctor will look for or try to prevent	Doctor will do	Factors for consideration
Syphilis	Test umbilical cord blood at birth	Known history of casual sex by either partner, prostitution, etc.
Gonococcal infection in the eyes	Silver nitrate drops into eyes as preventive	Known history of casual sex by either partner, prostitution, etc.
Inadequate thyroid function	Test blood for thyroid hormone	
Phenylketonuria* (PKU). (A disorder of the body's metabolism leading to intellectual impairment.)	Blood test	Test may need repeating.
Congenital† dislocation of hip	Physical examination. X-ray if suspected	
Congenital† heart disorders	Physical examination and history	X-rays and other tests may be necessary
Growth problems*	Measure length, weight, and circumference of head	Begin growth chart. Follow at later visits.
Parenting problems*	Counselling	Family history. Particularly unplanned children, problem families, etc.
Squint	Inspection of eyes	
Hearing problems	Observe response to being startled, unusual noise, character of cry	
Blood incompatibility	Blood test from umbilical cord at birth	
Accidents (at home and in vehicles)	Counselling	Need for seat belts and home safety precautions.
Cystic fibrosis	Examination of sweat	Especially if family history of this disease.
Iron deficiency (anaemia)	Blood test	Especially premature babies, twins or triplets, mother anaemic or on poor diet.
Hepatitis B	Give injection	Especially those in low socio-economic conditions

*See notes following
†Congenital disorders are conditions which are present at birth.

(3) Infants 2–4 weeks of age

Things doctor will look for or try to prevent	Doctor will do	Factors for consideration
Congenital displacement of the hip	Physical examination	X-ray if suspected
Disorders of the urine collecting system	Ask about force of urinary stream	
Growth problems	Physical examination. Length, weight and head circumference	Continue growth chart.
Parenting problems* (including child abuse)	Assess way parents and child interact	
Accident prevention (at home and in vehicles)	Counselling	Need for seat belts, etc. Home safety precautions.
Syphilis	Blood test	If mother at high risk.

(4) Infants 6 weeks to 2 months of age

Things doctor will look for or try to prevent	Doctor will do	Factors for consideration
Congenital heart disorders	Physical examination. X-rays, etc., if suspected	History.
Diphtheria, whooping cough, tetanus (and polio)	Immunisation	If child is in good health and no contrary features.
Hepatitis B	Immunisation at 6 weeks	
Growth problems and nutrition	Physical examination. Length, weight and head circumference	Continue growth chart.
Delayed development*	Use of standard tests for development assessment	Denver Test may be used as a supplement.
Parenting problems* (including child abuse)	Assess way parents and child interact	
Squint	Inspection of eyes	

*See notes following

(5) Infants aged 3-4 months

Things doctor will look for or try to prevent	Doctor will do	Factors for consideration
Diphtheria, whooping cough, tetanus and polio	Immunisation	Only if child in good health. Avoid whooping cough immunisation if child subject to fits.
Growth problems and nutrition	Physical examination. Length, weight, and head circumference	History. Continue growth chart.
Delayed development*	Standard tests of development	Denver Test may be used as supplement
Parenting problems* (including child abuse)	Assess ways parents and child interact	History, particularly unplanned children, problem families, etc.
Accidents (at home and in vehicles)	Counselling	Advice about restraints and home hazards

(6) Infants aged 6 months

Things doctor will look for or try to prevent	Doctor will do	Factors for consideration
Diphtheria, whooping cough, tetanus and polio	Immunisation	Only if child is in good health. Avoid whooping cough immunisation if child subject to fits.
Growth problems and nutrition	History, physical examination. Length, weight, and head circumference	Continue growth chart.
Delayed development*	Standard tests of development	Denver Test may be added as a supplement.
Parenting problems* (including child abuse)	Assess ways parents and child interact	History, particularly unplanned children, problem families, etc.
Hearing problems	Observe response to being startled, unusual noise, character of cry	
Measles	Immunisation	Only if child in good health. Avoid if child subject to fits. Some prefer to give at 12 months.

*See notes following

(6) Infants aged 6 mnths (cont.)

Things doctor will look for or try to prevent	Doctor will do	Factors for consideration
Hepatitis B	Immunisation, preferably at 5 months	Especially those in low socio-economic conditions.

(7) Infants aged 9 months

Things doctor will look for or try to prevent	Doctor will do	Factors for consideration
Growth problems and nutrition	History, physical examination. Length, weight, and head circumference	Continue growth chart.
Delayed development	Standard tests of development assessment	Denver Test may be added as a supplement.
Parenting problems* (including child abuse)	Assess ways parents and child interact	History, particularly unplanned children, problem families.
Accidents (at home and in vehicles)	Counselling	Advice about restraints and home hazards.
Anaemia due to a deficiency of iron	Blood test	Especially children from low-income homes.

(8) Infants aged 12–15 months

Things doctor will look for or try to prevent	Doctor will do	Factors for consideration
Measles	Immunisation	Only if child in good health. Avoid if child subject to fits.
Mumps	Immunisation	Only if health of child good. Not all authorities recommend as routine.
Rubella (German measles)	Immunisation	Only persons in good health. Some authorities do not give as routine at this age and give only to females 11–12 years.

*See notes following.

Infants aged 12–15 months (cont.)

Things doctor will look for or try to prevent	Doctor will do	Factors for consideration
Growth problems and nutrition	History, physical examination. Length, weight, and head circumference	Continue growth chart.
Parenting problems* (including child abuse)	Assess ways parents and child interact	History, particularly unplanned children, problem families.

(9) Infants aged 18 months

Things doctor will look for or try to prevent	Doctor will do	Factors for consideration
Diphtheria, whooping cough, tetanus, poliomyelitis	Immunisation	Fourth dose. Only if health of child is good. Immunisation against whooping cough often omitted at this age if given earlier.
Growth problems	History, height, weight and head circumference	Continue growth chart.
Problems of behaviour* or development	Assess how child and parents interact. Use standard development tests	Can use Denver Test as a supplement.

(10) Children aged 2–3 years

Things doctor will look for or try to prevent	Doctor will do	Factors for consideration
Growth problems	History. Height, weight and head circumference	Continue growth chart.
Problems of behaviour or development	Assess how child and parent interact. Use standard development tests	Can use Denver Test as a supplement.
Squint and focusing problems	Inspection. Visual chart test	

*See notes following.

Children aged 2–3 years (cont.)

Things doctor will look for or try to prevent	Doctor will do	Factors for consideration
Hearing problems	Physical examination.	History. Defective speech development.
Dental caries*	Physical examination	Best done by dentist.

(11) Children aged 4 years

Things doctor will look for or try to prevent	Doctor will do	Factors for consideration
Growth problems	Height, weight, and head circumference	Continue growth chart
Behaviour problems	Assessment	
Dental caries*	Physical examination	Best done by dentist.

(12) Children aged 5–6 years (school entry)

Things doctor will look for or try to prevent	Doctor will do	Factors for consideration
Diphtheria, whooping cough, tetanus and poliomyelitis	Immunisation	If other immunisation complete, sometimes polio only given at this age.
Growth problems	History, height, weight, head circumference, chest and arms	Continue growth chart.
Problems of behaviour or development	Assess how child and parents interact. Enquire about schooling	
Squint and focusing problems	Inspection. Visual chart test	
Hearing problems	Physical examination.	History. Defective speech.
Dental caries*	Physical examination	Best done by dentist

*See notes following

Children aged 5-6 years (cont.)

Things doctor will look for or try to prevent	Doctor will do	Factors for consideration
Accidents (at home and in vehicles)	Counselling	
Tuberculosis*	Tuberculin testing. Immunisation with B.C.G. if thought appropriate	Tb contacts. At-risk groups.

(13) Children aged 10-11 years

Things doctor will look for or try to prevent	Doctor will do	Factors for consideration
German measles (Rubella)	Immunisation of girls	If immunisation has not been done already
Growth problems	Height, weight, head circumference, chest and arms	
Behavioural or developmental problems*	Assess how parents and child interact	If earlier assessments suggest desirable.
Focusing problems	Visual chart test	
Hearing problems	Examination	History.
Dental caries* (and malplacement of teeth)	Examination	Best done by dentist.
Accidents (home, vehicle, and water)	Counselling	
Use of alcohol, use of tobacco, drugs	Counselling	
Sexual development		

(14) Adolescents aged 12-15 years

Things doctor will look for or try to prevent	Doctor will do	Factors for consideration
Growth problems	Height, weight, head circumference, chest and arms	

*See notes following.

Adolescents aged 12–15 years (cont.)

Things doctor will look for or try to prevent	Doctor will do	Factors for consideration
Accidents	Counselling	
Use of alcohol, use of tobacco, drugs	Counselling	
Sexual development		
Dental caries* (and malplacement of teeth). Gum disorders	Examination	Best done by dentist.
Inadequate nutrition	Check proteins in blood. Height, weight, head circumference, chest and arms	History. Especially adolescent girls.
Muscular wasting diseases	Amount of creatine phosphokinase in blood	Especially relatives of patients with muscular dystrophy.
Cancer of the neck of the womb (cervix)*	Papanicolaou smear	When first sexually active. Recheck 1–3 years.

(15) Men and women 16–44 years

Things doctor will look for or try to prevent	Doctor will do	Factors for consideration
Poliomyelitis	Immunisation	Booster to persons in good health.
Tetanus and diphtheria	Immunisation	Optional for diphtheria. Tetanus booster every 20 years for persons in good health.
Alcoholism, smoking, drugs, motor-vehicle accidents	Counselling	History.
Unwanted pregnancy	Contraceptives	
Family disturbance Marriage problems Sexual problems	Counselling	History.
Hearing problems	Examination	History
High blood pressure	Measure B.P.	At least every 5 years.

*See notes following.

Men and women 16–44 years (cont.)

Things doctor will look for or try to prevent	Doctor will do	Factors for consideration
Dental caries* Gum disease Cancer of mouth	Examination Encourage oral hygiene	
Rubella (German measles)	Immunise women at risk	If not immunised at younger age.
Cancer of neck or womb (cervix)*	Papanicolaou smear	First smear at start of sexual activity, then again after 1 year, thereafter every 3 years. More frequently if risk high.
Muscle-wasting diseases	Measure creatine phosphokinase in blood	Especially female relatives of known sufferers.
Diseases related to foreign travel	Immunisations as indicated depending on country visited	
Tuberculosis*	Tuberculin testing B.C.G. immunisations	Persons at special risk only.
Gonorrhoea	Swabs of neck of womb (cervix), urethra; culture of secretions from these sites and of early morning urine	Persons at risk, also pregnant women.
Thalassaemia (sickle cell blood disease)	Laboratory tests, screening	History. Asian, African and Mediterranean persons of parenting age, who, having been informed that no treatment is available, still wish to be screened.
Anaemia due to low level of iron and inadequate nutrition	Measure protein in blood. Concentration of pigment (haemoglobin) in blood	History. Particularly the lower socio-economic groups.
Cancer of the skin	Inspection. Counselling	High risk groups.
Cancer of bladder	Examination of cells in urine	High risk groups, including smokers.
Cancer of breast	Physical examination. Mammography or ultrasound	Annually for women over 30 years, especially high-risk persons.

*See notes following

(16) Women and men 45-64 years

Things doctor will look for or try to prevent		Time of search and action doctor will follow
Cancer of large bowel* and rectum	Test bowel motion for traces of blood	Approximately annually
Retirement distress	Counselling	
Cancer of breast*	Examination plus X-ray or ultrasound of the breast	Annually for women 45–59 years.
Inadequate functioning of thyroid gland (hypothyroidism)	Examination	Every 2 years in women past the menopause.
Osteoporosis	Check height	Annually all women after the menopause.
Plus all things recommended for men and women 16-44 years of age		

(17) Women and men 65-74 years

Things doctor will look for or try to prevent	Doctor will do	Factors for consideration
Tetanus and diphtheria	Immunisation	Booster every 20 years only persons in good health. Diphtheria optional.
Influenza	Immunisation	Annually. Not if allergic to egg protein.
Hearing problems	Examination	History.
High blood pressure*	Check B.P.	Every 2 years.
Dental caries* Diseases of gums Cancer of mouth	Examination. Advise daily oral hygiene	Annually.
Cancer of large bowel* and rectum	Test bowel motion for traces of blood	Annually.
Inadequate nutrition. Failure to cope with aging	Assess physical, social and psychological functioning	Every 2 years. Home visit often helpful.
Inadequate functioning of thyroid gland (hypothyroidism)	Examination	Every 2 years.

*See notes following.

Women and men 65–74 years (cont.)

Things doctor will look for or try to prevent	Doctor will do	Factors for consideration
Disorders related to foreign travel	Immunisation as indicated depending on country visited	
Tuberculosis*	Tuberculin testing B.C.G. if indicated	At-risk persons
Cancer of skin	Examination	
Cancer of bladder	Microscopic examination of urine	High-risk groups. Include smokers.
Cancer of neck of womb (cervix)*	Papanicolaou smear	3 yearly, or more often if judged desirable.
Osteoporosis	Check height	Annually all women.

(18) Women and men 75 years and up

Things doctor will look for or try to prevent	Doctor will do	Factors for consideration
Tetanus and diphtheria	Immunisation	Booster for persons in good health — every 20 years. Diphtheria optional.
Influenza	Immunisation	Annually. Not in persons allergic to egg protein.
Hearing problems	Examination	History.
High blood pressure	B.P. measurement	Every 2 years.
Cancer of large bowel* and rectum	Test bowel motion for traces of blood	Annually.
Cancer of mouth	Examination	Annually.
Increasing incapacity with age. Inadequate nutrition.	Assessment of physical, social and psychological function	Annually. Home visits very valuable.
Inadequate function of thyroid	Examination	Every 2 years.
Immunisations related to foreign travel	Immunisation	Varies with needs of particular countries.

*See notes following.

Women and men 75 years and up

Things doctor will look for or try to prevent	Doctor will do	Factors for consideration
Tuberculosis	Tuberculin testing B.C.G. immunisation	At-risk persons.
Cancer of skin	Examination	
Cancer of bladder	Microscopic examination of urine	High-risk groups. Include smokers.
Cancer of neck of womb (cervix)*	Papanicolaou smear	Every 3 years. More often in at-risk groups.
Osteoporosis	Check height	Annually all women.

*See notes following

2.3 Commentary on certain screening procedures

(1) Parents at risk of abusing their child

The careful doctor will be alert to emotional problems in the prenatal period, particularly with a view to preventing subsequent child abuse. Attention will be paid to parents who are clearly unhappy about the pregnancy and enquiries may be made about the parents' wishes with regard to the sex of the unborn child. If this is a matter of significance to the parents, the doctor may discuss whether this is related to the mother's need to please the father, or whether it is in some way to satisfy the mother's own needs. Discussion about these issues can be valuable.

If parents have unrealistically high expectations of the baby, who may be seen as a means of fulfilling needs in their own lives, they may later appear worried about minor delays in the development of the child, either physically or behaviourally.

They may be concerned that they cannot really cope with yet another child, or they may feel that there has been an insufficient gap since the last child. Such anxiety in the parents can lead to a deterioration in their relationship with other children in the family.

Some mothers try to convince themselves that they are not pregnant. They may refuse to discuss the pregnancy and take steps to avoid putting on weight. Such mothers may also make no plans at all for the arrival of the baby in the home. Depression about the baby is another warning sign. This may show as an otherwise unexplained disturbance of sleep, or reluctance to go out and to meet people. At worst there may be attempts at suicide or even successful suicide.

It may be appropriate for the doctor to ask such parents if they had ever given thought to having the pregnancy terminated and if so, why this was not done; or why, having thought seriously about it, they let the time slip by so that it would not be medically feasible. Allied to this is the question of whether the parents had ever thought of having the child adopted out and if they had, why they had not taken appropriate steps.

With single mothers and some couples, enquiries may be made about who is available to give the mother support and whether these people can be relied upon when needed. The extent to which helping agencies have been utilised may also be useful information.

If the mother feels isolated or apprehensive, this may be simply because of lack of understanding of what is happening to her or fear of the delivery. She may be concerned about the physical changes that her body is undergoing. It is even possible that rather than allaying these anxieties, as they should do, antenatal (i.e., prenatal) classes may be making them worse.

If the mother's demeanour shows no signs of joy or excitement at the prospect of the new baby, the possibility of later child abuse takes on an increasing importance.

If the mother is visiting the doctor more often than is strictly necessary, and particularly if she is producing many symptoms which seem to have little physical basis, the possibility of emotional problems is very high. Some patients develop an abnormal dependence on doctors or nurses.

Other matters that may warrant discussion, particularly with single mothers, are the living arrangements — whether these are suitable, whether she is on the phone and what is the availability of transport. Are there friends and relatives nearby that she can call upon when needed?

The doctor will probably also be interested in the home backgrounds of the parents and whether they were subject to child abuse themselves; what sort of discipline was administered and whether it was a stable home? The doctor may be interested to know if they plan to bring their own child up in the same way as they were brought up.

Note may be made of whether the parents can talk comfortably about these topics and whether they can look the interviewer in the eye as they do so. If the parents are thought to be at risk of causing child abuse, the doctor will either take responsibility for keeping a surveillance of the family or, as is more probable, refer them to an appropriate helping agency. Sometimes the doctor will seek expert confirmation from a specialist before taking this step. 'Parent Help' is the name of one organisation which works in this field and there are usually a number of parent support groups available.

If you consider yourself to be at risk of abusing your children, you should not be shy about informing your doctor, so that suitable help can be obtained.

(2) Screening the newborn child

The first days, weeks, months and even years after childbirth are difficult times for both parents, but particularly for the mother, who usually assumes the greater responsibility for the care of the child. It is also usually the mother who brings the child to the doctor.

Many doctors will use this opportunity not merely to check the physical development of the child, but also to assess the emotional progress of both child and parents. A great many questions may be asked; these will enable the doctor to explore these areas. Here are some of the questions which you may be asked if you have a young baby:

How are you managing with your new baby?
Is your baby as you imagined it would be?
Are you gaining confidence in managing the baby?
How does your spouse feel about the baby?
Does the baby seem satisfied after feeding?

(If breast feeding) Are your nipples giving any trouble?
Are you enjoying the new baby?
Do you talk to and cuddle the baby?
Is your spouse assisting with the care of the baby?

and later —

Do you find time to play with the baby?
Does your spouse find time to play with the baby?
Does your spouse feel jealous and left out of things?
Do you allow the child to separate from you for some time each day?
Do you think the baby is being spoiled?
How do other members of the household feel about the new baby?
What assistance are you getting in the care of the baby?
Do you think the baby enjoys you?
Do you get easily upset?
Are you irritable, depressed?
Are you getting enough sleep?
Is your baby the cuddly sort?
What difference is the baby making to your life?
Are you and your spouse agreeing on matters relating to the upbringing of the baby?
What sort of playthings are you providing for the baby?
How do you feel about your baby becoming a toddler?
Are you being criticised for the way you are bringing up the baby?
Do you need additional assistance in the care of the baby?

and later still —

Were there difficulties at the time of weaning (i.e., cessation of breast feeding)?
Are there feeding problems now?
Are you able to accept the demands made on you by the baby?
Do you find a need to punish the baby? If yes, what methods do you use?
Have you had any separations from the baby? How did the baby react?
How does the baby respond to your anger?
How do you respond to baby's anger or tantrums?
Does baby show affection? Do you find it easy to show affection in return?

(Adapted from *A Manual for General Practice* by Selwyn Carson, published by Beecham's Research Laboratories, New Zealand)

(3) Milestones in the young child's development
Here are a few milestones that give a rough indication of development.

Age	Movement	Behaviour
4–8 weeks	Lying on stomach, tries to lift head up. Eyes follow objects.	Watches mother's face. Starts to smile. Listens to bell or rattle.
2–4 months	Lying on stomach, rests on forearms. If held standing, sags at knees.	Laughs. Watches the movement of own hands. Reaches for objects.
5–7 months	Able to roll over. Holds bottle. No longer squints. Sits without support.	Says 'da'. Indicates food likes and dislikes.
8–12 months	Bears weight on legs when supported. Sits alone on floor. Grasps objects between finger and thumb.	Responds to 'No'. Babbles. Waves goodbye. Shows excitement. Uses 2–3 words with meaning
12–14 months	Crawls and sits well. Walks. Takes off shoes.	Says a few words. Understands a lot. Understands single commands.
18 months	Runs and jumps. Takes off socks. Many are clean and dry by day.	Obeys single orders. Points to nose, eyes and hair when asked to do so.
2 years	Puts on shoes, socks, and pants. Washes and dries hands. Goes up and down stairs alone. Some dry at night.	Talks constantly. Makes marks with pencil. Makes tower of 5 blocks. Knows 4 parts of the body.

(4) Bacteriuria (bacteria in the urine)

Most of the problems mentioned in the foregoing screening tables are self-explanatory and obviously meet most, if not all, of the criteria recommended by the World Health Organisation. Thus examination of pregnant women for evidence of bacteria in the urine is of great importance, because during pregnancy, infection of the urine is believed capable of causing permanent kidney damage, as can infection in childhood. Infection in adults, except when pregnant, seems to be remarkably benign as far as long-term effects are concerned and studies done on some people who have experienced much inconvenience and pain as a result of recurrent infections of their urine over many years have found little or no abnormality of their kidneys or bladder.

(5) Phenylketonuria (PKU)

There is a simple test which is done on a sample of blood from newborn babies, which is capable of diagnosing this fortunately very rare condition. People suffering from this condition have an abnormality of their makeup which leads to them passing an excess of a substance called phenylalanine in their urine. The condition is an inherited one which is treated by a strict diet, particularly avoiding proteins which are broken down in the body of sufferers to phenylalanine. If this is achieved, the patients will usually develop normally, but untreated, the patients are mentally retarded, have small heads and develop eczema. They are also known for their bad tempers. Because of their mental retardation they usually need to be placed in an institution and are very costly to maintain.

(6) Congenital displacement of the hip (CDH)

This displacement (or *dislocation* as it is usually called) is relatively common. If identified early and given suitable treatment, the sufferer will usually develop a normal hip, whereas if left undiagnosed and untreated, a degenerative disease (i.e., osteoarthritis) usually supervenes. Sometimes the symptoms do not appear until many years after birth, but by then the damage is done.

(7) Dental caries

This diagnosis is usually made by a dentist. Dental decay is common and may require little more than a look in the mouth to identify. Sometimes X-rays are taken. Severe caries can have a profound effect on the ability to chew solid foods and can lead to malnutrition (i.e., inadequate or unsatisfactory diet). The treatment is straightforward and successful but not always acceptable to the patient.

(8) Cervical smears (i.e., Papanicolaou or 'Pap' smears)

The cervix is the lower part of the womb (uterus). It contains the opening (os) which enables spermatozoa from the male to enter the body of the uterus. It is an area which seems to be particularly liable to develop cancer (i.e., carcinoma of the cervix). By gently scraping the surface of the cervix it is possible to obtain a sample of the cells which can then be examined under a microscope with a view to identifying any which are atypical and thus suggestive of early carcinoma. Most authorities take the view that this test is worthwhile and encourage regular smears from the time a woman is first sexually active.

As with so many screening programmes, cervical smears were advocated before the natural history of the early pre-cancerous changes which occur at the entrance to the uterus had been properly evaluated. As a result, we have only fragmentary knowledge of whether these early changes always develop into cancer and if they do, how long it takes before this occurs. If we had this information we would know better how frequently these smears should be done.

There are also difficulties in assessing whether the cost of mass screening is justifiable in terms of the numbers of lives saved and amount of ill health prevented. Certainly there appears to have been a reduction in the number of women developing cancer of the cervix, as a result of screening programmes.

The treatment of abnormal smears has changed greatly over the years. At one time even very early changes in the cells of the cervix were considered sufficient justification for a *hysterectomy* (i.e., removal of the womb). Then followed the era of *conisation*, a procedure which involved the coring out of the affected part of the cervix. This had the effect of removing the abnormal cells but often resulted in women being excessively prone to miscarriages, as the cervix lost its effectiveness as a means of holding the unborn baby in place (i.e., cervical incompetence).

Today it is more usual to destroy the abnormal cells by freezing or burning and thereafter to examine the affected area on a regular basis. If there is evidence that cancer has established itself, procedures such as conization, hysterectomy and radiation of the cervix are still used.

Abnormal changes in the cells of the cervix seem to be becoming more common again and some attribute this to the changes in sexual habits which appear to have accompanied the widespread acceptance of the contraceptive pill. There is some suggestion that there is a relationship between genital warts and changes in the cervical cells. Others implicate also the viruses of genital herpes. Debate centres on:
(i) The age at which screening should start.
(ii) The frequency with which screening should be done.
(iii) Whether screening should be offered to all women or simply those who are known to be in special 'at risk' categories. These include:
(a) Those who have started sexual activity very early.
(b) Those who have had multiple partners.
(c) Persons of lower socio-economic class.
(d) Persons with a history of genital warts or genital herpes.
(e) Those who have had large numbers of children.
(f) Those with low standards of personal hygiene.

There seems to be little or no risk to women who have never had sexual intercourse.

Unfortunately, those who are at greatest risk seem to be the very ones who are least likely to cooperate in a screening programme. The usual recommendation is that initial screening should take place soon after the commencement of an active sexual life, one year later, and thereafter once every three years. Any women who are found to have minor abnormalities in their smears, not justifying active intervention, are recommended to have annual smears, as are those women listed above as being at special risk.

Many doctors when they do a cervical smear also take the opportunity to do a full internal examination of their patients. This involves inserting the two gloved fingers of one hand into the vagina and with the other hand, examination of the lower abdomen. In this way the doctor is able to ascertain the position of the uterus in the pelvis, feel for any irregularities or abnormalities of the cervix, determine the size of the uterus and whether there are any lumps or bumps (e.g. fibroids) in it and also whether there is present any abnormality of the ovaries (e.g. cysts) or the fallopian tubes and adjacent structures. Some believe this examination is more important than the smear itself and often treatable complaints are discovered at such times.

(9) High blood pressure (hypertension)

The test for this, done with an instrument called a *sphygmomanometer*, is a very simple one and presents no danger or embarrassment to patients. High blood pressure appears to be a good target for screening as the test is cheap and there seems to be an effective treatment.

Furthermore, there are usually few if any symptoms or signs until the condition is far advanced. Unfortunately the treatment is not without side effects and there is some doubt about how useful it is in reducing the incidence of heart attacks. Recent evidence, however, seems to support the view that it reduces the likelihood of the patient having a stroke. (See section on treatment of blood pressure.)

Usually *hypertension* is found by the process described as 'Case finding'. Sometimes attempts have been made at mass screening of populations but although the diagnosis is made quite frequently, many of those so identified do not seem to follow the matter up with their doctors even when advised to do so.

Debate centres around
(a) the level at which blood pressure should be considered abnormal in various age groups, and
(b) whether in mild cases the disadvantages of the treatment (i.e., side effects such as lassitude, dry mouth and sometimes impotence) outweigh the benefits.

Blood pressure is further discussed in other sections of this book. (See pp. 151–2 and pp. 243–8.)

(10) Cancer of the breast

Breast cancer is very common in women, with one in 17 suffering from it at some time in their lives. It is generally considered that the earlier it is found, the better the outlook. There are differences of opinion about the effectiveness of treatment. Apparently there are several types of cancer and some authorities take the view that in many cases there is early spread to other parts of the body (*metastases* or *secondaries*) even when the growth is still very small. With these types it is thought that even if the cancer is removed early, those elements which have spread are likely ultimately to grow and lead to the death of the patient. Other varieties seem to be much less virulent and the growth can become quite large before any spread occurs. Some are so slow growing that sufferers may die of something else before the growth has a chance to do its deadly work.

Regrettably, we do not have satisfactory ways of determining the presence of very early spread and once spread is detectable, it is usually, but not always, well advanced. As a result, it is commonly considered best to remove the growth in the breast. In addition the armpit area (i.e. axilla) which is where the earliest spread usually seems to occur, is sometimes irradiated with X-rays or other cell-destroying radiation in the hope of eliminating any tumour cells which may have lodged there.

Breast cancer is affected by certain chemical messenger substances within the body (i.e. *hormones*) and in some cases steps are taken to suppress the secretions of the pituitary gland or the ovaries which help in the production of these hormones. In advanced cases actual removal of the ovaries can be helpful.

Breast cancer is usually silent (i.e. without symptoms) until it is quite advanced and as it is thought to have a better outlook if it is found early, it has been considered a suitable target for screening programmes.

We do not know how long it takes from the very first development of cancer cells until the growth is clearly and easily felt by examining fingers. This means that we do not know how frequently the examination needs to be done. Certainly there are sophisticated new methods of detection by using X-rays, and also *ultrasound*, which enable the cancer to be identified much earlier than formerly and with much less radiation. Many authorities believe that the widespread use of these new techniques would lead to earlier detection and treatment of breast cancer and that as a result the mortality from this disease would fall.

Unfortunately the tests are complicated and expensive and the number of women who can be examined by one machine in one day is limited to about 50. For these reasons, in most countries such screening is not yet practicable on a large scale. An alternative is manual examination by a doctor or other trained professional. Actually the ideal would appear to be the combination of manual examination and mammography. Many doctors make a point of offering this examination to women at the same time as they have a cervical smear and internal examination.

However, even this may not be sufficiently frequent to pick up early growths and as a result some believe that regular self-examination of the breasts is desirable. Considerable publicity has been given to the techniques of this procedure and to the desirability of monthly examination, but the number of women who do breast self-examination conscientiously seems to be small. It is recommended that the examination should be done shortly after the monthly period has ceased. Immediately prior to the period, the breasts are often rather firm and have a natural tendency to lumpiness; after menstruation this largely disappears. If anything abnormal is found on this examination, a doctor should be consulted. An early cancer is likely to feel similar to a dried pea surrounded by sponge rubber although it can of course be either smaller or larger. Advice should also be sought if at any time there is an unexplained discharge from the nipple or any bleeding. Happily only about 1 in 20 breast lumps prove to be cancerous.

Mammography (X-ray of the breast or ultrasound)

Many recommend that rather than doing mammography on all women randomly, it is probably still better to reserve this resource for those women who are at greatest risk of breast cancer. These are:

1. Women who have their first baby after 30 years of age.
2. Women who have had no children.
3. Women who have already had cancer in one breast (approximately 15 per cent will develop cancer in the other breast).
4. Women who have a mother or sister with breast cancer.
5. Women whose periods cease at 54 years of age or older.
6. Women who already have other non-malignant lumps in their breasts.
7. Women whose breasts have been exposed to many X-rays.

The risk of developing breast cancer increases with increasing age, the condition being relatively rare before the age of 30.

In the future mammography services may become more generally available and it may be feasible to widen the net.

How to perform a breast self-examination

Position 1: Stand or sit before a mirror with your chest uncovered. Let your arms hang at

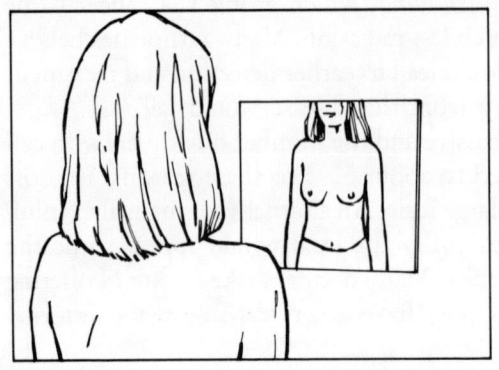
Position 1

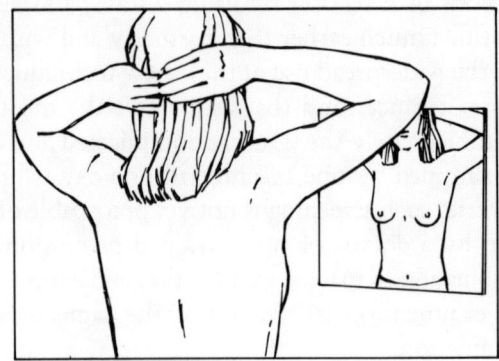
Position 2

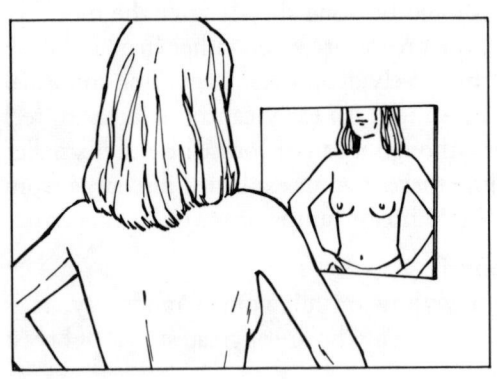
Position 3

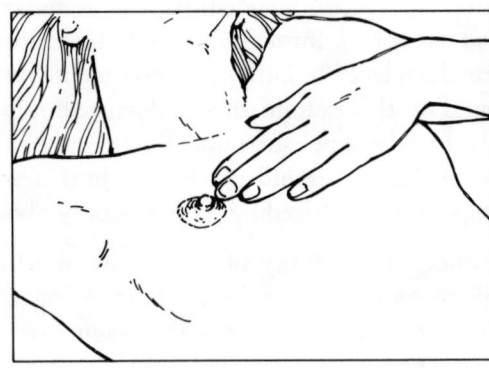
Position 4

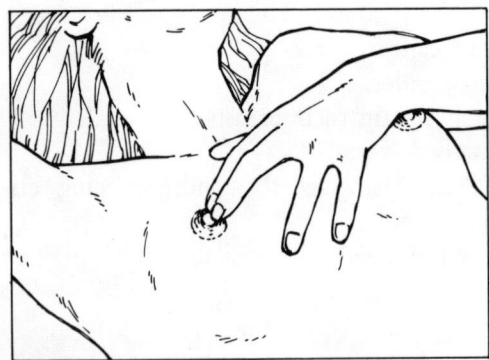
Position 5

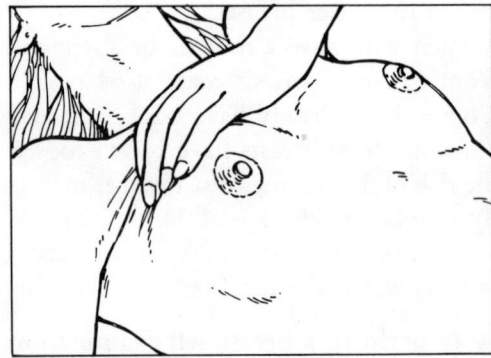
Position 6

your sides. Become familiar with the size and shape of your breasts so that you will be able to detect any changes.

Position 2: Raise your arms above your head and observe whether there is any alteration from the normal size and shape.

Position 3: Place your hands on your hips; press in and down firmly, tightening the muscles in the upper part of your body. Any abnormal dimpling or puckering of the skin, or pulling in of the nipple, will be visible.

Position 4: Now lie on your back with a small pillow or folded towel under your right shoulder. Raise your right arm above your head. Imagine your breast to be divided into six sections, radiating from the nipple. With the fingers of your left hand held flat, press your right breast gently from edge to nipple, starting at the top and working systematically over each section. This is called *palpation*.

Position 5: After palpating each section of your breast, use two fingers to examine the nipple area.

Position 6: Now lower your right arm to rest your hand on your right hip, and palpate the armpit area.

Remove the pillow, place under your left shoulder and examine your left breast in the same manner with your right hand.

(11) Cancer of the lung

Routine screening examinations for this cancer are seldom justified because the results of treatment are so poor. The number of people who recover completely from cancer of the lung after an operation is very small indeed. Let smokers be warned!

(12) Tuberculosis

Chest X-rays of people who are known to have been exposed to this disease, or communities that are believed to have a special susceptibility, can still be justified as a cost-effective screening procedure. In most western countries the number of cases picked up is very small now that there are effective treatment programmes available. Furthermore, because of these treatments, the disease does not present the same terrors as hitherto. There are also skin tests which can be done to determine whether a person has ever developed a resistance to tuberculosis.

Such skin tests are often given to adolescents, and those who show no evidence of having come into contact with tuberculosis bacteria are given the opportunity of inoculation with B.C.G. This inoculation is with a live but attenuated strain of tuberculosis. The strain is named *Bacillus calmette guerin* and the term attenuated refers to the fact that as a result of special techniques, its ability to produce tissue damage is reduced to almost negligible levels. Despite this, resistance is produced and as a consequence the tubercle bacillus proper is less likely to gain a foothold in the body.

(13) Cancer of the bowel

This is also a very common cancer which sometimes is not evident until it has reached a fairly advanced stage. The usual early signs are changes in the bowel habits, e.g. a person who has always had very regular bowels suddenly becomes constipated, or a person who has always had normal, well-formed solid bowel motions experiences persistent bowel looseness.

Sometimes there is bleeding from the bowel associated with the passage of the motion. Sometimes there is excessive mucus present. Abdominal pain and weight loss and even nausea may be features. The patient may be anaemic. Should any of these symptoms persist for any length of time, a visit to a general practitioner is indicated. Some people recommend that after about 40–45 years of age every adult should have their bowel motion checked each year for traces of blood. There are some fairly simple chemical tests which are capable of picking up such traces of blood from small samples of bowel motion (*faeces*). Such samples are usually collected on three or more separate days and then handed in to the laboratory for testing. If there is no trace of blood in the faeces, it makes it much less likely that there is a growth in the bowel, although it does not disprove it entirely. Most growths bleed a little.

Of course, this test is not very useful if there are also bleeding piles (haemorrhoids) or some other reason for bleeding in the bowel. The diet for a few days prior to the test should be watched (remembering that it takes approximately 48 hours for food to pass through the body) as certain things, including large amounts of ascorbic acid (Vitamin C) seem to be capable of causing the test to be falsely negative. Your doctor can advise you of any special precautions that need to be taken before embarking on the collection of samples.

Although a negative test is reassuring, positive tests cause anxiety and may make it necessary to do other investigations to elucidate the cause. False positives are fairly common and some doctors do not favour the test for this reason.

2.4 The emotions and disease

'Health and cheerfulness mutually beget each other'
— Joseph Addison, *The Spectator*, No. 25.

Just what part do the emotions play in the causation of ill health? Certain facts appear to be fairly well established, and one of these is that if we are tired or depressed, we are more prone to ill health. People who have a really buoyant, positive approach to life seem to be much less susceptible. Some would say that emotion plays a part in the production of almost all illness and certainly the opposite applies, for when we have fallen victim to an illness, this has an effect on our emotional state. Some people respond to illness with anger, others with depression. Few, if any, feel better for it, although sometimes illness can provide a wonderful excuse to avoid something distasteful.

At least one very unpleasant condition is said, at times, to give its sufferers a sense of wellbeing (euphoria). This is multiple sclerosis, otherwise known as MS. As a result, some of these patients may appear to be less concerned about their plight than might ordinarily be expected.

The effect of life events on an individual's health

Two researchers, Thomas Holmes and Richard Rahe, have attempted to quantify the effect of various life events on an individual's health. Their results were derived from a close study of 5000 people. Some of the events included are unexpected and would be regarded as desirable and certainly are not usually regarded as stressful. The determining factor seems to be *change* in the life pattern. It has been found that if the total for any 12 months, when all the life events are scored and added up, equals or exceeds 300, there is an 80 per cent chance of a major change in health in the following 12 months. If the score is between 150 and 299, there is a 50 per cent chance of a change in health and between 100 and 149 a 37 per cent chance.

This phenomenon of ill health following great emotional upheaval is particularly well recognised in relation to the death of a husband or wife. The incidence of illness in the surviving partner, in the year after a bereavement, is much greater than that in the unaffected population. Doctors who are aware of these increased risks in their patients can use this information and take steps to help them to identify the earliest signs of ill health, or better still, advise their patients against changes in their lifestyle which would increase their risks.

Here is the list of life events and the value assigned to each. Of course, we all react a little differently and an event which has a profound effect on one person may have a somewhat lesser effect on another.

Stressful situations capable of leading to ill health
(Holmes and Rahe Social Readjustment Rating Scale)

Event	Mean Value	Event	Mean Value
Death of a spouse	100	Son or daughter leaving home	29
Divorce	73	Trouble with in-laws	29
Marital separation	65	Outstanding personal achievement	28
Gaol term	63	Wife begins or stops work	26
Death of a close family member	63	Begin or end school	26
Personal injury or illness	53	Change in living conditions	25
Marriage	50	Revision of personal habits	24
Fired at work	47	Trouble with boss	23
Marital reconciliation	45	Change in work hours or conditions	20
Retirement	45	Change in residence	20
Change in health of family member	44	Change in schools	20
Pregnancy	39	Change in recreation	19
Sex difficulties	39	Change in church activities	19
Gain of new family member	39	Change in social activities	18
Business readjustment	39	Mortgage or loan for lesser purpose (car, TV, etc.)	17
Death of close friend	37	Change in sleeping habits	16
Change to different line of work	36	Change in number of family get-togethers	15
Change in number of arguments with spouse	35	Change in eating habits	15
Mortgage or loan for major purpose (home, etc.)	31	Vacation	13
Foreclosure of mortgage or loan	30	Christmas	12
Change in responsibilities at work	29	Minor violations of the law	11

There are certain conditions where the association between emotional disturbances and illness are apparently very clear cut and these are sometimes referred to as *psychosomatic* diseases. (The 'soma' is the body and the 'psyche' refers to the mind.)

There are other disorders where there is probably very little psychological influence. In between are some conditions where it is thought psychological influences may play a part, but just how great a part remains uncertain. Cancer would be one such condition. In fact the division of disorders into those which are psychosomatic and those which are not has come to be seen as unhelpful for the very reason that the emotions play such a large part in so many. However, as an example we can list some disorders in a sort of spectrum according to the degree to which emotional influences are thought to play a part:

Small involvement	Some involvement	Considerable involvement	Major involvement
Leptospirosis	Influenza	Hypertension	Hyperventilation
Measles	Coryza	Asthma	Globus hystericus
Paget's disease	Glandular fever	Neurodermatitis	Irritable colon

Small involvement	Some involvement	Considerable involvement	Major involvement
Renal calculus	Atopic eczema	Rheumatoid arthritis	Tension headache
Osteoarthritis	Psoriasis	Anorexia nervosa	
Worms, etc		Thyrotoxicosis	
		Peptic ulcer	
		Migraine	
		Type A behaviour heart disease	

Whole-person care Sometimes you may wonder why it is that your doctor asks you personal questions concerning certain aspects of your life. This is usually because the doctor is endeavouring to provide whole-person care, and is not content merely to treat the presenting problem which may be the symptom of a major family or work upheaval and its consequent anxieties.

Hyperventilation

This is the medical term for *overbreathing*. Some people, when they are in a state of great anxiety, respond by breathing faster or more deeply. Not only is this a natural reaction to such situations, but often people are advised to take deep breaths in order to steady themselves. Such advice, if acted upon, may be helpful where a person has been breathing very rapidly, but of course, if persevered with too long, can itself cause symptoms.

The person who hyperventilates, for whatever reason, expels an excessive amount of carbon dioxide from the lungs and hence from the bloodstream. Carbon dioxide is produced when the oxygen which is inhaled is utilised by the body. In effect, the carbon dioxide is the waste product of the chemical reactions involved in gas exchange in the lungs, and it has to be removed or it will accumulate in the body and the person concerned will become very drowsy. Although it is essentially a waste product, the carbon dioxide does have its uses. First, it has the power to combine with water in the bloodstream to form a weak acid, and this plays an important part in keeping the acid/alkali balance of the blood normal. Its other function is to act on certain receptors at the base of the brain which have the ability to stimulate the rate of breathing, according to the concentration of carbon dioxide in the blood. If this stimulus is lost, the person loses his or her automatic breathing movements and may cease to breath altogether until further carbon dioxide accumulates.

Some swimmers deliberately hyperventilate before diving so as to increase the time before the body automatically requires them to take further breaths. This may enable them to remain under water for a longer time, but is nevertheless a hazardous thing to do.

In those circumstances where a person hyperventilates in response to anxiety, the breathing is usually obviously abnormal and the person begins to experience some unusual and frightening symptoms which often further increases the anxiety and leads to even more rapid breathing. Ultimately some people lose consciousness altogether, but before they do so they may experience a variety of symptoms. These may include dizziness, faintness, headache, pins and needles in the hands and feet and often characteristically, around the mouth. The chest may feel tight and there may be frequent sighing and yawning. There may be muscle cramps and the muscles may twitch, particularly if they are tapped. Often there is sweating, the mouth and throat may feel dry; the patient may swallow air and subsequently belch or may develop a bloated abdomen, swollen with air. Sometimes the patient is conscious of irregular, rapid or heavy heartbeats (palpitation) and there may be aches in the chest wall.

If the condition is prolonged, the person may feel very weak, may sleep poorly and have difficulty with concentration.

Air hunger With all these symptoms it is not surprising that many people are greatly alarmed. Some even believe that they are having a stroke or a heart attack. A usual complaint is of being unable to get enough air into the chest. Minor degrees of this problem are probably commoner than we suppose. Severe cases are obvious and usually respond remarkably to the reassurance of doctors who are confident of their diagnosis. Sometimes it is not entirely a nervous disorder, and there is a disease process present which produces the symptoms which are responsible for the anxiety in the first place.

Once patients have been reassured, they can often control their breathing voluntarily, but if all else fails they can be told to breathe into a paper bag held tightly around the nose and mouth. In this way they will inhale again most of the carbon dioxide they have breathed out and before very long the normal balance of oxygen to carbon dioxide in the lungs and the bloodstream will be restored. The circumstances which have led to the onset of the hyperventilation can then be fully explored.

Globus hystericus

This is really a problem with swallowing, which is particularly likely to develop in people who worry about their health when they are under stress. It is a feeling of a lump or obstruction in the throat, even though expert examination shows that there is no physical abnormality. Reassurance after adequate examination is often enough to make it go away. A few of the cases which had been thought to be entirely nervous in their origin have actually proved to be the result of some regurgitation of acid from the stomach. Doctors always have to be very cautious about attributing symptoms entirely to nervous origins.

The irritable bowel

The alimentary tract (the pathway that the food which we eat takes through the body) seems peculiarly sensitive to emotional stimuli. Most of its activity is entirely involuntary (i.e. automatic, and independent of an individual's control). However, it does seem to respond to numerous stimuli.

The lower part of this tract — the so-called 'large bowel' — responds to a variety of irritants and this is the mechanism by which many laxatives (medicines given to cope with constipation) work. Substances such as senna (from senna pods) and danthron act principally by stimulating the bowel into greater activity. When the activity is excessive, diarrhoea is produced. For some people, even worry is enough to stimulate the bowel into action, as many students know at examination time. Where the anxiety is chronic, the stimulation of the bowel may also be chronic and some individuals regularly have one, two or more loose motions every day. It would seem also that certain foodstuffs are capable of irritating some bowels. We are all different in our responses, and a substance which is tolerated perfectly well by the majority of people may act almost like a poison in others. The same applies to medicines.

Unfortunately the various irritants that are referred to above often lead to bowel spasm and this can be painful. Sometimes the spasm, rather than causing diarrhoea, actually slows down the action of the bowel, thus leading to constipation.

The pain of irritable colon can be very persistent and usually has a colicky nature (i.e., intermittently, but regularly rising to a crescendo and then diminishing or going away completely). It is likely to occur in a variety of places in the abdomen and is seldom in the same place for more than a few hours. Nevertheless, it may mimic a number of abdominal conditions, including appendicitis. Often it is associated with the swallowing of air which in turn may lead to belching of wind (eructation) and the passage of wind from the back passage (flatus). The irritated bowel tends to produce more mucus than normal and the patient may be alarmed by the excessive amounts of this colourless or white, somewhat thick material which may be found on the toilet paper after the passage of a bowel motion.

If blood as well as mucus is present, the problem is more serious than an irritable bowel and should always be thoroughly investigated.

The onset For many people with an irritable bowel, the problem seems to start with a bowel infection. Presumably while the bowel is still recovering from this, other irritating factors come into play, factors which perhaps would not normally have caused problems but which now assume importance. As a consequence, many believe that the condition is 'multifactorial'. Thus we may have any or all of the following contributing:

> Infection
> Emotion — usually anxiety
> Food irritation
> Food allergy
> Inadequate bulk in the diet

and possibly others.

Many sufferers from irritable bowel seem to have an underlying fear of cancer of the bowel and sometimes the condition seems to go into remission for quite some time after a thorough investigation, including X-rays.

The most important part of the treatment of the condition is again adequate reassurance and this often means a full examination and appropriate tests. Spasm of the bowel, which, as stated, is often painful, seems to be reduced if the bowel contains a reasonable amount of bulky residue. Diets which have a high level of residue, such as those containing fibre (see p. 100), can be effective here. Unfortunately, for many people moderate amounts of bran (a good source of fibre) produce an unacceptable quantity of gas, which before it is passed as wind may aggravate the pain due to the bowel spasm. There are other, even more inert, bulk-producing agents, of which Isogel is one. This is made from the husk of the ispaghula plant. It is available in granule form and these granules absorb fluid and form a gelatinous mass. The substance is quite harmless, although it has occasionally been known to lead to blockage of the bowel in persons who already have a partial blockage from other causes.

Isogel is often used by people who are prone to constipation. Not only does its bulk help to make the bowel work more efficiently, but also its physical characteristics assist in preventing the bowel motion from becoming too hard. Some people have great difficulty in swallowing Isogel, but it can be sprinkled on a breakfast cereal or quickly stirred into water and drunk. Others prefer to place the spoonful of granules on the back of the tongue and then swallow it with a gulp of water, as is the practice with tablets. It is desirable that it should be taken with plenty of fluid as otherwise it will absorb water from the bowel and this can be even more constipating. In fact Isogel can be used to help control a mild diarrhoea, and in this case it is usually taken with a minimum of fluid.

A similar substance to Isogel is Metamucil, while Granocol is really Isogel combined with a mild irritant to further stimulate bowel action.

Other treatments There are other agents which can play a part in controlling an irritable bowel. These include some of the antispasmodics (see Section 4 on medicines), some derivatives of opium, which reduce the activity of the bowel, and even tranquillisers, which may help to relieve any underlying anxiety.

Although we often refer to the 'irritable *colon*' because the colon or large bowel is the part most often involved, it is probably more accurate to refer to the 'irritable *bowel*', for the abnormality in the contractions of the bowel which are responsible for the symptoms may be experienced almost anywhere in the alimentary tract. Even globus hystericus, referred to earlier, may be a manifestation of disordered contractions of the oesophagus (gullet). Other people may get pain in the central lower chest as a result of spasm of the lower end of the oesophagus. This is particularly likely to occur if the valve-like mechanism at the junction of the stomach and oesophagus is not working well and some of the acid from the stomach gets a chance to wash back on to the oesophagus, thus damaging its lining.

Unfortunately, taking antispasmodics in this complaint may relax the valve-like mechanism even further and so facilitate the regurgitation of acid on to the oesophagus. Should the acid get up to the throat or mouth, the sufferer becomes very aware of its presence, and this is described as 'water brash' or 'heartburn'. The fluid has a sour, rather acrid taste, and there is likely to be a burning feeling in the mouth as well as in the oesophagus.

Other disorders where emotion plays a role

Two other conditions where emotion plays a major role are *tension headache*, which is discussed in another section of this book (see p. 137) and *anorexia nervosa*, which is referred to in Chapter 2.5 on diet (p. 88).

In those conditions where emotional influences are listed on pp. 78–9 as having a *considerable* involvement, the relationship is much less clear cut, but seems well established in most cases. However, usually other factors are of equal or greater importance. Some of these conditions will be discussed in other sections of this book.

As far as those conditions listed as having *some* emotional content is concerned, the evidence is even less secure. Many doctors have observed that colds and other viral infections such as influenza seem more likely to occur when people are feeling depressed and 'run down'. It is interesting that glandular fever (infectious mononucleosis) is particularly prone to occur in young people at exam time.

The real cause of many skin conditions remains obscure, but there is good evidence that some, such as atopic eczema, worsen when the patient is below par. The doctor who makes such judgements has to be careful, of course, that the sensation of suboptimal health is the cause of the worsening and is not, in fact, a reaction to the worsening. Sometimes this is very hard to determine and makes research in these conditions difficult.

Finally there are the conditions in which emotion plays almost no part at all as far as can be determined. A few examples of these are included in the list.

The treatments discussed here are designed to give symptomatic relief only. The best answer to such disorders lies in identifying the problems which are the background to them and then trying to resolve these. (See also Chapter 4.1, Emotional and mental problems, pp. 190–203.)

2.5 Diet and health

'So I think it is very nice for ladies to be lithe and lissome,
but not so much that you cut yourself if you happen to embrace or kissome'.
— Ogden Nash (1902-71)

There is a widely held view, which has more than an element of truth, that, 'You are what you eat'. Attitude to diet tends to vary from those who take the view that most people will instinctively find their way to getting all the necessary nutrients, to those who believe that everything we eat should be rigidly studied and controlled. The truth probably lies somewhere between the two extremes. A balanced diet must be suited to the individual's nutritional requirements. Additionally it must be correct in *quantity* and *quality*.

Quantity

The energy content of a diet is measured in kilocalories. One kilocalorie = 4.2 kilojoules. Each person requires a number of kilocalories to keep their body functioning. Only certain nutrients contribute to the kilocalorie content of the diet. These are *proteins*, which are mostly in meat, nuts, milk, fish, eggs; *carbohydrates*, which are the sugars and starches; and *fats*, some of which are listed later in this chapter.

One gram of carbohydrate used by the body provides 4 kilocalories (1 teaspoon of sugar weighs 5 g and provides 20 kilocalories), 1 gram of fat 9 kilocalories and 1 gram of protein 4 kilocalories. These kilocalories can be likened to the petrol that a car requires. Just as a certain amount of petrol can take a car a certain distance, so a certain number of kilocalories will keep the body going for a certain time. Once those kilocalories are used up, the body can go no further unless it draws on energy stores in the body, mostly in the form of fat. When this occurs, fat and other substances are used up and the weight drops. Thus, regardless of whether a person has a glandular disorder or not, if the kilocalories in the food which is eaten are less than those used in daily living, the weight of that person must fall. Were this not so, the body would have to be seen as a sort of perpetual motion device, defying the laws of thermodynamics.

These simple facts form the basis of all reducing diets and highlight the part that diet must play in weight reduction. If a person is not losing weight on a diet which is carefully designed to give fewer kilocalories than that person's basic kilocalorie needs for everyday life, there can be only one explanation — that person is not keeping to the diet. There were no overweight people in the German prisoner-of-war camps when food was severely restricted during World War II.

Sometimes difficulties arise in tailoring a diet to an individual's needs. Some people's basic needs for kilocalories seem to be lower than others so that their diet must be stricter than others. Occasionally this appears to be related to a more efficient utilisation of food by the body, but more often it seems to be due to less muscle activity. Whatever we are doing, there is always some muscle activity, but for some folk this movement when at rest is very slight, whereas for others, who might be considered fidgety people, it is likely to be much greater. Studies have shown that most overweight people have fewer of these muscle movements than those who are lean. Obviously deliberate exercise, whether in the course of daily work or sport, will also have an effect on kilocalorie utilisation, and some people keep their weight down by virtue of regular strenuous exercise. The average energy requirements for moderately active men and women is shown in the table below.

Approximate daily energy requirements for moderately active people (in kilocalories)

Men	Average	Range	Women	Average	Range
19–22 years	2900	2500–3300	19–22 years	2100	1700–2500
23–50 years	2700	2300–3100	23–50 years	2000	1600–2400
51–75 years	2400	2000–2800	51–75 years	1800	1400–2200
76+ years	2050	1650–2450	76+ years	1600	1200–2000

The amount of exercise necessary to reduce body weight by half a kilogram is remarkably large. Furthermore, some claim that exercise leads to an increased appetite, making it hard to avoid undoing some of the benefit obtained. Probably the best approach to weight reduction is a combination of diet and exercise, with the greater emphasis on diet.

Another reason for overweight

A few people, for various reasons, accumulate fluid in their tissues. This fluid is known as *oedema* and the amount is usually small. This is not fat and usually it can, if necessary, be removed by the use of diuretics (q.v.).

It is true that when first starting on a weight-reducing diet, the breakdown of fatty tissues leads to the production of water which may lead to a temporary increase in weight, which can be very disheartening to a person who is trying very hard and needs some evidence of success. Such people need to know that the weight gain is temporary only, or at least will not be excessive, and that a fall can be anticipated in a short time if they persevere.

The regular use of diuretics in the management of patients who are overweight is not indicated and not really helpful unless there is some other problem as well. Furthermore, being overweight increases the chances of developing diabetes and as most diuretics also represent a risk factor for diabetes, they are better avoided if possible.

Other medical problems associated with overweight
1. An increased tendency to high blood pressure.
2. Varicose veins.
3. Possibly coronary artery disease and stroke.
4. Osteoarthritis.
5. Back problems.
6. Skin irritation.
7. Gallstones and gallbladder disease.
8. Hiatus hernia.
9. Constipation.
10. Poor wound healing after operations.
11. Cancer of the uterus
12. Chest disorders.
13. In women, increased tendency to menstrual problems.
14. Breast cancer.

Overall there is a reduced life expectancy.

Recommended weights
Here is a table of recommended weights so that you can check to see how you measure up. (Courtesy of 'Health Information' Series, No 87, issued by the New Zealand Department of Health.)

Note: Measurements are made without clothing and shoes.

Men				Women			
cm	(in)	kg	(lb)	cm	(in)	kg	(lb)
165	(65)	62 ± 5	(137 ± 11)	155	(61)	50 ± 4	(112 ± 9)
170	(67)	66 ± 5	(146 ± 12)	160	(63)	54 ± 5	(118 ± 10)
175	(69)	70 ± 6	(155 ± 14)	165	(65)	57 ± 5	(126 ± 10)
180	(71)	74 ± 7	(163 ± 15)	170	(67)	60 ± 5	(133 ± 10)
185	(73)	78 ± 7	(171 ± 15)	175	(69)	65 ± 5	(140 ± 11)

Appetite-reducing substances
There are a number of substances which have an effect on the appetite. Thus alcohol, insulin, certain steroids, thyroid hormone, sulphonylureas (used in the treatment of diabetes), certain antidepressants and tranquillisers and the antihistamines can all increase the appetite, whereas bulk agents, such as methylcellulose and Isogel (which take up space in the stomach), glucagon (a drug which releases glucose, i.e. sugar, stored in the liver), indomethacin (an anti-inflammatory agent), morphine and digoxin (used in heart disease), all tend to diminish the appetite.

Certain substances have been developed specifically for the purpose of reducing appetite. Many of these are related to amphetamine and although it is claimed that they have little or no tendency to habit formation, I prefer not to use them. Amphetamine itself is a stimulant which gives those who take it a feeling of great energy and wellbeing. It also makes them more wakeful — in drug-user circles it is known as 'speed'. Habituation, once acquired, is hard to break. Apart from these hazards, the principle behind the use of drugs for weight reduction seems hard to sustain. For most people an abrupt loss of weight associated with a radical but temporary change of diet serves little purpose. Once the former dietary regime is re-established or the tablets are discontinued, the patient rapidly returns to the previous weight level.

A lifetime eating pattern

The aim of any dietary programme for weight loss must be to develop a habit of eating less and in my view this should start from the commencement of the diet and be regarded as a lifetime regime. There should be a slow and steady fall of approximately 0.5–1.0 kg per week, over a period of months rather than a sudden steep fall over a period of days or weeks. Once the target weight is achieved, advice should be sought about slight modifications to the diet which will enable the weight to be maintained permanently at the lower level.

The best diets are those which are tailored to the individual's needs or lifestyle. Most of us have evolved a pattern of eating which remains constant year in and year out. Few are prepared to make major changes in that pattern, so the secret is to modify in small ways the existing diet.

The habit of skipping meals does not seem to be helpful. The majority of my overweight patients seem to go without breakfast and often they have only a small nibble of food at lunchtime. By the evening they are feeling very virtuous and consider they have been so well disciplined that they deserve an ample dinner. This pattern of eating seems to encourage obesity and I always advise such people to have three small meals each day and avoid snacks between meals — but again, old habits die hard.

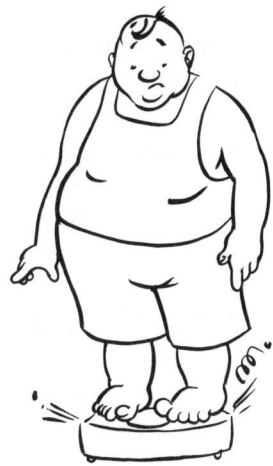

Before starting weight reduction, it is a good idea to keep a diary of everything that is eaten, and the quantity (preferably the weight) of what is eaten. If this is done over a period of several weeks, a dietitian can work out the total kilocalorie content of the food, and can modify the kilocalorie content to a level that is consistent with height and build, yet designed to lead to weight reduction. In this way a personalised diet can be implemented which has a lot in common with the current diet.

Follow-up by the doctor or the dietitian is important. Many patients seem to feel that such follow-up is unnecessary, but very few who omit follow-up visits actually seem to lose weight. The continuing interest of a second person provides a necessary stimulus and also affords an opportunity for intervention if all is not going well. In addition some people are helped by group therapy such as is provided by 'Weight Watchers' and 'Over-eaters Anonymous'.

In my experience, almost every overweight person, when tackled about their weight by a doctor, will agree that they should lose weight, many will say that they would really like to lose weight, but unless there is a real, expressed determination, very few people will persevere with a diet for any length of time.

Anorexia nervosa and bulimia Unfortunately a few people, usually women, are so obsessed with their weight that they take dieting to extremes. Some such people have a condition known as *anorexia nervosa* and this is believed to be essentially an emotional disorder. Numerous explanations have been offered, and certainly subconscious anxieties (e.g. relating to pregnancy) seem to be present. Most appear to have a distorted body image and believe themselves to be becoming obese, even when they are quite slim. As a result of their dieting, certain changes occur in the pituitary gland which leads to a cessation of menstrual bleeding and the occurrence of excessive hair on the limbs. Once the condition has developed, it is extremely difficult to re-establish normal eating patterns — and some sufferers eventually die of malnutrition.

An allied condition which seems to have been fashionable lately, is bulimia, where the patient deliberately induces vomiting or diarrhoea after meals. Both these conditions usually require specialist treatment and are often associated with depression.

Food quality is important

It is always wise to seek medical advice before embarking upon any diet. This is partly because the quality of the food eaten is most important or else malnutrition may ensue. Most authorities believe that *for every kilogram of body weight in adults there should be a daily intake of 0.8 g of protein.* Thus a 70 kg person should require approximately 56 g of protein which is equivalent to 600 ml of milk, 125 g of meat and 4 slices of bread. Young children, whose bodies are growing, need much more proportionately so that in infancy it is likely to be 3.5–2.5 mg/kg; from 4–6 yrs, approximately 3 g/kg; from 10–12 yrs 2 g/kg and from 13–19 years, 1.6 g/kg.

In passing, it can be mentioned that a baby requires 150 ml of fluid each day for every kilogram of weight (2½ oz per lb of body weight). Breast milk is a perfect food for babies, containing precisely the right nutrients despite sometimes giving the appearance of being watery. Cow's milk, after it is diluted with water — as it needs to be for young babies — contains insufficient kilocalories so that supplementary sugar is added to give it the necessary kilocalorie content.

Some people are sufficiently motivated to work out their own diet once they are told how many kilocalories they should have. Such people can vary their diet tremendously by substituting different foods or different quantities of food so long as the total kilocalories in any one day do not exceed the total permitted.

Choosing one's own food from a kilocalorie chart should not be attempted by those on very strict diets in the region of 800 kilocalories daily, as it is very easy on such a diet to get insufficient essential food substances. In fact, people on really strict diets should be under close medical and/or dietetic supervision.

In diets containing 1200 kilocalories or more, the food is usually sufficiently varied to provide most essential nutrients.

The following is a list of kilocalorie food values which can be used by people looking for extra variety in the diet. Such analyses are often based on the *weight* of foodstuffs, and to be used effectively, the dieter should weigh all items of food until really reliable estimates can be achieved. This list of energy values of commonly used foods is simpler but leaves more to judgement. It comes from 'Health Information' Series, No 87, issued by the New Zealand Department of Health.

Approximate energy value of some commonly used foods

Beverages	Kilocalories
Beer, 200 ml (7 oz) glass	100
Carbonated drinks, 180 ml (6 oz)	75
Cocoa made with ½ milk, sweetened, 1 cup	90
Coffee and tea, black (no sugar)	Nil
Lemon juice, unsweetened	Nil
Milk, 200 ml (7 oz) glass	140
Orange juice, 200 ml (7 oz) glass	90
Sherry (dry), port, etc., 60 ml (2 oz)	60
Skimmed milk, 200 ml (7 oz) glass	70
Soda water	Nil
Spirits, 18 ml (1 nip)	60

Breads and cereals	
Bran, All Bran, ¼ cup	50
Bread, brown or white, fresh or toasted, 30 g (1 oz)	70
Cornflakes, 1 cup	105
Flour, 2 tablespoons, 30 g (1 oz)	100
Macaroni (cooked), ¾ cup	100
Porridge, ¾ cup	100
Rice (water boiled), ½ cup	100
Ry Vita, 1	30
Scones, plain, 1 average	160
Water biscuits, 1 small	22
Wheatgerm, 1 tablespoon	16

Dairy products and fats	
Butter, 1 tablespoon	106
Cheese, 1 segment	100
Cream, 1 tablespoon	50
Egg, 1 whole	80

Dairy products and fats (cont.)	Kilocalories
Egg, 1 fried	135
Ice cream, plain, 60 g (2 oz)	120
Margarine, 1 tablespoon	106
Milk — condensed, unsweetened, 1 tablespoon	30
condensed, sweetened, 1 tablespoon	70
skimmed, 600 ml (1 pint)	200
whole, 600 ml (1 pint)	400
powdered, skimmed, 1 tablespoon	21
Vegetable oil, 1 tablespoon	125
Yoghurt, plain, 1 carton, 240 ml (8 oz)	50
Yoghurt, flavoured, 1 carton, 240 ml (8 oz)	200

Cakes, pies, etc.	
Biscuit, sweet (no icing)	80
Cake, iced, plain, 1 piece	300
Doughnut	210
Fruit cake (light), 1 piece	140
Fruit pie, 1 serving	250
Gingerbread, 1 piece, 60 g (2 oz)	200
Lemon meringue pie, 1 serving	280
Milk cereal pudding, ½ cup	150

Fruits	
Apple, 1 medium	70
Apricots, 2 to 3	50
Bananas, 1 medium	70
Berries, ¾ cup	50

Fruits (cont.)	Kilocalories
Cherries, 10 large	45
Dates, 3 to 4	75
Figs, dried, 2 small	60
Grapefruit, 1 medium	40
Grapes, 20 medium	60
Mango, ½ medium	76
Orange, 1 medium	60
Pawpaw (papaya), 1 small slice	30
Peach, 1 medium	50
Pears, 1 medium	80
Pineapple, canned, 1 slice	45
Plums, 2 medium	60
Prunes, 3 medium	54
Raisins, ¼ cup	80
Rhubarb, chopped, 1 cup	16
Tamarillos (tree tomatoes), 2 medium	40

Nuts

Almonds, 12 to 15	83
Brazil, 2	87
Coconut, 2 tablespoons	85
Peanuts, 10	50
Walnuts, 4 large	100

Vegetables

Low kilocalorie value: asparagus, cabbage, carrot (grated), cauliflower, celery, chives, cucumber, kale, lettuce, marrow, mint, mushrooms, parsley, peppers, radish, shallot, silver beet, spinach, tomato, watercress, white turnip.

Moderate kilocalorie value: (Values are for a ½ cup serving of cooked vegetables).

Broccoli, brussel sprouts, carrots, choko, onions, swede, turnips	30
Beetroot, parsnip, peas, pumpkin	50

Starchy vegetables

Broad beans, ½ cup	80
Kumara, boiled, 1 medium, 120 g (4 oz)	150
Kumara, roasted, 1 medium	250
Potato, mashed, ½ cup	85

Vegetables (cont.)	Kilocalories
Potato, boiled, 1 medium, 120 g (4 oz)	100
Potato, roasted, 1 medium	200
Potato, chips, fried, 8	220
Sweetcorn, ½ cup	90
Sweetcorn, 1 ear, 13 cm long	145
Taro, cooked, 100 g (3½ oz)	110

Note: For vegetables baked in fat, add 100 kilocalories per serving.

Meats (without gravy)

Bacon, lean, 1 small piece	60
Beef or mutton, roast, medium serving	300
Chicken, 1 medium portion	130
Lamb chop, small, lean, grilled, 1	200
Liver, fried, 1 medium serving	200
Pork, loin chop, 1	300
Sausage, pork, 1	140
Gravy, 2 tablespoons	30

Fish and shellfish

Fish fillets, steamed, 1 serving	110
Oysters, 6 medium	70
Sardines, 3 medium	60

Salad dressing

French, 1 tablespoon	60
Mayonnaise, 1 tablespoon	95

Soups

Clear soups, ¾ cup	Negligible
Cream soups, ¾ cup	150

Sweets, jams, etc.

Chocolate fudge, 1 piece, 25 mm square	100
Chocolate, plain, 30 g (1 oz)	150
Honey, jam, or jelly, 1 tablespoon	60
Peanut butter, 1 tablespoon	106
Potato chippies, 8–10 large	100
Sugar, 1 tablespoon	50
Syrup and treacle, 1 tablespoon	60
Yeast extracts	Negligible

Remember to include alcoholic drinks in your daily diet tallies. (If necessary, see list in National Heart Foundation's *Controlled Diets for the Overweight*.)

I am also including here a series of diets recommended by the National Heart Foundation for weight reduction. They are best used under medical supervision.

Weight reduction diet — 1000 kilocalories per day

BREAKFAST
Fruit juice (unsweetened) OR half grapefruit
1 slice bread or toast (thin), with thinly spread margarine
1 egg, OR slice bacon, OR small yoghurt, OR small portion cereal
Grilled tomatoes
Tea or coffee (no sugar)

LUNCH (OR TEA)
1 cup clear soup
Lean meat, OR chicken OR fish (60 g)
Salad from unrestricted vegetables (see p. 92) *but* use vinegar or lemon juice as dressing, *not* mayonnaise
OR slice of wholegrain bread
1 tablespoon low-fat cottage cheese
Tea or coffee (without sugar), OR unsweetened fruit juice

DINNER
1 cup clear soup OR tomato juice
Lean meat, OR chicken, OR fish (90 g)
Vegetables from unrestricted list (see p. 92)
1 potato (medium-sized, boiled or baked)
2 tablespoon peas or other starchy root vegetable
1 piece of fruit
Skimmed milk from daily allowance of 300 ml

Weight reduction diet — 1200 kilocalories per day

BREAKFAST
As for 1000 kilocalorie menu, but in addition you may have:
1 slice bread or toast
OR 1 bread roll with thinly spread margarine
OR ½ cup breakfast cereal (or cooked porridge) with skimmed milk, *no* sugar

LUNCH (OR TEA)
1 cup clear soup
Lean meat, OR chicken, OR fish (60 g)
Salad from unrestricted vegetables, plus 2 thin slices of bread and 1 piece of fruit
OR ¼ cup cooked spaghetti and ½ cup unsweetened stewed fruit and 1 pottle fat-free yoghurt
Tea or coffee, no sugar, OR unsweetened fruit juice

Weight reduction diet — 1200 kilocalories per day (cont.)

DINNER
1 cup clear soup OR tomato juice
Lean meat, chicken, fish (100 g)
Vegetables from unrestricted list
2 potatoes (medium-sized, boiled or baked)
2 tablespoon peas
1 serving fruit (fresh or cooked without sugar)
Skimmed milk from daily allowance of 300 ml

The portions below are roughly equivalent in energy and can be exchanged in the foregoing diets:

½ thick slice of bread
1 thin slice of bread
3 small or 2 large water biscuits
½ cup cooked porridge
½ cup cornflakes or rice bubbles
3 teaspoons All Bran
1 Weetbix
¼ cup cooked spaghetti, noodles or rice
2 rounded tablespoons cooked peas, corn, yams, kumera, beetroot
1 medium piece raw fruit (½ banana)
½ cup stewed fruit (without sugar)

Unlimited use of the following foods is allowed:

Unrestricted vegetables: asparagus, beans (butter, french, runner), broccoli, brussel sprouts, cabbage, carrots (small serving), cauliflower, celery, chives, chokos, cucumbers, egg plant, red and green peppers, leeks, lettuce, marrow, mushrooms, onions, puha, pumpkin, radishes, silver beet, spinach, tomatoes, turnips, watercress.
Fruit: green gooseberries, lemons, rhubarb, rockmelon, watermelon.
Miscellaneous: beef and chicken stock, gelatine, herbs, pepper, spices, vinegar, diabetic jellies (artificial sweeteners).
Unlimited drinks from the following are allowed: water, tea, coffee, soda water, bouillon, unsweetened tomato juice.

Additional points: Use high-fibre foods. Eat fruit (apples with skins on), vegetables (potatoes in jackets). Use unrefined cereals, All Bran, porridge, Weetbix (commercial muesli is too high in energy). Use more wholemeal and wholegrain bread.

Don't fry in fat or oil or roast vegetables. All other cooking methods are suitable — grilling, roasting (inside cuts of meat only), stewing or steaming. Avoid thickened sauces and gravies. Use lean meat only — trim and skim off all fat.

Avoid all fat and oil except allowance of margarine; all fried food, nuts, cream, pastry; sugar in any form — glucose, brown, raw or white, golden syrup, honey, jam, marmalade, sweets, sweetened condensed milk; biscuits, cakes, pastries, pies, sugar-coated breakfast cereals; fruit if cooked, tinned or preserved in sugar; ice cream, salad dressing (unless low calorie).

Quality foods are essential

Below is a list of important nutrients which must be a part of any diet.

Nutrient	Source	Effects of deficiency
Essential fatty acids	Vegetable oils (corn, sunflower, safflower)	Cessation of growth, skin problems
Sodium	Widely distributed: pork, fish, beef, cheese, potato chips	Low blood pressure
Potassium	Widely distributed: milk, bananas, raisins, prunes	Muscle weakness, disturbances of heart rhythm. Occasionally sudden death
Calcium	Milk, cheese, yoghurt, meat, fish, eggs, cereals, fruits, beans, vegetables	Muscle twitching
Phosphorus	Milk, cheese, meat, fish, cereals, nuts	Weakness of muscles
Magnesium	Nuts, cereals, seafoods, green leaves	Irritable muscles
Iron	Beef, kidney, liver, beans, peaches	Anaemia
Iodine	Seafoods, iodised salt, dairy products	Thyroid enlargement
Fluorine	Tea, coffee, some water supplies	Tendency to dental decay. Possibly loss of calcium from bone
Zinc	Widely distributed: many vegetables	Growth retarded
Copper	Widely distributed: offal meat, oysters, nuts, peas, whole grain cereals	Anaemia
Cobalt	Green vegetables	Possibly anaemia
Chromium	Widely distributed: brewer's yeast	Possibly a tendency to diabetes

Note: If any of the conditions in the last column appear in an individual, it should not be assumed that dietary deficiency is necessarily the underlying cause of that condition; there may be many other reasons. Thus, if the thyroid is enlarged, it does not always mean that giving iodine will remedy the condition.

Vitamin	Source	Effects of deficiency
A	Fish liver oil, liver, egg yolk, butter, cream, green vegetables	Night blindness and other eye problems
D	Fish liver oil, butter, egg yolk, liver, ultra-violet irradiation	Inadequate calcium in the bone

Important nutrients (cont.)

Vitamin	Source	Effects of deficiency
E	Vegetable oil, wheat germ, leafy vegetables, egg yolk	Anaemia
K, K_1, K_2	Leafy vegetables, pork, liver, vegetable oils. Intestinal bacteria	Bleeding
B_1 (thiamine)	Dried yeast, wholegrains, meat, nuts, potatoes	Beriberi. Heart disorders.
B_2 (riboflavin)	Milk, cheese, liver, meat, eggs	Skin, mouth and eye problems
Niacin (nicotinic acid)	Yeast, liver, meat, fish, peas	A disorder called pellagra
B_6 (pyridoxine)	Yeast, liver, offal meats, wholegrain cereals, fish, peas	Anaemia, skin problems
Folic acid	Green leafy vegetables, fruit, liver, other offal meats, yeast	Anaemia
B_{12}	Liver, kidney, eggs, milk	Pernicious anaemia
Biotin	Liver, kidney, egg yolk, yeast, cauliflower, nuts	Skin and tongue disorders
C	Citrus fruits, tomatoes, potatoes, cabbage	Bleeding, loosening of teeth. Scurvy.

Food allergies

Medical opinion about the importance of food allergies varies from the obsessional to the nihilistic, with a few doctors believing that almost every complaint can be attributed to food allergy and others denying its existence. Few, however, would doubt that certain urticarias (i.e. allergic rashes) are caused by food, and occasionally asthma and migraine may be precipitated. Proteins are amongst the most allergenic (i.e. allergy-producing) substances, so milk, meat, fish, cheese and eggs are frequently thought to be implicated.

Among the conditions in which food allergies are thought sometimes to be a contributing factor are eczema, urticaria, asthma, migraine, hyperactivity, irritable bowel and even ulcerative colitis.

It is seldom possible to identify a food allergy by the use of skin tests and usually the most successful approach is to give sufferers a few weeks on a diet which is very low in foods known to have a tendency to cause allergic reactions. Such diets are very restrictive and if persevered with for more than a few weeks can easily lead to malnutrition. As allergies may persist in the body for some weeks, it may be necessary to continue with a diet for 2–3 weeks before any improvement is obtained.

If improvement is apparent, the procedure is to introduce gradually various foods known sometimes to cause allergic reactions. It is desirable to continue each new introduction for at least a week before accepting that it is not harmful. Of course if an obvious allergic response occurs at any time, one should not persevere with that item.

Some foods which very seldom cause allergies
Tea and instant coffee (powder type); no milk, no lemon.
Sugar, salt, treacle, 'golden' syrup.
Lamb, mutton, rabbit.
Leaf vegetables, e.g. cabbage, brussel sprouts, lettuce, celery, carrots. (*Avoid broccoli, cauliflower and spinach*)
Bananas, pears.
Sago and sago flour.

Possible allergy-causing foods   The following is a list of foods which may be a cause of allergy, and these may be cautiously introduced to the diet, one group at a time.
1. *Grains*, particularly wheat and foods containing wheat, rye, oats, barley, rice, corn and corn oil
2. *Milk* and milk products. (Dried milk may possibly be tolerated even when fresh milk causes problems. The same applies to butter and cheese.)
3. *Egg and poultry*
4. *Fish*
5. *Beef, pork and other meats*
6. *Onions and garlic*
7. *Nuts and fruits* — particularly peanuts
8. *Yeast* and derivatives such as Marmite, Vegemite and Bovril
9. *Shellfish* (squid comes into this category)
10. *Potatoes* and other root vegetables
11. *Peas*
12. *Foods which have artificial flavourings, colourings or preservatives.*

Remember that *aspirin*, which is a *salicylate* (see p. 145) can potentiate many allergic reactions, making worse an existing allergy. Some foods contain salicylates. *Tartrazine* is a common cause of allergies. It is used as a colouring agent. A list of foods containing tartrazine can be found on p. 144.

Antibiotics are used in animal husbandry and traces get into the meat and sometimes the milk. Although the quantity absorbed is small, a few people who have severe antibiotic allergy will suffer reactions from this source.

Any dietary experiments such as have been described here should only be attempted under the guidance and supervision of a doctor or a dietitian.

A daily record of foods eaten and any reactions observed should be meticulously maintained and, of course, while the study is in progress, no antihistamines or other allergy-preventing medication should be consumed as this will confuse the results.

2.6 Special diets

Low-cholesterol diets

The evidence that the cholesterol that we eat has an influence on the level of cholesterol in the bloodstream is increasing and the majority of heart specialists seem to agree that our diets should be designed to try to reduce the level of cholesterol.

However, there are other components to the fatty substances in the blood, and two which are recognised as having special significance are respectively, *low-density lipoproteins* (LDL) and *high-density lipoproteins* (HDL). These substances seem to play a part in causing changes in the blood vessels (i.e., atheroma, see p. 46), but their actions appear to be in opposition. Thus current evidence suggests that a high level of high-density lipoproteins actually protects the vessels from atheroma, whereas a high level of low-density lipoproteins is believed to be harmful.

The level of cholesterol is measured in S.I. units known as millimoles per litre of blood and the level recommended as desirable is 5.2 millimoles/litre or less. In a similar way, the recommended level of high-density lipoprotein is 1.10 millimoles/litre or more.

Some authorities maintain that it is the ratio

$$\frac{\text{Total cholesterol (millimoles/litre)}}{\text{High density lipoprotein (millimoles/litre)}}$$

that is of primary importance, and claim that one should aim for a figure of 4.5:1. It is suggested that an even lower ratio of 3.5:1 is probably the ideal.

The following things are known to increase HDL: very strenuous exercise, significant weight reduction in those who are overweight, oestrogens, alcohol.

The following appear to reduce HDL: being overweight, cigarette smoking, beta blockers, progestagens, thiazide diuretics.

Current recommendations suggest that not more than 30 per cent of our kilocalorie intake should be in the form of fat and that the total cholesterol intake for one day should not exceed 200 mg. (*Note*: 1 egg contains 300 mg.) See table, p. 100.

As a corollary, it is suggested that 60 per cent of the dietary kilocalories should be in the form of carbohydrate and 10 per cent of the dietary kilocalories should be in the form of protein. Other suggestions are that the daily intake of food should include 30 g of fibre (see table, p.100) and not more than 5 g of sodium chloride (common salt) daily. (See table, p. 101.)

A fish diet seems to be beneficial and this may be why the Japanese and Eskimos are relatively immune to coronary heart disease. The best way to prepare the fish is to steam it or grill it. Some believe that 30 g of fish daily may be enough to halve an individual's risk of death from coronary heart disease.

Basic rules for a good diet
The Heart Foundation has suggested ten basic rules for any diet:
1. Have a varied diet to maintain normal body weight.
2. Be sparing in the use of all fat. Avoid meat fat, lard and dripping. Reduce the use of butter. Grill rather than fry. Use olive oil or polyunsaturated oil for cooking as a substitute for saturated fat.
3. Eat fish at least twice a week if possible.
4. Be sparing in the use of sugar.
5. Use bread, rice, peas or beans daily; select wholegrain bread and cereals where possible.
6. Use low-fat milk (0.1 per cent) or reduced-fat milk for adults in place of whole milk.
7. Be sparing with salt. (See table, p. 101.)
8. Be sparing in the use of instant foods that are rich in saturated fats, sugar and salt. (See tables, pp. 98–101.)
9. If you take alcohol, do not exceed 2 single drinks a day.

The Pritikin Diet
Nathan Pritikin, a non-medical health enthusiast in the United States, has claimed to be able to reduce atheroma by diet and exercise and has written books on the subject. The essence of the advice given is a very low-fat diet with low sugar content and low salt. Pritikin set out clearly the foods that he felt fulfilled the desired criteria. His regime is stricter than those given in the 10 basic rules suggested by the Heart Foundation.

Pritikin recommended that as a meat dish, fish cooked without fat was suitable, as was chicken and turkey, without the skin and with any fat removed. Very lean beef was also considered acceptable and many people would also allow veal. For grains it was suggested whole grains such as brown rice were desirable.

Pritikin also encouraged the following:
Bread: use of whole wheat, rolled oats, breads made without fat, whole-wheat pasta, pitta bread, flat bread and crisp breads.
Legumes: all beans, peas and lentils, but not soya beans.
Fat and oils: nil, except those that occur naturally in the grains, vegetables and fruits recommended.
Fruits and vegetables: all fruits except avocados and olives; up to 5 items of fruit per day. Any amount of vegetables so long as they are eaten raw or steamed or baked or cooked without butter, oil, margarine or salt. Thirty grams of dried fruit per day and 125 ml of fruit juice.
Dairy products: up to 225 g per day of skimmed milk. Powdered skim milk, cheese made from skim milk, yoghurt made from skim milk (maximum 60 ml per day).

Sweet: fruit (but avoid if tinned or prepared in syrup).
Drinks: decaffeinated coffee, herb teas.
Spices: vinegar, fresh or dried herbs.

Pritiken advised people to avoid:
Meat: lamb, pork, goose, ham, sausages, bacon, smoked meat, salmon, shellfish, tuna.
Grains: any bread products made with fat, sugar or eggs, bleached white flour, soya flour (too much protein), biscuits and scones.
Legumes: soya beans, all nuts, seeds such as sunflower seeds or sesame seeds.
Fats and oils: butter, margarine, all oils either saturated or unsaturated, fat on meats.
Fruits: avocados and olives (rich in fat)
Dairy products: eggs, whole milk, cream, yoghurt, most cheeses, tinned milk.
Sweets: sugar, sugared drinks, including coffee and tea; chocolate or anything containing sugar.
Salty savouries such as crisps.
Any sauces containing cream or butter.

Pritikin's is a very strict regime and if adhered to closely, it will almost certainly lead to weight loss. The basic principles appear sound, although I am not aware of any conclusive studies concerning its effectiveness. It will be noted that Pritikin recommends strict limitation of all fat, regardless of whether it is saturated fat or polyunsaturated fat.

Anyone wishing to pursue this regime would be well advised to obtain a copy of the book *The Pritikin Promise*, which also gives recipes and advice on exercise. They should also discuss the plan with their family doctor. Among other problems, there is the possibility that prolonged adherence to such a diet might lead to the development of osteoporosis as a result of reduced calcium intake. (See p. 187.)

Food analyses

The following are listings of some of the foods which are richest in fat, together with the percentage which is polyunsaturated. Also listed are foods rich in cholesterol, fibre, calcium (see section on menopause), potassium (see section on diuretics) and sodium (i.e. salt).

Foods high in fat (grams per 100 g portion)

	Grams	Percentage polyunsaturated		Grams	Percentage polyunsaturated
Vegetable fat	100.0	7.0	Margarine	81.0	17.3
Sunflower oil	99.9	63.1	Mayonnaise	78.9	40.5
Cod liver oil	99.9	0	Brazil nuts	66.9	36.4
Olive oil	99.9	8.1	Bacon	65.0	10.0
Corn oil	99.9	56.0	Dried coconut	64.9	0.9
Safflower oil	99.9	72.1	Walnuts	64.0	74.2
Soyabean oil	99.9	60.1	Hazel nuts	60.9	37.8
Lard	99	10.1	Dried almonds	54.2	19.9
Butter	81.0	4.9	Peanut butter	49.4	24.1

Foods high in fat (cont.)

	Grams	Percentage polyunsaturated		Grams	Percentage polyunsaturated
Peanuts	48.7	28.7	Camembert cheese	22.8	0
Cashew nuts	45.7	6.6	Tunny (fish)	20.9	0
Egg powder	41.2	0	Ham (boiled)	20.6	2.0
Potato chips	39.8	0	Hamburger	20.3	0
Cream cheese	37.7	2.6	Beef sausages	18.4	0
Chocolate	32.3	0	Lamb (leg)	18.0	2.8
Cheddar	32.2	3.1	Soyabeans	17.7	60.4
Lamb (chop)	32.0	2.2	Avocado	17.0	11.8
Egg yolk (raw)	31.9	21.0	Tongue	15.0	0
Ham (raw)	31.0	0	Caviar	15.0	0
Pie crust	31.0	0	Salmon (Atlantic)	13.6	38.9
Cream	30.4	2.6	Olives	12.7	7.9
Whole dried milk	27.5	2.5	Chicken (roasted)	12.6	0
Pork loin	26.0	0	Corned beef	12.0	0
Eel	25.6	0	Wheatgerm	10.9	26.6
Rump beef	25.3	0	Beef (lean)	8.2	0
Cocoa powder	24.5	1.7	Veal	6.0	6.7
Sardines in oil	24.4	0	Venison	3.6	8.3

It is believed that a significant component of polyunsaturated fat is desirable as this seems to help to keep down the level of cholesterol in the blood. On the other hand, if there is also a high cholesterol level present in the food, this may undo the benefit. Thus cod-liver oil in quantity could be considered undesirable on two counts. First it has no polyunsaturated component and secondly it has a high cholesterol content. Sunflower, safflower, corn and soyabean oils are all considered to be good because of their high content of polyunsaturated fat.

Egg yolks have considerable polyunsaturated fat but also much cholesterol.

Olive oil forms an important component of the diet in Spain and Italy, two countries where the incidence of coronary artery disease is low. This is in spite of a low polyunsaturated fat content. Why should this be? The answer is uncertain, but olive oil and peanut oil contain a considerable percentage of yet another type of fat — mono-unsaturated fat — and some work suggests that this may help protect from atheroma. Most previous research has suggested that mono-unsaturated fat is neutral, being neither good nor bad.

In summary, after reviewing the current literature, the following would appear to be the best available advice.

1. Keep the total intake of fat down to less than 30 per cent of the total kilocalorie requirements.

2. In choosing fats, try and choose those that incorporate a reasonable proportion of polyunsaturated fat. If possible, polyunsaturated fats should represent about 30 per cent of the total kilocalories provided by fats (i.e., about 10 per cent of kilocalories overall).

3. Keep the total daily cholesterol content of the diet below 200 mg. (See table, p. 100.)

4. Maintain an intake of about 30 g of fibre daily. (See table, p. 100.)

Foods rich in cholesterol (mg per 100 g portion)

Beef brain	2360	Bacon fat	220
Egg powder	2140	Chicken liver	200
Egg yolk (raw)	1600	Beef tripe	150
Cod liver oil	850	Beef (average)	120
Goose liver	490	Cream cheese	120
Whole egg (raw)	460	Sheep liver	120
Beef liver	320	Smoked raw ham	110
Caviar	300	Lard	100
Butter	280	Cheddar cheese	100

Foods rich in fibre (grams per 100 g portion)

Dried apricots	24.0	Quinces	6.4	Chives	3.1
Dried coconut	23.5	Hazelnuts	6.1	Brussel sprouts	2.9
Almonds	14.3	Loganberries	5.7	Cabbage	2.8
Soyabean flour	11.9	Currants	5.3	Gooseberries	2.7
Dried figs	10.3	Peas	5.2	Parsnips	2.5
Whole wheat flour	9.6	Walnuts	5.2	Wheatgerm	2.5
Parsley	9.1	Soyabeans	4.9	Popped corn	2.2
Brazil nuts	9.0	Broad beans	4.2	Strawberries	2.2
Dried dates	8.7	Blackberries	4.1	Cauliflower	2.1
Wholemeal bread	8.5	Broccoli	4.1	Avocados	2.0
Horseradish	8.3	Leeks	3.9	Celery	1.8
Dried prunes	8.1	Cress	3.7	Persimmon	1.5
Peanuts	8.1	Dried lentils	3.7	Cashew nuts	1.4
Raspberries	7.4	String beans	3.4	Peppers	1.2
Dried yeast	6.9	Carrots	3.1	Jams	1.1
Dried chestnuts	6.8				

Note: These figures can only be a guide to content. Few people would be eating 100 g of many of these foods.

Foods rich in calcium (mg per 100 g portion)

Nonfat dried milk	1300	Molasses	273
Swiss cheese	1180	Sweetened condensed milk	262
Parmesan cheese	1140	Turnip tops	260
Whole dried milk	909	Canned whole sockeye salmon	259
Cheddar cheese	750	Hazelnuts	250
Roquefort cheese	700	Almonds	234
Torula yeast	424	Almonds sweetened with chocolate	228
Camembert cheese	382	Soyabeans	226
Canned whole sardines	354	Dried brewer's yeast	210
Pressed caviar	276	Parsley	203

Note: Figures above for calcium could be misleading as availability of calcium varies according to the body's ability to utilise it.

Foods rich in potassium (mg per 100 g portion)

Torula yeast	2046	Parsley	880	Peanut butter	670
Dried soyabeans	1900	Potato chips	880	Spinach	662
Dried apricots	1700	Dried chestnuts	875	Hazelnuts	618
Soyabean flour	1660	Dried lentils	810	Baker's compressed yeast	610
Dried potatoes	1600	Dried dates	790	Garden cress	606
Tomato purée	1600	Fennel	784	Pecans	603
Molasses	1383	Wheatgerm	780	Dried coconut	588
Dried onions	1383	Dried figs	780	Beet tops	570
Non-fat dried milk	1335	Roasted peanuts	740	Tinned sardines	560
Whole dried milk	1330	Dried raisins	725	Dried apples	557
Kidney beans	1310	Dried prunes	700	Horse radish	554
Dried peaches	1100	Dried almonds	690	Sweet potatoes	530
Pistachio nuts	972	Buckwheat flour	680	Mushrooms	520
Dry cocoa powder	900–3200	Lima beans	680	Garlic	515
		Brazil nuts	670		

Orange juice and bananas are also good sources of potassium, but it is less concentrated in these foods.

Foods rich in iron (mg per 100 g)

Torula yeast	20.0	Full fat soyabean flour	8.4	Dried peaches	6.0
Pork liver	19.0	Dried soyabeans	8.4	Dried split peas	6.0
Dried brewer's yeast	17.3	Pistachio nuts	7.3	Mussels	5.8
Dry cocoa powder	12.5	Raw egg yolk	7.2	Oysters	5.5
Pressed caviar	11.8	Molasses	6.7	Dried apricots	5.5
Sheep liver	10.9	Beef liver	6.5	Calf liver	5.4
Wheatgerm	9.4	Dried broadbeans	6.3	Pine nuts	5.2
Egg powder	8.7	Parsley	6.2	Dried salted beef	5.1
Dried lentils	8.6	Kidney beans	6.1	Venison	5.0

Note: Figures above could be misleading as availability of iron varies according to body's ability to utilise it.

Foods rich in sodium (salt) (mg per 100 g)

Salted dried beef	4300	Tomato ketchup	1042	Peanut butter	607
Raw smoked ham	2530	Cooked crab meat	1000	Tomato purée	590
Green olives	2400	Pickled herring	1000	Plain piecrust	568
Pressed caviar	2200	Margarine (salted)	987	Canned sockeye salmon	522
Medium fat bacon	1700	Boiled ham	876	Egg powder	519
Pretzels	1680	Smoked eel	798	Canned sardines	510
Brown mustard	1307	Parmesan cheese	755	Breads (various)	500–580
Bologne sausages	1300	Port sausages	750	Pancakes (enriched flour)	425
Canned corn beef	1300	Smoked herring	720	Dried whole milk	410
Salami	1260	Mayonnaise	702	Potato chips	340
Camembert cheese	1150	Cheddar cheese	700	Fennel	331
Canned spiced ham	1150	Cornflakes	660	Lobster	300
Beef sausages	1130	Sauerkraut	650		
Self-raising wheat flour	1079	Swiss cheese	620		

Plus many canned vegetables to which salt may have been added.

2.7 Fitness and exercise

'Consider Man, who may well become extinct
Because he forgot how to walk and learned how to fly before he thinked.'
— Ogden Nash (1902–71)

As a result of the many labour-saving devices now available, the activities of daily living are often inadequate to supply the body with the sort of exercise that it needs to function efficiently. It is widely believed that this contributes to ill health, and such conditions as heart disease, low back pain, obesity and disorders related to muscle tension have all been blamed on inactivity.

The following statements and recommendations have been made by the Department of Health, British Columbia.

What is fitness? In general terms, fitness can be related to one's capacity to enjoy life to the full. More specifically, it can be broken down into the three S's: 1. Strength, 2. Suppleness and 3. Stamina — the most important of which is stamina (endurance fitness).

No one gets fit overnight and only fools and fanatics try. If you assault your body with sudden bouts of unaccustomed exercise it will talk back to you in a language you can understand; pain. You cannot turn back the clock, and if you try to perform as you did when you were at school, you may be reminded of your age by a pulled muscle or other physical breakdown.

Try the 'half-as-much' approach If you think you might be able to jog around the golf course in ten minutes, take 20.

If it is just possible for you to swim 20 laps of the pool, limit yourself to 10.

Five easy sit-ups will be better for you initially than struggling to do 10.

Strength and suppleness Certain activities seem to be basic to most major exercise programmes. These fundamental movements include: 1. bent knee sit-ups, 2. arm circling, 3. trunk twisting, and 4. seated toe touching.

Other exercises can be added to suit individual preferences. All movements should be performed slowly and smoothly, and the number of repetitions gradually increased.

When to increase? In your 20s two weeks of 'half-as-much' without any problems means that you can gradually start to increase. In your 30s wait three weeks, in your 40s try four weeks of 'half-as-much', and so on.

Stamina

Using the half-as-much principle, your endurance activity should begin at a relatively easy level. There are several ways of assessing how your body is responding to sustained activity. One of these is *heart-rate counting*.

How to measure your heart rate The pulse can be felt through gentle pressure on one side of the neck about 25 mm behind the Adam's apple or, preferably, in the hollow of the wrist just above the thumb. Use the index and middle fingers and press lightly. Simply stop your activity, *take your pulse for 10 seconds and then multiply by six* which will give you your approximate pulse rate in beats per minute.

The table below provides a guide as to the sort of heart rates you might aim for when you begin exercising. Be content to work at the lower 'Fit Start' heart rate initially, and then as your condition improves, gradually begin to increase the vigour and volume of your activity until your heart rate is reaching the 'Keep Fit' levels. Enter and exit quietly. Begin your activity session easily so that the heart rate gradually increases towards your target, and finish the session with a cool down of light activity to assist the circulation as the heart rate goes back to normal.

Fit start		Keep fit	
Age	*Heart rate*	*Age*	*Heart rate*
20–29	118	20–29	146–164
30–39	112	30–39	138–156
40–49	106	40–49	130–148
50–59	100	50–59	122–140
60–69	94	60–69	116–122

Obviously, one formula cannot fit everybody and there might be some individual variations, but don't believe you are so different that your body does not need time to adjust to the pleasure of vigorous activity.

An endurance exercise programme

Frequency: 3–5 times per week
Intensity: Work up to and sustain a target heart rate (for your age) during exercise.
Time: Once your body is accustomed to exercise, attempt to keep moving for at least 15 minutes (even if it means slowing down a little).
Type: Any endurance exercise — walking, jogging, swimming, cycling, skipping, vigorous ball games, etc.

A 'physical activity readiness' questionnaire

The following physical activity readiness questionnaire is designed to help you help yourself. Many health benefits are associated with regular exercise, and the completion of the questionnaire is a sensible first step to take if you are planning to increase the amount of physical activity in your life.

For most people physical activity should not pose any problem or hazard. The questionnaire has been designed to identify the small number of adults for whom physical activity might be inappropriate or those who should have medical advice concerning the type of activity most suitable for them.

Common sense is your best guide in answering these few questions. Read them carefully and see if any apply to you.
1. Has your doctor ever said you have heart trouble?
2. Do you have pains in your heart and chest?
3. Do you often feel faint or have spells of severe dizziness?
4. Has a doctor ever said your blood pressure was too high?
5. Has your doctor ever told you that you have a bone or joint problem such as arthritis that has been aggravated by exercise, or might be made worse with exercise?
6. Is there a good physical reason not mentioned here why you should not follow an activity programme even if you wanted to?
7. Are you over age 65 and not accustomed to vigorous exercise?

If you answered 'yes' to any question and you have not recently done so, you should consult your family doctor *before* increasing your physical activity and/or taking a fitness test. Tell the doctor what questions you answered 'yes' to on the questionnaire.

After medical evaluation, seek advice from your doctor as to your suitability for:
unrestricted physical activity, probably on a gradually increasing basis;
restricted or supervised activity to meet your specific needs, at least on an initial basis. Check in your community for special programmes or services.

If you answered the questions accurately and the answer was 'no', you have reasonable assurance of your present suitability for:

A graduated exercise programme A gradual increase in proper exercise promotes good fitness development while minimising or eliminating discomfort.

An exercise test Simple tests of fitness may be undertaken if you so desire, but postpone activity if you have a temporary minor illness, such as a common cold.

An exercise 'safety code'

Here is the British Safety Council's Sportsman's Safety Code:
1. The benefits of exercise come from a regular graduated programme. Decide which sport or activity you would like to adopt and establish that it is possible, in practical terms, for you to maintain regular participation.
2. There is nothing to be gained from over-exertion. A gentle progression to extend your limits is the best way.

3. The body needs time to regain agility and suppleness — unfamiliar movements are likely to cause sprains and strains.

4. The warm-up period before any sport is vital. Top professionals would not neglect it. A few simple stretching and loosening exercises even before jogging are essential. (See below.)

5. Unused muscles are bound to ache but acute pain could be a warning sign of a heart attack or serious injury and should not be ignored.

6. Wear suitable clothes and the right protective equipment where required — with particular attention to footwear.

7. Do not undertake the 'hazardous' sports (e.g. climbing, canoeing, pot-holing) except under expert guidance and tuition.

8. All sports equipment should be of the highest possible quality, be well maintained, and be checked regularly.

9. As far as possible, participate in your sport with others, joining clubs or associations, or forming small groups (e.g. jogging party). This will give you access to expertise, provide encouragement for flagging enthusiasm, and create an automatic supervision.

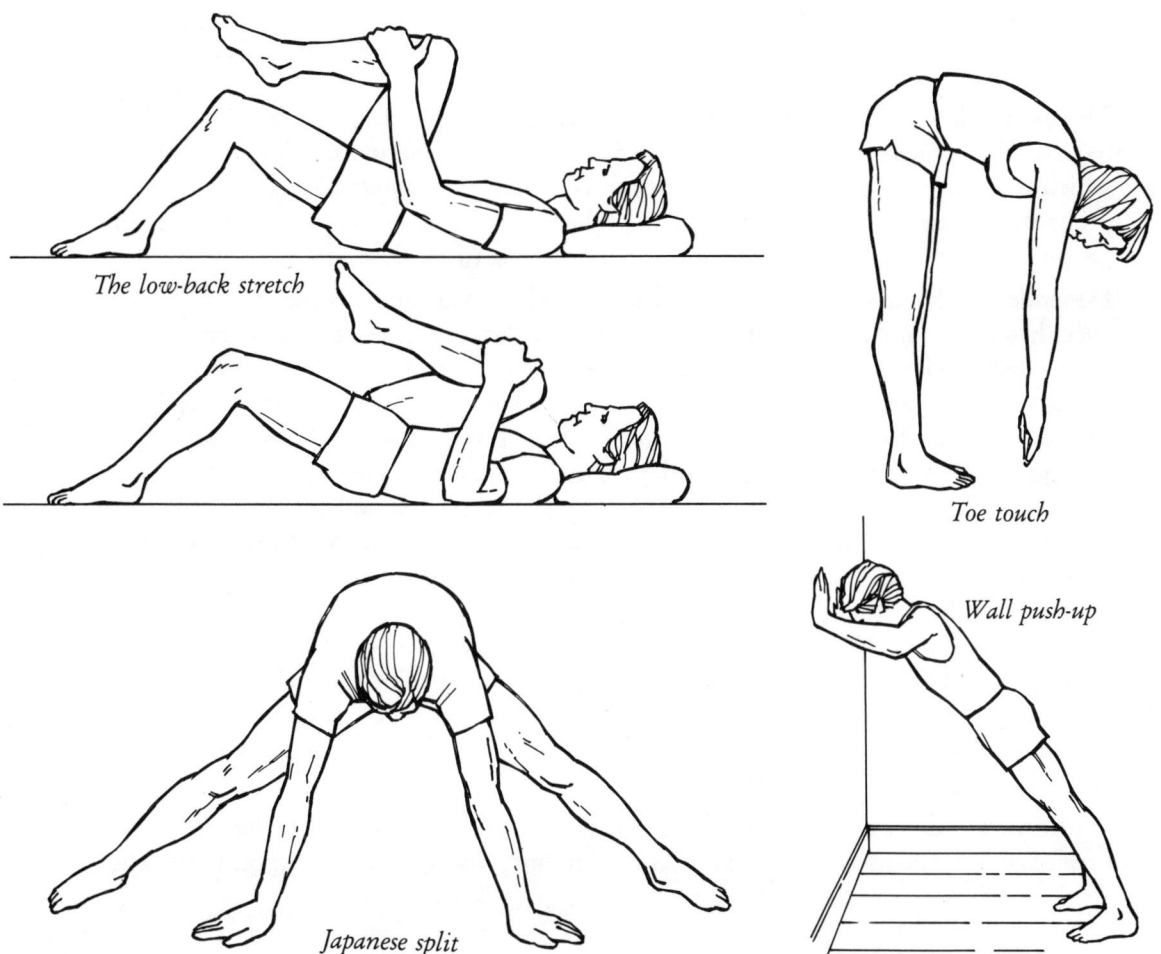

The low-back stretch

Toe touch

Japanese split

Wall push-up

2.8 Alcohol and tobacco — threats to health

'Wine is a mocker, strong drink is raging'
— Proverbs 20, Verse 1

'Hellish, devilish and damned tobacco, the ruin and overthrow of body and soul.'
— Robert Burton (1577–1640)

The use of alcohol and tobacco are two features of the western lifestyle which are known to have severely deleterious effects on health. Almost every culture has developed some agent which is effective in relieving the symptoms of stress. This universal need for stress relief is probably the reason why both alcohol and tobacco are inclined to cause dependence in some people — a dependence which to some extent seems to be dose related.

Dependence Some personalities would appear to have a greater tendency to develop dependence than others and it seems that a few individuals may become alcoholics very quickly and with relatively few drinks. Most, however, have to work at their addiction.

The same, of course, is true of the opiates. Few people, if any, develop a dependence as the result of three or four injections of morphine given to relieve pain or anxiety. If the injections are continued over several days, however, the incidence of dependence increases alarmingly. In a similar way, the more alcohol that is drunk, and the more frequently, or the more cigarettes that are smoked, the harder it is to live without these crutches. These two must be among the most dangerous tranquillisers known to man.

In general the road to dependence on alcohol would seem to be a longer one than is the case with narcotics. However, this road may be greatly foreshortened by the combination of alcohol with other drugs which have themselves a potential for dependence. Many tranquillisers fall into this category and it is believed that regular use of drugs like diazepam (Valium) in combination with alcohol can lead to serious dependence in half the time that it takes with alcohol alone.

Withdrawal Once acquired, both alcoholism and tobacco smoking are very hard habits to break and unfortunately it is by no means uncommon to be dependent upon both. The term 'addiction' is really not a good one. It is better to speak of 'dependence'. Dependence is often thought of as being either physical or emotional, but usually it is a combination of the two. Physical dependence is present when the withdrawal of the offending agent leads to physical symptoms. Thus the patient with a physical dependence on alcohol may experience an unwelcome shakiness, hallucinations (i.e., seeing things which are not really present), and even fits. An emotional dependence would be manifested by a sense of needing alcohol in order to get through the day or to make some aspect of life seem tolerable. Emotional dependence usually comes first, and the physical dependence develops later, but the two are seldom separable. When a physical dependence is allowed to develop unchecked and then the source of the dependence is abruptly withdrawn, the process is described as 'cold turkey'. Unless carefully monitored this can be very dangerous and should only be attempted by experienced professionals.

The sudden withdrawal of tobacco by smokers is not fraught with danger, but the person concerned may be very jittery and irritable and may make life a misery for those who share the same house and workplace.

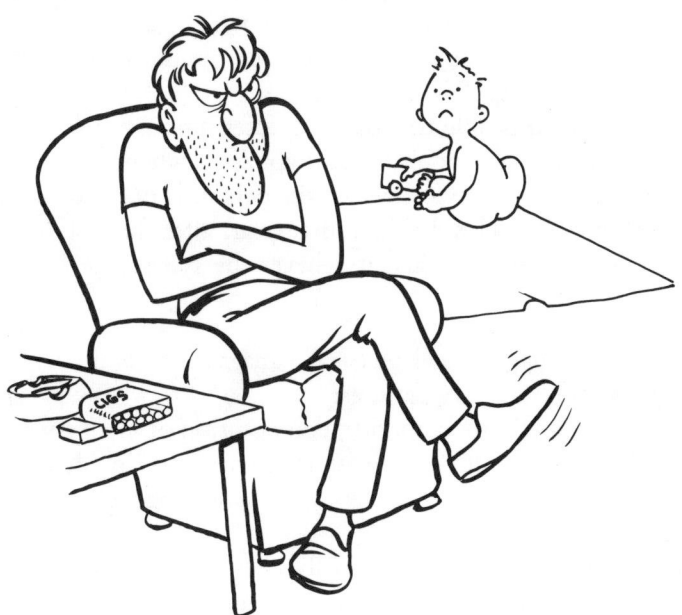

As with all drugs of dependence, once the initial break is made and the withdrawal symptoms dealt with, it is absolutely vital that the offending agent is not used again; a single cigarette or a single glass of alcohol and the patient is back to the beginning and almost inevitably will follow the first with more, and the sorry sequence is repeated.

Unfortunately the behaviour of the person undergoing withdrawal may be so disruptive that before the process is complete, relatives and friends may be pleading with him or her to resume the habit and give them some peace.

It is said that approximately 15 per cent of alcohol users become dependent, whereas the figure for tobacco users is nearer 60 per cent.

(1) Alcoholism

Definitions There have been many definitions of alcoholism but limited agreement. Many incorporate the concept of compulsion to drink and emphasise the physical and psychological dependence.

The World Health Organisation (WHO) states that *'alcoholics are those excessive drinkers whose dependence upon alcohol has attained such a degree that it shows a noticeable mental disturbance or an interference with their bodily and mental health, their interpersonal relations and their smooth social and economic functioning or who show the prodromal signs of such development. They therefore require treatment.'*

Another definition comes from Rutgers University Centre of Alcohol Studies. *'Alcoholics are those who are unable to consistently choose whether they shall drink or not and who if they drink are unable to consistently choose whether they shall stop or not.'*

Unfortunately alcoholism is on the increase, especially amongst young people and some studies have shown that up to 25 per cent of the patients in medical wards of the public hospitals have alcohol problems. The features which suggest alcoholism in any patient are:

1. The person becomes aware of a compulsion to drink and of being unable to control his/her drinking.
2. The person is able to tolerate greater amounts of alcohol without signs of intoxication.
3. Withdrawal symptoms become apparent when the person is without alcohol for any time. This is often first noticed when the person is noted to be very tremulous (shaky) first thing in the morning. This shakiness disappears after the first drink. Early morning drinking rapidly becomes a feature because it relieves the symptoms.

Physical damage Later physical damage to the brain may supervene. This takes many forms but the following are features:

1. Loss of intellectual capacity, deterioration of memory and judgement, mood disturbances.
2. A tendency to invent stories to compensate for deficiencies in memory (confabulation).
3. A paralysis of some of the eye muscles together with some difficulty in walking (inco-ordination).
4. Delirium tremens (DTs) usually does not occur for many years. It is precipitated by withdrawal of alcohol. Often the patients do not know where they are or what the day is. They may think they see or hear things which in reality are not present (hallucinations). They are very restless, sleepless and sweating, and have a rapid heart beat.

Psychological disorders also occur, while some experience a combination of physical and psychological features. Thus there may be an inability to perform the sexual act (i.e. impotence). There may be depression and even suicide, abnormal and unjustified jealousies, usually suspecting the partner of unfaithfulness. Often more prolonged hallucinations are experienced than occur in delirium tremens. Physical damage to other parts of the body is widespread. Stomach ulcers, liver damage (cirrhosis), varicose veins of the oesophagus (gullet) and inflammation of the pancreas affect the organs of digestion. Loss of sensation in the hands and feet (peripheral neuropathy) and damage to muscles (myopathy), including the heart (cardiomyopathy), are some of the other problems that occur. In addition to this, there are often the effects of vitamin deficiencies.

Toxicity Most countries have an organisation that provides surveillance of the medicines which pharmaceutical companies make available for the treatment of disease. There is little doubt that if alcohol had only recently been discovered and was presented to an organisation such as the Federal Drug Administration in the USA it would be returned to the manufacturers with the statement that it was too toxic to be introduced.

The at-risk person Many efforts are being made to identify those people who are at special risk of alcoholism and suggestions have been made that the tendency is inherited or that there is some abnormality in the chemical makeup of such people, and certainly these may be factors. In my view the person who is at risk is the person who needs to drink to forget or to relax, particularly those who are depressed, agitated or heavily stressed, and especially if such drinking becomes a regular pattern in their lives. Thus I would feel that the person who drinks every day is at considerably greater risk than the person who drinks only on some days.

Associated features A doctor when examining patients will be alert to the possibility of an alcohol problem in persons showing a tendency to any of the following:
Suffering from stomach symptoms of nausea, morning vomiting, stomach ulcers, inflammation of the pancreas and liver damage.
Mental disorders such as depression, loss of memory, vagueness.
Frequently change jobs (or have bad work records) or who are known to be accident prone.
Have children who have psychological problems or who often present with illnesses of psychological origin.
Are shy, sensitive and self-conscious.
Are separated or divorced.
Are homosexual.
Have a criminal record.
Come to the surgery smelling of alcohol.

Certain occupations also seem to carry a greater risk, particularly those which involve working in the alcohol or alcohol-related industries, e.g. persons serving in bars. The professions are not exempt and alcoholism is by no means uncommon among doctors. Men are more than four times as likely to develop alcoholism as women, although with the dropping of traditional taboos on females drinking, this proportion will probably decrease.

A self-test The following is a way by which readers may themselves assess whether they have a drinking problem:
1. Do you lose time from work because of drinking?
2. Is drinking making your home life unhappy?
3. Do you drink because you are shy with other people?
4. Is drinking affecting your reputation?
5. Have you ever felt remorse after drinking?
6. Have you got into financial difficulties because of your drinking?

7. Do you turn to 'lower' companions and an inferior environment when drinking?
8. Does drinking make you careless of your family's welfare?
9. Has your ambition decreased since drinking?
10. Do you crave a drink at a definite time daily?
11. Do you want a drink the next morning?
12. Does your drinking cause you to have difficulty sleeping?
13. Has your efficiency decreased since drinking?
14. Is drinking jeopardising your job or business?
15. Do you drink to escape from worries or trouble?
16. Do you prefer to drink alone?
17. Do you sometimes have complete loss of memory because of drinking?
18. Has your doctor ever treated you for drinking?
19. Do you drink to build up your self confidence?
20. Have you ever been to hospital or an institution because of your drinking?

If the answer to more than two or three of these questions is 'yes', you have a drinking problem and maybe you are an alcoholic.

The CAGE test Here is another test along the same lines as the above.
1. Have you ever felt you should *Cut* down on your drinking?
2. Have people *Annoyed* you by criticising your drinking?
3. Have you ever felt *Guilty* about your drinking?
4. Have you ever had a drink first thing in the morning to steady your nerves or get rid of a hangover? (*Eye-opener*)

Two or three positive responses suggest alcohol dependence.

People who have developed the habit of drinking every day should be encouraged to try going three or four days without alcohol and to observe their reactions. If they find themselves excessively irritable or if the compulsion is too great and they give up with the rationalisation that they could do it if they felt it was worthwhile, then they are probably well on the way to alcoholism. If, on the other hand, they are scarcely conscious of any difference in themselves, one can reasonably assume that dependence has not yet developed.

It is said that those patients do best who have a proper understanding and acceptance of their problem; have a home; get support from a family and are able to keep a job; are able to control sudden urges and put off anticipated pleasures, and are able to form meaningful long-term relationships.

Acceptance One of the greatest difficulties health professionals have is in being able to convince alcoholics that they really have this problem and that they need help. It is unusual for patients to approach a doctor and announce that they need help, but acceptance of the problem is the vital first step to successful therapy.

Once the doctor is sure about the nature of the problem, it is often necessary to confront the patient with the facts and then usually tell the patient directly that he or she is an alcoholic. Sometimes this is best achieved by putting it in the form of a question, 'Do you think you could be an alcoholic?' If the patient replies negatively, the doctor may well have to spend further time explaining the reasons why that diagnosis is probable or even certain. With other patients, a doctor may consider it best to make a definitive statement from the beginning — 'All the evidence points to your being an alcoholic,' or something similar.

A common phenomenon is the spouse who protects his or her partner out of a misguided loyalty. Some can never accept that the other's drinking has got out of hand. Many alcoholics will not accept help until they have reached the stage where they feel alone and unsupported. Sometimes their non-alcoholic partner must leave home before the message really gets through and sometimes professional helpers have to recommend this unpalatable course if no progress is being made. Such medicine may be hard to take because with it the family must also swallow its pride.

Scapegoating Many alcoholics tend to be scapegoated and become the butt of all the animosity of friends and relatives.

If the alcoholic then recovers, this focus for the release of aggression disappears and can lead to emotional disorders in the rest of the family. Thus it is not uncommon for the wife of an alcoholic who has had to take all the responsibility for the family and cope with the aberrant behaviour of her husband, to become severely depressed when he gives up the alcohol and effectively becomes a member of the family again. This is a classic example of how important it is that doctors should wherever possible provide whole family care.

Community attitudes towards alcoholism

In terms of prevention, the biggest problem is to try to alter the community's attitude toward alcohol.

Our social mores are such that it is widely thought of as inhospitable to entertain without providing alcohol — usually to excess! The host or hostess who does not keep on topping up guests' glasses despite being aware that they have had as much as is good for them, is often considered mean. Worst of all is the popular conception that it is unmanly not to drink, and furthermore not to drink heavily. Advertisements for alcoholic beverages are designed to associate alcohol

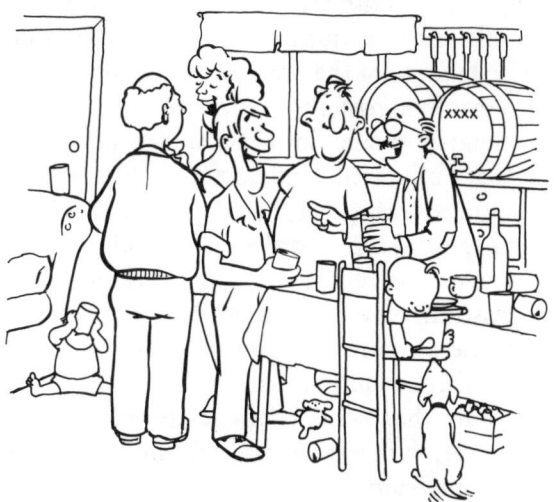

with a macho image in men, and a sexual attraction and femininity in women. The reality is usually quite the reverse.

The antics of the intoxicated are commonly displayed as being amusing and this too is counter-productive. Robert Benchley once said, 'Drinking makes such fools of people and people are such fools to begin with, that it is compounding a felony.'

For the established alcoholic, group therapy seems to provide the best results and the general practitioner can usually advise about where this is obtainable. It has been shown that increasing the price of alcohol is also an effective way of discouraging excessive use.

Alcoholics Anonymous

In general the most effective group therapy seems to be that provided by A.A. (Alcoholics Anonymous), but psychiatric clinics and hospitals may be better suited to the needs of some patients. Where 24-hour surveillance proves necessary, that extension of group therapy — the therapeutic community — may be a satisfactory answer. A therapeutic community is created when a number of people having similar problems live together as a group for mutual support and emotional development.

Patients often have to be convinced that they cannot fight alcoholism alone. Even then some patients seem unable or unwilling to succeed, despite much well-meaning support. A substance known as disulfiram (Antabuse) can be taken on a daily basis by those so motivated. If, after taking this, the patient drinks alcohol, it is converted in the body to formaldehyde which is a toxic substance capable of causing nausea and vomiting. A recent development is a long-acting preparation of disulfiram which is given by injection and is slowly released into the bloodstream.

Total abstinence

Almost all workers in this field believe that patients must be told that they can never drink again once they have got over their withdrawal symptoms and that they must be supported in their determination to adhere to this principle. If they weaken in this resolve it is sometimes due to a lack of understanding of the problem by family or friends, who are often not prepared to alter their own drinking patterns in order to assist the patient's attempts at abstinence. Failures and their attendant disappointments are frequent and the family must be prepared for these. It is right that both family and doctor should make known their disappointment to patients but little purpose is gained by adopting a scolding, puritanical attitude as often this will lead to further drinking in order to conceal chagrin.

A positive approach is imperative, reinforcing past decisions and encouraging the patient to try again. It is always most important that those involved demonstrate their interest and concern by expressing genuine pleasure in a patient's continued success in achieving abstinence. This is known as 'positive reinforcement'.

Patients must be made aware that alcoholism is a chronic disorder and that no one can claim a complete cure. However, with appropriate help and total abstinence, many alcoholics seem to achieve permanent remission.

Al-Anon objectives

Al-Anon is the organisation which has been set up to assist the families of alcoholics by —
1. helping solve problems due to alcoholism in the home;
2. the sharing of experience, strength and hope with others in similar circumstances;
3. improving their own emotional health and spiritual growth; and
4. providing a more wholesome environment for the whole family, including the alcoholic, whether drunk or sober.

The organisation has adopted a checklist of the qualities of a mature adult which is worthy of study by all.

The mature adult is one who —
1. does not automatically resent criticism because it is realised that it may contain suggestions for self improvement;
2. knows that self-pity is futile and childish — a way of placing the blame for disappointments on others;
3. does not lose temper readily or 'fly off the handle' over trifles;
4. keeps a cool head in emergencies and deals with them in a logical, reasonable fashion;
5. accepts responsibility for acts and decisions and does not blame someone else when things go wrong;
6. accepts reasonable delays without impatience, realising that one must adjust oneself to the convenience of others;
7. is a good loser, accepting defeat and disappointment without complaint or ill temper;
8. does not worry unduly about things for which nothing can be done;
9. does not boast or 'show off' but when praised or complimented, accepts with grace and appreciation, without false modesty;
10. applauds others' achievements with sincere goodwill;
11. rejoices in the good fortune and success of others without petty jealousy and envy;
12. listens courteously to the opinions of others and when they hold opposing views, does not enter into hostile argument;
13. doesn't find fault with 'every little thing' or criticise people who behave in ways that are not approved;
14. makes reasonable plans for activities and tries to carry them out in orderly fashion; does not do things on the spur of the moment without due consideration;
15. shows spiritual maturity by:
accepting that there is a superior power and that that power plays an important part in his or her life;
realising that he or she is part of mankind as a whole, that others have much to give and that there is an obligation to share with others one's own gifts;
obeying the spirit of the golden rule: 'Do unto others as you would have them do unto you.'

The acceptance that there is a power greater than oneself is a feature also of the credo of Alcoholics Anonymous and a stumbling block for some prospective members. For those of atheistic leanings, this 'power' is liberally interpreted. Thus it could be thought of as the power of a group as a whole, which is widely believed by those who have studied group dynamics to exceed the sum of the power of the individuals who comprise the group. Hence the references below to 'God as we understand Him (or Her)'.

The 12 steps of Alcoholics Anonymous

1. We admitted we were powerless over alcohol . . . that our lives had become unmanageable.
2. We came to believe that a power greater than ourselves could restore us to sanity.
3. We made a decision to turn our will and own lives over to the care of God as we understood Him (or Her).
4. We made a searching and fearless moral inventory of ourselves.
5. We admitted to God, to ourselves and to another human being the exact nature of our wrongs.
6. We were entirely ready to have God remove all these defects of character.
7. We humbly asked Him (or Her) to remove our shortcomings.
8. We made a list of all persons we had harmed and became willing to make amends to them all.
9. We made direct amends to such people wherever possible, except when to do so would injure them or others.
10. We continued to take personal inventory and when we were wrong, promptly admitted it.
11. We sought through prayer and meditation to improve our conscious contact with God as we understood Him (or Her), praying only for knowledge of His (or Her) will for us and the power to carry that out.
12. Having had a spiritual awakening as a result of these steps, we tried to carry this message to others and to practise these principles in all our affairs.

(2) Smoking

Thus far most attention has been devoted to alcohol in this chapter. Smoking is another example of health-damaging dependence.

Physically tobacco smoking is no less dangerous than alcohol, perhaps more so. The smoking of tobacco has the advantage that it does not lead to intellectual impairment or a deterioration in social skills. The dependence, however, is almost as difficult to break.

As Mark Twain said, 'Stopping smoking is the easiest thing I ever did: I ought to know because I have done it a thousand times.'

There is now much evidence available about the hazards of smoking. One author has estimated that for each cigarette smoked, an average of 5.5 minutes of life is lost. A 25-year-old man who regularly smokes 40 cigarettes each day will reduce his life expectancy by 8.3 years.

It is well known that, on average, women live longer than men. One recent study went so far as to suggest that in the past a major reason for this has been the differences between males and females in smoking habits.

Heart attacks We tend to hear most about the risks to smokers of developing lung cancer, but probably a greater risk is from heart attacks and this is compounded in women on the contraceptive pill.

Pipe and cigar smokers are at slightly less risk than cigarette smokers but the risk is still greatly enhanced when compared with non-smokers.

Where there are other risk factors such as a high level of cholesterol in the blood or high blood pressure, the risks tend to be multiplied and increase markedly. This risk is increased even further if smoking commenced very early in life, continued for many years and the person concerned inhales deeply. When a person ceases to smoke the risks of dying of heart disease reduce by half in the first year, but it takes at least 10 years before the risks return to the same level as a non-smoker.

Other physical problems Apart from heart attacks, what are the other problems attributable to smoking?

1. *Blockage of the blood vessels to the extremities (i.e. atherosclerosis or atheroma)*. This occurs particularly in the legs and can lead to gangrene, often requiring amputation of the limbs. The same condition can occur as a complication of diabetes. One of the earliest symptoms of this problem is pain in the calves on walking. Sufferers come to realise that after they walk a certain distance they develop a severe pain which, if they stand still, slowly abates, only to return again when they have once again completed a similar distance. As time passes the distance that can be accomplished without pain tends to diminish. This condition is known as *intermittent claudication*.

2. *Disorders of the blood vessels to the brain*. This usually takes the form of a 'stroke', known in medical parlance as a *cerebrovascular accident* or CVA. The result is usually paralysis of one side of the body, although sometimes it is more localised. Sometimes the stroke occurs in a part of the brain which does not have anything to do with movement. In such cases there may be very little evidence of the stroke, or alternatively there may be signs of intellectual impairment which again may be mild or severe and sometimes can be very bizarre. An example of the latter would be patients who refuse to recognise one half of their body and who, when asked to wash or dress themselves, do so on one side only, completely ignoring the other.

3. *Lung cancer*. Lung cancer can occur in non-smokers, but 80–85 per cent of cases occur in smokers. In the USA this is the leading cause of death from cancer. What many smokers do not realise is that the treatment for this condition is still singularly ineffective, even when it is detected early. Occasionally a patient with lung cancer is cured, but this is the exception, and those people who continue to smoke with the idea that provided they have regular chest X-rays and other medical checks, they will escape the consequences, are deluding themselves. However, even if a cure for lung cancer were discovered tomorrow, the other consequences of cigarette smoking would be enough to justify massive campaigns against smoking, in the interests of health promotion.

4. *Cancer of the throat*. Here again smoking is a major cause and smoking associated with heavy alcohol intake seems to increase the risk even further. Filter cigarettes may reduce this risk very slightly. Pipe and cigar smoking appear to confer no reduction in risk.

5. *Cancer of the mouth*. The situation is much as for cancer of the throat. The chewing of smoking tobacco and snuff dipping can also cause cancer of the mouth.

6. *Cancer of the gullet.* Smoking and alcohol are believed to play a part in many of these cases.

7. *Cancer of the bladder.* Many of the cases of this cancer are believed to be due to smoking.

8. *Cancer of the pancreas.* The risk of this relatively rare cancer is doubled in smokers as compared with non smokers.

9. *Lung disease.* The effect of smoking is seen particularly in relation to the amount of air which the lungs can expand to contain, and the ability to expel air without obstruction on breathing out. When these functions are regularly impaired the patient is said to have *chronic obstruction respiratory disease* (CORD). It is usually associated with marked breathlessness. In its advanced stages there is usually damage to the structure of the lung and a compensatory dilatation of the terminal air passages; this is known as *emphysema*. The risk of these problems is increased about 30 times in heavy smokers. It would seem that the irritation from cigarette smoking produces inflammation of the lining of the tubes of the lungs (bronchi and bronchioles) which leads to the secretion of thick mucus (phlegm or sputum). The presence of this leads in turn to impaired lung function and particularly obstruction to the free flow of air in and out of the lungs. In addition these secretions make an excellent place for bacteria to settle and multiply and when this occurs in the medium-sized tubes of the lung (bronchi), the condition of chronic bronchitis results.

10. *Stomach ulcer.* Ulcers of the stomach have been shown to be significantly more frequent among smokers when compared with non smokers.

Passive smoking This is the situation in which people who are not actually smoking themselves, inhale the smoke of other people who are smoking. There are some who take the view that they don't mind if smokers destroy themselves — that, they say, is their privilege if they have a mind to do so — but they are concerned if they affect the health of others.

There is no doubt that people working in enclosed spaces alongside smokers do breathe in appreciable amounts of carbon monoxide (a poisonous gas), nicotine and substances known to produce cancer.

Passive smokers in one study were shown to have concentrations of carbon monoxide in their bloodstream equivalent to smoking five cigarettes. Another researcher discovered that the nicotine content of the body of non-smokers working alongside smokers could be equal to the nicotine content of the bodies of light smokers (1–10 cigarettes/day) after an exposure of four hours.

Recently it has been demonstrated that breathing other people's smoke increases the risk of lung cancer in non-smokers (US Surgeon General, 1986.)

In adults the most frequent evidence of passive smoking are irritation of the eyes, headaches, nose symptoms and cough. In some people respiratory allergies and even asthma may be precipitated.

Chest infections: Possibly of even greater concern is the increase in the number of chest infections (bronchitis and pneumonia) in children under the age of two when their parents are smokers. This is particularly evident when both parents smoke. Wheezing and asthma is also more common among the children of smoking parents. Asthmatic children of smokers are said to show improvement when their parents give up smoking.

Heart problems: People who are prone to heart pain (due to diminished oxygen supply to the heart) often find that their attacks occur more easily after exposure to cigarette smoke. The carbon monoxide reduces the oxygen carrying capacity of the blood.

Danger to the unborn: In the unborn, smoking by the mother increases the risk of the baby being born before it is due (prematurity) and leads to a lower birth weight. After birth there is a greater risk of death of the baby as a consequence of the low birth weight.

Strategies

What can be done to reduce the incidence of smoking in the community? Many strategies have been employed and considerable knowledge acquired. Present efforts tend to concentrate on prevention, e.g. education of children in how to cope with peer pressure, and on the eradication of the impression that smoking is a grown-up, macho and sophisticated thing to do; reduction or elimination of advertising for smoking; education on risk factors and how to promote positive health; increasing the tax on tobacco; individual efforts by physicians and health-related personnel to use their influence to dissuade people from starting smoking.

For those who already smoke, efforts are directed at:
1. Education concerning the health hazards of smoking.
2. Education concerning alternative means of coping with nervousness and embarrassment. (Many people smoke because it gives them something to do with their hands when talking to others.)
3. Provision of substitutes which are less dangerous, such as nicotine chewing gum (Nicorette).
4. Providing group activity comparable to Alcoholics Anonymous.
5. Public pressure so that smoking becomes widely regarded as an antisocial activity — smoke-free weeks and the like.
6. Pressure from health professionals on an individual basis and the employment of a variety of other techniques which seem to work for some people, such as hypnotism and acupuncture, or even mouth sprays which make the smoking of cigarettes a distinctly unpleasant experience.

Remember: 40 per cent of heavy smokers (more than 25 cigarettes per day) will die before reaching 65, compared with only 15 per cent of non smokers. The average loss of life for a 20-per-day smoker is 5 years, while for a 40-per-day smoker life expectancy is reduced by 8 years. Thus the average regular smoker's life is shortened by about 5.5 minutes for each cigarette smoked — approximately the same time that it takes to smoke it.

KICK THE HABIT

Here is a 'Kick the Habit' cigarette smoking pattern sheet. Each time you take out a cigarette, mark on this sheet —

1. The time at which you smoke the cigarette.
2. The occasion (e.g. breakfast, coffee break, TV, party, etc.)
3. The amount of need you feel for it on a scale of '1' for little or no need to '5' for greatest need.
4. The amount of cigarette smoked (e.g., ½, ¼, etc.)

Fill out one of these sheets every day in which you smoke.

Cigarettes on day _____

Time	Occasion	Need	Amount smoked
1.			
2.			
3.			
4.			
5.			
⋮			
46.			
47.			
48.			
49.			
50.			

REASONS FOR STOPPING SMOKING

1. _____
2. _____
3. _____
4. _____
5. _____
6. _____
7. _____
8. _____
9. _____
10. _____

The following advice is adapted from the Canadian Tuberculosis and Disease Association 'Kick the Habit' Kit: *'Helpful hints for quitting smoking'*.

If you are still smoking:

1. Keep a daily smoking pattern sheet as shown opposite. Inspect the record every evening and resolve to cut out the less important cigarettes, for instance, all number 1s. If this proves to be easy, start on the number 2s.

2. Carry your pattern sheet with 'Reasons for stopping smoking' with you. Look at it often and add to it. If you feel you have overwhelming reasons why you *should* smoke, put these down, too.

3. Write down any observations, gimmicks, or shortcuts that help you overcome your urge to smoke.

4. If you are keen to stop smoking, **stop buying cigarettes and get rid of the cigarettes you have stocked up.**

5. Switch brands. Go to a brand you dislike.

6. Do not carry matches or a lighter.

7. Put all ashtrays aside.

8. Put your pack of cigarettes in a place where you must make an effort to reach it. You should *know* that you are reaching for a cigarette; you should ask yourself whether you really want or need this cigarette. If you decide you do, go ahead and smoke.

9. Buy sugarless gum, sugarless confectionery, or ginger and carry it with you. Use it instead of a cigarette. (Never with it!)

If you are no longer smoking, carry out points 2 and 3 above, plus:

10. Drink plenty of water; keep a full cup at your desk.

11. Breathe deeply once in a while, particularly when the urge to smoke is great.

12. Get up, walk around the room briskly, stretch. In general, keep busy. Remember it can be done and thousands have given up before you.

13. Avoid the company of persons who smoke, particularly those who disapprove of quitting or would be apt to kid you about it; instead spend your time with non-smokers.

14. If your spouse, boyfriend or girlfriend, or other members of your household, smoke, try to make them join you in quitting.

15. DON'T CHEAT. If you find you cannot give up smoking at this time, don't worry and don't feel guilty. But above all, don't cheat! Remember that each smoker has to find the one reason which is meaningful to him or her to stop smoking.

Remember — *'It's a matter of life and breath!'*

SECTION THREE

Some common problems and their causes

(Based roughly on the 31 most common problems presenting to general practitioners, in the order of their frequency of appearance)

3.1 Sore throats

Although these are seen so commonly in the doctor's surgery, there are still many things which remain unknown about sore throats. Of course, many sore throats do not even get to the doctor. Some are very mild and disappear quickly, others are part of the development of certain other condition such as the common cold. Most are probably caused by viruses and so are unresponsive to antibiotics. About one in five of severe sore throats are caused by bacteria known as *streptococci*.

Streptococci

Streptococci are unpleasant bacteria because, apart from causing sore throats, they can also lead to rheumatic fever or to nephritis, which is an inflammation of the kidney. These conditions are fortunately rare as they are capable of causing some serious long-term effects and even, in severe cases, death.

Some families seem to have a special susceptibility to rheumatic fever or nephritis and research suggests that rheumatic fever is common in people who are living in rather poor social circumstances. Nevertheless, it can occur in any family.

Rheumatic fever This condition seldom develops for the first time in children under five years of age or adolescents over 15 years of age, but if young people do suffer from it, they probably remain liable to recurrences of the disorder, in association with reinfection by the streptococcus, for the rest of their lives.

The most obvious feature of rheumatic fever is the hot, swollen and painful joints that the sufferer develops. The trouble often seems to flit from one joint to another. Usually when the condition has come under control, the joints return to normal. Less obvious is the effect that the disorder has on the heart, where there may be damage to the valves, making the action of that organ much less efficient. It also makes the valves of the heart susceptible to other infections.

Although some cases of rheumatic fever appear to develop without a preceding sore throat, there is evidence that when the sore throat does occur, it needs to be present for nine days at least before there is a risk of rheumatic fever developing. Most sore throats, including those which are caused by streptococci, clear up spontaneously in less then seven days, so it is certainly not necessary for all patients with sore throats to have antibacterial agents.

It is a pity that it is so difficult to diagnose the nature of a sore throat from the appearance of the throat. When the doctor looks inside the mouth the back of the throat generally looks much the same regardless of the cause of the problem. If the lymph nodes in the neck, just below the corner of the jaw, are swollen and tender, the chance of a streptococcal infection is greater, but other organisms can produce an almost identical picture.

If the tonsils are covered with a white layer, looking a bit like blobs of ice cream, the problem is more likely to be glandular fever (i.e. infectious mononucleosis). If Amoxycillin (a form of penicillin) is given for this, it will certainly not kill the viruses responsible and almost invariably it will bring the patient out in a generalised, measles-like rash. This is a curious reaction which is not an allergy, and the patient can be given penicillin again in the future if there is a need for it.

Nephritis This, the other unpleasant complication of streptococcal infections, is quite different. Unlike rheumatic fever, there is no clear relationship to the duration of the infection. In fact it would seem that if you are a susceptible person, any infection by a nephritis-producing strain of streptococcus, however brief, will produce the reaction in the kidneys which is manifested as nephritis. In other words, it is an 'all or none' situation.

In this instance, the only argument for treating the sore throat is the possibility that the offending streptococcus may, if not removed, be transmitted to other people.

Not all streptococci are quite the same and some variations seem to have a greater tendency to cause nephritis than others, just as some people seem to be more susceptible than others. Occasionally such a strain of streptococcus becomes rampant in a community and there is a small epidemic of nephritis. Most cases, however, seem to arise independently of an epidemic (i.e. sporadically). Another form of streptococcal infection which seems to be a more usual prelude to nephritis than sore throat is the common 'school sore', otherwise known as impetigo. This condition does not cause rheumatic fever.

Penicillin treatment

Happily the streptococcus remains very sensitive to penicillin in any form — even the cheapest — but there is reason to believe that in any individual the treatment should be continued for at least ten days in order to eradicate these bacteria completely. Because some people are not as conscientious as they should to be about taking medications once the symptoms are gone, some doctors prefer to give an injection of long-acting penicillin. They can then be sure that the patient gets adequate treatment.

Once a person has had one attack of rheumatic fever, there is always the risk of another as a result of further infection with the streptococcus. As a result, such people are advised to continue taking a small dose of penicillin every day, indefinitely — probably for the rest of their lives. This will prevent further damage to the heart. Again, because so many people find it difficult to remember to take a tablet every day, some authorities believe that this penicillin should also be administered by periodic injections of long-acting penicillin.

Allergies Some people are allergic to penicillin and so cannot be given this very valuable medicine. There are a number of alternatives which may be given, of which erythromycin is the best known. Cephalosporin is another. There is argument among doctors as to whether taking penicillin for a streptococcal sore throat — probably unnecessary unless there is a special risk of rheumatic fever — makes any difference to the duration of the sore throat. In fact it has facetiously been stated by some researchers that if you leave such a sore throat it will be better in seven days, whereas if you treat it, it will be better in a week!

Unfortunately no two people and no two sore throats are the same and so a satisfactory controlled trial is difficult to carry out. However, it should not be impossible to get this information using modern research techniques but it highlights how much we still have to learn about even very common complaints.

Some doctors will prescribe penicillin or some other antibiotic for every sore throat that is presented to them. Their patients run the risk of developing an allergy to penicillin or of encouraging the development of resistant strains of bacteria (but not of streptococci, which so far have developed no resistance to penicillin). Many doctors will consider whether the patient is 'at risk' of rheumatic fever, and take into account how long the throat has been sore. If the throat has been sore a week or longer, they may decide to do a throat swab, the results of which are usually available in 24 hours. If a streptococcus is found as a result of the swab, they will then institute a ten-day course of penicillin. If a streptococcus is not found, it is reasonable to continue to watch and wait for the sore throat to subside spontaneously. Meantime, it is usually possible to provide some medication which will make the sore throat more tolerable. Soluble aspirin dissolved in water can be used as a gargle, resulting in some reduction in pain. Should the doctor suspect some other condition, such as infectious mononucleosis, a blood test may be ordered.

Post-nasal discharge

It is worth noting that some sore throats seem to occur as a result of infected material from the nose passing down the back of the nose into the throat. This is referred to as 'post-nasal discharge'. Where this is a frequent problem the sufferer may also experience recurrent attacks of tonsillitis. (See section on nasal congestion, p. 156.)

People who sleep with their mouths open often wake to find that their throat is dry and even a little sore. Occasionally sore throats are caused by fungal infections (thrush). Usually this infection involves the gums and the roof of the mouth as well. If this occurs, the treatment should be an antifungal agent.

Mouth ulcers Another problem, which tends to be recurrent, is mouth ulcers. These are usually seen as small white patches in the crevice between the gums and the cheek. They can be very sore. The usual form is called an 'aphthous ulcer' and the cause remains uncertain. Some people seem to get benefit from sucking small pellets of hydrocortisone or one of its derivatives, in contact with the ulcer. Eventually they go away, regardless of what is done.

3.2 Back problems

The frequency of back problems would seem to confirm the belief of many that mankind has not yet fully adjusted to the upright position. There are many misconceptions about the spine and probably the greatest is that the vertebrae slip and slide about like so many beads on a string. Some people talk glibly about vertebrae being slipped into place. Even 'slipped disc' is a misnomer — 'squashed disc' would probably be a more accurate term.

Injury

The majority of back problems are related to injury, either acute or chronic. In acute situations the sufferer can usually describe a particular incident which has apparently been responsible for the trouble. Commonly this is due to lifting inappropriately. Chronic conditions are more likely a reaction of the vertebral column (i.e. backbone) to the repeated minor insults produced by poor posture. Sagging beds have a particularly bad reputation, and I have known people who have suffered for weeks from sciatica become virtually pain free within a few days of starting to sleep on a very firm mattress, or even on the floor.

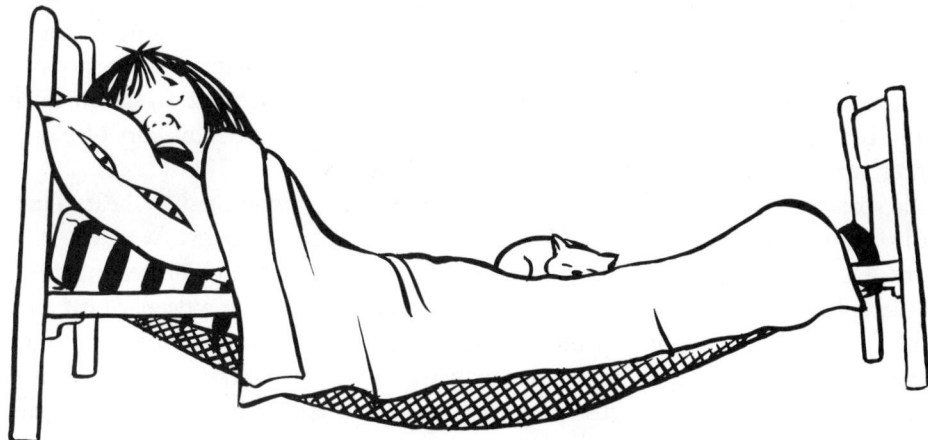

It would seem that sitting or lying in a position which places an unnatural strain on ligaments or muscles ultimately leads to some relaxation of these structures, with consequent pressure on nerves or other pain-producing tissues. Often it would appear that the abnormal movement or abnormal pressure leads to tissue swelling, as when a joint is sprained. This swelling is not outwardly visible but presses on pain-sensitive structures. It is only when this swelling has subsided, and the pressure has thus been released, that the patient becomes pain free. Usually this inflammation of the tissues will disappear most rapidly when the back is rested. Manipulation can make the problem worse.

Sometimes in these circumstances there is slight bony movement, causing pressure on nerves, and in such cases careful manipulation will at times lead to a dramatic improvement.

Underlying disorders

The exact mechanism of many back problems is difficult to ascertain and the most important thing is for the doctor to try to make sure that there is no serious underlying disorder present. Very occasionally a back problem can be due to a disorder of the bony structure itself. Thus the bone may have lost its calcium (which gives it strength) in a condition called *osteoporosis*. This can lead to a squashing of the vertebrae, with a consequent loss of height. This is seen most often in elderly women and is the reason why some of them actually get shorter as they get older. (See section on the menopause, pp. 186–7.) In fact, regularly checking a person's height is a valuable way of gauging whether the condition is active or not.

Sometimes there can be deposits of cancer present in the bone. These are likely to be the result of pre-existing cancer, particularly in the prostate gland, the breast or the thyroid. Occasionally there are deposits resulting from abnormal blood components. The best known condition leading to this is multiple myeloma. If these deposits go undiagnosed and manipulation is attempted, the results can be disastrous. When there is any doubt about diagnosis, certain blood tests and X-rays can help to sort things out. Nevertheless, the majority of back problems respond well to conservative treatment and do not require extensive investigation.

Muscle pains When muscles are under prolonged strain, they often go into painful spasm, which is the name given to an involuntary, but usually painful, tightening of the muscles. Cramp is a particularly severe form of spasm which sometimes seems to arise spontaneously. Bad posture can often provide the abnormal muscle tensions which lead to spasm. Such spasm is responsible for many aches and pains. Students often experience this sort of pain in their back after sitting tensely writing exams for several hours.

Muscle spasm is usually relieved by relaxation and this is promoted by heat. This is why hot baths and spas have such a reputation for relieving aches and pains. Warmth from whatever source is likely to promote relaxation and an electric blanket or heater may be helpful. Physiotherapists have special equipment which apparently provides a deeper heat and is even more effective. Some work on a principle similar to a microwave oven. Most use radiation in the high frequency range, so we have shortwave diathermy, ultrasonics, etc. It is believed that these devices do more than just provide heat and probably help to break up unwanted fibrous tissue which could cause adhesions and disperse substances which have accumulated as a result of tissue damage.

The non-steroidal anti-inflammatory medicines (NSAIDS — see section on medication) are also believed to be useful where there is a need to disperse the products of tissue damage.

Predisposition Most back problems will settle down in time — but sometimes improvement is quite slow. Some people seem to have a particular predisposition to back troubles and they have to learn to be very careful at all times. In fact, because back problems are so common, we should all take the trouble to learn good lifting habits.

The most important lesson to learn is that, whenever possible, lifting should be done with a straight back. One should crouch down and then, maintaining a straight back and with head up, take the weight through the knees and hips, gradually moving to the erect posture. As they say, one should 'never use one's back like a crane'. It is also important that the feet should be correctly positioned. One should maintain a wide base and have a foot pointing in the direction in which it is intended to move. The arms should be kept close to the body and the elbows tucked in. A good grip with the hand or hands is also essential; don't try to lift more than is reasonable for one person; do not overreach when placing high loads; pulling is preferable to pushing; do not stand too far away from the object to be lifted; do not hold for prolonged periods an out-of-balance, heavy load.

When sitting, the small of the back should always be well supported. Much furniture fails to provide this support.

Work surfaces Many work surfaces are at the wrong height for the people working at them. Thus a sink bench should be set lower for a person who is short than for one who is six feet tall. Unfortunately some designers assume that all people are the same height and abide by rules that are made for Mr or Mrs Average — a very rare person.

Firm mattress For most back pains, lying on the back with a firm mattress is the most effective treatment. The patient should be in the position of maximum comfort. Sometimes a pillow in the small of the back is helpful, but only one pillow under the head should be permitted. Local heat is likely to be helpful as are NSAIDS (non-steroidal anti-inflammatory drugs), of which aspirin is amongst the best known and still one of the most effective.

When there is sciatica (i.e. pain due to pressure on the sciatic nerve which runs from the back to the buttock and right down the leg), the ability to raise the leg to a position at right-angles to the body is impaired. Progress can be measured by checking how near the patient gets to achieving such a right-angle. In some backaches which fail to respond to rest and physiotherapy, injections of hydrocortisone into key positions may be helpful, while some doctors seem to get good results with acupuncture.

Exercises designed to strengthen the muscles which straighten the back may make the patient somewhat less susceptible to problems.

Other causes

Of course, not all backaches are due to disorders of the back itself. Occasionally kidney disorders and gynaecological disorders (i.e. disorders of the female organs) can cause pain in the back. Rarely, back pain seems to be primarily the result of an emotional problem.

Any backache that is associated with prolonged numbness and tingling in the legs or buttocks must be thoroughly investigated and treated with special concern, as it is possible that the spinal cord and spinal nerves are involved.

The examination

In the evaluation of backache, you can expect your doctor to take a detailed history and then to examine the back thoroughly, looking for any abnormal curvatures in the spine either from side to side (i.e. scoliosis) or from forward to back. An exaggerated forward stoop is a *kyphosis* and an exaggerated extension of the back is known as a *lordosis*. All of these can disturb the centre of gravity of the back and place abnormal strains on the supporting structures. In particular, a very marked lordosis may, over a period of time, cause a small forward displacement of some vertebrae, known as spondylolisthesis.

The back should then be put through its full range of movements, most clothes having been removed. A search will be made for tender spots along the course of the spine and adjacent to it. Knee jerks (i.e. reflexes) and ankle jerks should be checked if the pain is in the lower back, while the reflexes in the arms should be studied if the pain is in the neck region. A check should also be made for any area of the body where there is numbness or other loss of sensation.

Often an examination of the back passage (rectum) with a gloved finger is indicated, and in women a gynaecological exam may be thought desirable. X-rays are sometimes requested and also blood tests. If the trouble is only in the neck, the examination may be confined to that region and to the examination of the shoulders and arms. If kidney trouble is a possible cause, a urine examination may be required. Of course neck and back problems can be part of a generalised joint problem, e.g. gout or rheumatoid arthritis, and in this case the examination may have to be even more extensive.

3.3 Coughs

Coughs are caused by irritation of the respiratory (i.e. breathing) passages. They are an important means by which unwanted substances are expelled from the body. Sometimes these unwanted substances are irritating fumes, dusts or even food which has become displaced and has not gone down the oesophagus. On other occasions the cough is produced in an attempt to rid the body of sputum (phlegm) which has accumulated in the tubes leading to the lungs. This sputum is mostly mucus which has been produced by the lining of these tubes. It is very profuse when there is infection or spasm of the tubes, as in bronchitis or asthma. Even cold air can cause the production of mucus and induce coughing. People seem to vary in the sensitivity of their throats.

The smoke from tobacco is one of the commonest causes of irritation.

We all get coughs from time to time, but most go away after a few weeks.

Mucus is naturally white or colourless and relatively watery. If the sputum produced becomes discoloured or thick, it usually means that it has become infected with bacteria and if this persists for more than a few days and shows no sign of clearing, it may be an indication for an antibiotic. Sometimes discoloured sputum is due to a virus and antibiotics will not help. A cough without sputum or with only a little clear mucus seldom requires treatment with an antibiotic.

Prolonged cough Do not be surprised if some irritation of the throat leading to frequent coughing persists for up to six weeks after treatment with an antibiotic. So long as the sputum is clear, this is usually of little consequence as it just represents a degree of residual irritation. Many patients return to the doctor expecting more antibiotics because the cough has not gone. In these circumstances further antibiotics will often do more harm than good.

Another reason for prolonged cough is an underlying wheeziness. Some people suffer from mild spasm of the tubes leading to the lungs (i.e. bronchi). This is known as *bronchospasm*. It can be so mild that the patient is unaware of being wheezy, but is conscious of a persistent cough. Most doctors these days possess a simple device that gives a measure of the amount of air which can be breathed out in a brief period of time. If this amount of air is seriously reduced, it strongly suggests that spasm of the bronchial tubes, together with secretions, are restricting the free flow of air. When this is obvious it is given the name 'asthma'. (See section on shortness of breath, p. 152.) When a troublesome cough is due to bronchospasm it will usually respond to medicines called *bronchodilators* (see p. 153–4).

Cough medicines Cough medicines tend to be of two types. There are those which are designed to loosen up the sputum and so make expectoration easier, and there are those which are designed to depress the centre in the brain which is designated the 'cough centre' and make it less sensitive to the messages which it receives from the throat and bronchial tubes. There is a danger here, for if the depression is too great, secretions which ought to be removed by coughing may remain and aggravate any existing blockage, increasing the opportunities for infection.

However, in many sufferers, persistent coughing is of limited value and rather exhausting. For this reason, medicines which are capable of diminishing the frequency and severity of cough are often prescribed. The best agents are derived from opium but have little potential for habit formation. Traditionally, codeine has been used, but latterly preparations such as pholcodine, which is much less constipating, have been popular.

Rarely cough is due to serious disease such as tuberculosis, cancer or pneumonia, and it is for this reason that anyone who has an unexplained cough should have their chest thoroughly examined by inspection, percussion (i.e. tapping) and listening with the stethoscope (i.e. auscultation). If the doctor is in any doubt, an X-ray may be ordered. Blood tests are sometimes desirable, but sending a sample of sputum to the laboratory is seldom helpful except in the diagnosis of tuberculosis and a few obscure infections.

Bronchitis

Bronchitis is a somewhat formidable term. It really means inflammation of the bronchial tubes. In fact, any cough with infected sputum which is not due to tuberculosis or another rare condition — bronchiectasis — is designated as bronchitis. Where it is very persistent and occurs repeatedly, it is referred to as chronic bronchitis. If there is chronic bronchitis there is usually some irreversible lung damage, so it is wise not to permit a cough which produces discoloured sputum to go too long untreated.

Chronic bronchitis is more likely to occur in people who smoke or who work in dusty or cold environments. When masks are provided in the workplace, as they should be where dangerous dusts or fumes are present, they should always be worn.

Sinusitis

People with infected sinuses usually have some of the infected mucus from their noses passing down the back of their noses into the throat. In the daytime this material is usually coughed up, but when we are asleep at night our cough responses are less active and sometimes some of this infected material gets into the bronchial tubes and lungs. In the throat this material can produce tonsillitis, and in the lungs it may give rise to bronchitis or even pneumonia.

Another cause of congestion and irritation in the lungs is what is known as heart failure. This really means that the left side of the heart, which pumps blood around the body, is under strain and as a result there is some back pressure in the lungs. This leads to an accumulation of fluid at the base of the lungs, usually accompanied by breathlessness and cough. Commonly when this occurs the sufferer has had high blood pressure or has had a heart attack (i.e. myocardial infarct), but there are other causes such as the later stages of rheumatic fever.

This is another reason why the heart and lungs should be carefully examined in a patient with a cough which has caused sufficient anxiety to lead to a consultation with a doctor.

One interesting but rare cause of cough is wax in the ears. For some unexplained anatomical reason, there is an area within the ear canal which, when touched, leads to a reflex cough. If a piece of wax moves about in the ear canal it can lead to repeated coughing. Similarly, attempts to remove wax may lead to paroxysms of coughing.

3.4 Abdominal pain

Everybody suffers from this at some time in their lives and the causes are many. It is a condition which lends itself particularly to the symptom description outlined in the section on going to the doctor, pp. 24-5.

Thus a clear history of how and when the pain started, its site, any change in position of the pain, any radiation, together with factors which make it worse or give relief, are very important. Some indication of the type of pain is also desirable, e.g. is it burning, stabbing, dull, etc. Associated symptoms such as flatulence, vomiting, diarrhoea, fever and the like, can also afford a clue.

Renal colic

A *colic* is a pain which gradually worsens, reaches a peak and then eases off, all this occurring on a regular basis. It is usually produced by obstruction of one of the many tubular structures within the body. The pain is caused by the contractions of the tube in an effort to be rid of the obstruction.

The most severe abdominal pain is probably that of *renal colic* due to a stone forming and lodging in the *ureter*, which is the tube that conveys urine produced in the kidney to the bladder. The pain often seems to start in the loin and travels down the abdomen into the groin and in males it often seems to be felt also in the testicle. The pain is usually so severe that it causes the sufferer to writhe. The small stone sometimes manages to pass out of the ureter and into the bladder, with immediate relief of symptoms. However, further pain may occur lower down as it passes along another tube (the *urethra*), finally being expelled and plopping to the bottom of the toilet pan. If this occurs, it is always worthwhile trying to retrieve the stone (referred to as a 'calculus') so that it can be given to the doctor for analysis. There are several different types of stone and information about the constituents may help the doctor to plan further treatment to prevent a recurrence.

Biliary colic

Another cause of colic — although sometimes the pain seems to be constant rather than colicky — is the presence of a stone in the *bile ducts* which are the tubes leading from the *gallbladder* (a repository for bile) to the lower outlet of the stomach. This pain is referred to as *biliary colic*. When the bile is prevented from escaping it goes back through the liver and gets into the bloodstream and is one cause of the yellowing of the skin known as jaundice. The commonest cause of jaundice, however, is hepatitis. This too can cause abdominal pain, but the mechanism is rather different. Sometimes gallbladder pain is felt in the shoulder region rather than the abdomen.

Acidity

Many people get abdominal pain which is apparently due, in the first instance, to the effects of stomach acid on the lining of the stomach. In normal people the stomach lining has considerable ability to resist the effects of the digestive juices which normally act on the food which we eat. However, if the acid level in the stomach is excessive, some damage can occur. There are probably other factors at work as well and researchers are even wondering if certain infections may not play a part in the production of stomach ulcers.

Ulcers Excessive acid production seems to be the fate of some people, regardless of what they try to do to prevent it, but cigarette smoking, alcohol consumption, tea and coffee are some of the agents which seem to make matters worse. Anxiety can also play a part, as can an excess of acid foods in the diet. If the acidity persists unchecked, ulcer formation may occur. Such stomach ulcers are grouped together as 'peptic ulcers', and when they occur in the *duodenum* (i.e. that part of the gastro-intestinal tract immediately beyond the stomach itself), they are known as *duodenal ulcers*, while if they occur in the body of the stomach they are known as *gastric ulcers*.

It would seem that duodenal ulcers have a closer relationship to excess acid production than gastric ulcers. Unfortunately most of the anti-inflammatory agents which we use have a deleterious effect on ulcer healing and may even precipitate an ulcer. Even a medicine as common as aspirin can be very damaging in a susceptible person.

Relation to meals In duodenal ulcers, the pain usually has a clear relationship to food intake. Commonly food in the stomach provides relief of pain, which may last a greater or lesser time. Normally it takes about two hours after food goes into the stomach for it to pass into the next part of the alimentary tract, so the pain is especially likely to return two or more hours after a meal. Actually patients with duodenal ulcers seem to empty their stomachs rather faster than average. The pain of duodenal ulceration, which is often worse at night, is usually located 25 to 50 mm below the sternum (i.e. breastbone). This area of the abdomen is often referred to as the 'epigastrium'.

In some cases it can be very difficult to differentiate the pain of duodenal ulcer from that of gastric ulcer. As a rule, in gastric ulcer the relationship to meals is less clear cut, the response to anti-acid medication is less certain and there is a greater chance of weight loss.

Either condition can occasionally exist without the patient having any symptoms. On the other hand, sometimes an ulcer can be so severe as to perforate a blood vessel and cause profuse bleeding, while at other times it can perforate the stomach itself — both serious conditions. The diagnosis of peptic ulcers is usually made using a *barium meal X-ray*. (Barium or its substitutes are opaque to X-rays and so enable the outline of the stomach to be visualised on

X-ray films.) There is also an instrument called a gastroscope which can be passed through the mouth and inserted into the stomach. This allows a specialist to see the ulcer directly and also to take samples of the ulcer wall to check whether there are any signs of cancer or other disease processes present.

Regurgitation At the junction of the oesophagus (i.e. gullet) and the stomach, at about the level of the diaphragm (i.e. the muscular partition that separates the abdominal contents from the chest), there is a valve-like mechanism which is responsible for preventing the regurgitation of stomach contents on to the oesophagus. Sometimes part of the stomach protrudes into the chest because there is a defect (i.e. hiatus) in the diaphragm. Such a situation is referred to as a *diaphragmatic* or *hiatus hernia* and often it is associated with a poorly functioning valve. When this occurs the stomach contents can flow into the oesophagus and irritate its walls. The oesophagus is much less able to resist the effects of acid than the stomach and the patient usually experiences a burning sensation behind the lower end of the sternum (i.e. breastbone). This is known as *heartburn*. This pain is in the chest and so should not be included in this section, except that it is relevant to the discussion on stomach acid. The condition is affected by gravity and is much more likely to occur if the sufferer bends over or lies down.

Acid risings When the stomach contents are still very liquid, as after taking a drink, the patient may also notice the sensation of sour stomach fluids coming up the back of the throat. This is sometimes referred to as *water brash* or *acid risings*. Probably everyone experiences this at some time in their lives, but when there is a hiatus hernia it can be very frequent. Symptoms of hiatus hernia are often worse when people are overweight and the effects of dieting will sometimes produce dramatic improvement. It is recommended that people with this problem should not lie flat and even a couple of bricks placed under the head of the bed, so that the patient sleeps on a slight slope, can be helpful. As far as possible, any bending should be avoided. Sometimes it is beneficial to avoid drinking too much fluid prior to lying down.

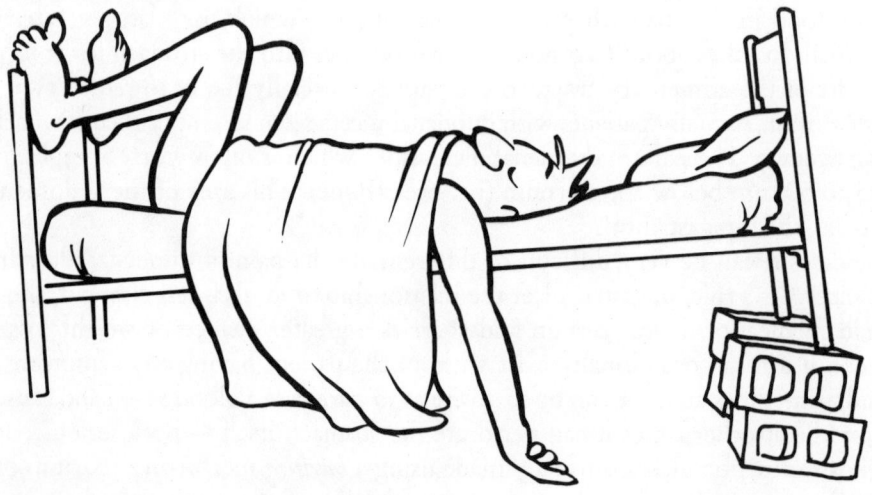

Reducing acid Where acid plays a part in the causation of disease, symptoms can often be reduced by neutralising the acid. Some foods are better for this than others and milk can be helpful if nothing else is available. Most people eventually take acid-neutralising tablets or mixtures, but these do not always lead to ulcer healing.

More recently there have been developed tablets which actually influence the production of acid and these are usually very successful in getting rid of symptoms and healing ulcers. Cimetidine (Tagamet) comes into this category and so does ranitidine (Zantac). The evidence that changes in diet make much difference to ulcer healing is not good. Unfortunately people who are susceptible to ulcers are very prone to recurrences. Many ulcers seem to be precipitated by alcohol, and anyone who has one should have their alcohol intake reviewed by their doctor as sometimes the ulcer is the first clue to the presence of alcoholism. (See p. 109.)

Appendicitis

Most people, when they experience a pain in the abdomen, worry about the possibility of appendicitis. This disorder seems to be a product of the western lifestyle and it is seldom seen amongst primitive races. The suggestion is that the low residue diet that is so common in the west plays a part. The problem presents as an inflammation in the vestigial organ known as the appendix, which has no known function in humans and so can be removed without disadvantage to the sufferer. Sometimes blockage of the appendix plays a part and this can be due to a seed, a small fragment of hard faeces or even worms.

The onset of the condition is often abrupt and the patient may in the first instance experience central abdominal pain. Usually the pain eventually moves to the lower right hand corner of the abdomen, with maximum tenderness about two-thirds of the way between the umbilicus (tummy button) and the most prominent part of the bony pelvis. The pain may vary in intensity, but there is commonly an underlying constant component so one can say that it is unusual for the pain to go away completely and then return again. If the appendix is significantly inflamed, there is likely to be tenderness in the tissues overlying the appendix and the patient is reluctant to allow an examining hand to compress the abdomen. Often pressure on the immediately opposite side of the abdomen increases the pain in the appendix region. The bowels are usually constipated (although occasionally there is diarrhoea) and there is a low-grade temperature. Very seldom does the temperature exceed 38.5°C. The tongue of the patient is usually furred.

The examining doctor will feel the abdomen carefully and then will usually insert a gloved finger into the back passage. In this way a tender appendix residing behind the bowel may be detected. In most cases a blood test and a urine test are also desirable. If appendicitis is present there will be an increase in the white cells of the blood and the urine test is done to ensure that the pain present is not due to an infection in the urine masquerading as appendicitis.

Appendicitis is a surgical emergency and most cases require prompt surgery. This cannot be commenced until the stomach is empty of its contents. Thus, if you suspect appendicitis, it is wise not to offer the patient food or fluid until after the doctor has decided whether or not an operation is likely, otherwise the waiting time for surgery will be prolonged.

The *worst* thing that you can do for the patient is to offer a laxative (i.e. a medicine designed to make the bowels work). This can sometimes cause so much bowel activity that the appendix ruptures. If this occurs, pus will be spilt into the abdominal cavity, probably leading to a very serious *peritonitis* (i.e. an inflammation of the lining of the abdominal cavity).

Lymphadenitis There is a condition of the lymph nodes in the abdominal cavity, probably caused by a virus infection, which presents itself in very much the same way as appendicitis, and quite a few of these cases undergo surgery because appendicitis is suspected.

Sometimes appendicitis can be atypical and present in ways that are quite different from the description given above.

Irritable bowel

These days many people suffer from what is described as an *irritable bowel*. Some doctors use the term *spastic colon* to refer to the same condition. This is also discussed in the section on disorders in which the emotions play a significant part. (See p. 80.) There seem to be several factors at work in this condition and these include stress, previous irritation from infection, probably food allergies and even the overuse of laxatives. The pain is usually related to muscle tightening (spasm) of the large bowel (colon). As a consequence, it seldom appears in the same place twice. The pain is often intermittent (i.e. colicky) and may mimic a variety of other conditions. Some patients experience an associated looseness of the bowels, often passing large, watery and almost explosive bowel motions, while others are troubled by constipation. Flatulence is often a problem, and after the bowel motion there is frequently the passage of some clear or whitish mucus, but never blood. If blood is present there must be some other condition coexisting.

Relief may be obtained by increasing the bulk of the food residues. This may be achieved by eating more high-residue foods (see p. 100), particularly grains, or by introducing bran into the diet. There are also some preparations which may be taken medicinally and which absorb water within the bowel and as a result swell up and provide bulk. Isogel is one such substance and Metamucil is another.

Some people get help from the use of medicines designed to prevent muscle (in this case, bowel-wall muscle) spasm (see pp. 153–4). Others again find that their symptoms abate with a short course of a tranquilliser, but this should be a last resort.

If some sort of bowel allergy or an abnormal sensitivity to some ingredient of the diet is present, removal of that substance from the diet may make a remarkable difference. However, such removal should be done under medical advice as there is a danger of the patient becoming deficient in essential nutrients if important foods are removed by the over-zealous dieter. (See also section on diet, pp. 88–9, 93–5, 97.)

Diverticulitis

In older people a much more common condition is *diverticulitis*. As a person ages there seems to be a tendency for the muscular wall of the large bowel to lose some of its strength and as a result the inner lining of the bowel may bulge out, creating pockets (or diverticulae) in the bowel wall. These make an ideal place for small collections of faeces to lodge. As time passes it would seem that these create some irritation and infection and this manifests itself as abdominal pain, usually on the left side of the abdomen. The condition is believed to be more common in people who are heavy users of laxatives (i.e. medicines for the treatment of constipation), and fortunately it usually responds to antibiotics.

Sometimes the inflammation is very extensive and can even lead to bowel blockage and/or bleeding. If the outer wall of the bowel is also involved, it may actually perforate or cause the bowel to adhere to other adjacent structures. Surgery is sometimes necessary. Many people have a few diverticulae in the bowel but it is only when they become infected that the patient experiences pain and fever.

There are of course many other less common causes of abdominal pain and if a pain persists one should always see a doctor. (Refer also to sections on diarrhoea and menstrual disorders.)

3.5 The common cold (coryza)

This is arguably the most common infection known to mankind, and there are probably about 24 different viruses involved. Doctors are often chided because they cannot cure this disorder but as with most viral infections, we are almost powerless to do anything about it. Happily, the common cold is usually a short-lived infection with only about a one degree rise in temperature. Often there is a sore throat and always nasal congestion. It is probably spread via the nasal secretions and carried in the air we breathe, particularly after a person who has the infection has talked, coughed or sneezed. The sufferer is infectious only for the first 24 hours. Whether one acquires the infection probably depends primarily on the dose received and one's overall resistance at the time. Thus people who are tired, run-down or depressed are probably more susceptible. Exposure to cold temperatures can probably also help to reduce resistance and this I suspect is the origin of the name.

Secondary infection Although the viral infection is short lived, lasting only a day or two, many people continue to have blocked noses and a drip down the back of the nose into the throat (post-nasal drip) for a long time. This is usually due to a secondary invasion of the nasal passages by bacteria. It would seem that the profuse mucous discharge produced by the virus makes an attractive site for the multiplication of bacteria. When this occurs, the mucus becomes discoloured — usually yellow, brown or green — and also becomes thicker. This discharge may also infect the throat and if it slips down into the lungs, as it is particularly likely to do when the patient is asleep, it may provide the beginnings of an infection of the tubes leading to the lungs (i.e. the bronchi) known as bronchitis, or even an infection in the lungs themselves, known as pneumonia.

These same bacteria may be passed into the tubes which travel from the back of the nose to the middle ear (i.e. eustachian tubes), usually as a result of blowing the nose too vigorously or possibly even sniffing too forcibly. Once in the middle ear, these bacteria can multiply and cause inflammation. This is known as *otitis media*, which simply means inflammation of the middle ear. (See also p. 149.) If the drainage of the nose is poor, the bacteria can go on building up inside the nasal cavities, and in severe cases this results in a painful increased pressure in these areas and usually a high temperature. These nasal cavities are known as the sinuses so this inflammation is called *sinusitis*.

Antibiotics Some doctors prescribe antibiotics for patients with a viral cold. There can be no real reason for this at this stage except that it might be thought that antibiotics will prevent the secondary infection by bacteria that so commonly occurs. Unfortunately the evidence that such treatment prevents bacterial infection is not good, and in fact some researchers have suggested that it makes matters worse.

With proper care, many colds do not lead to secondary infection and in these cases the antibiotics would be given unnecessarily. Even when bacterial infection has supervened, many people fight off the infection without the need for antibiotics and possibly improve their resistance to future infection at the same time. However, persistent cough with the production of discoloured sputum (i.e. phlegm) or acute otitis media, or acute sinusitis, when they develop are usually considered to require antibiotic treatment. These conditions are commonly associated with a higher temperature, as is also 'influenza', another viral condition which may start in much the same way as a cold.

Treatment

For a viral cold and influenza, the best treatment is to keep warm, ensure an adequate intake of fluids — water is quite satisfactory, although not very nourishing — and perhaps take some measures to relieve the symptoms.

Some people seem to get relief from agents designed to reduce the congestion of the nose — various drops are available, but there are also tablets and sprays. The sprays and drops should be used infrequently, as there is some tendency to 'rebound'. This is the term that is used for the enhanced congestion which often seems to follow an hour or so after the use of such agents. Otrivine seems less likely to cause rebound congestion than the others. Some authorities say that drops are always preferable to sprays as they penetrate better.

A cough mixture may be of some use if the throat is sore and irritable, particularly if the cough is dry, i.e. not producing any sputum. Aspirin or paracetamol taken as a warm gargle can be comforting.

The doctor will probably want to make sure no other condition is present. Usually an examination of the throat, nasal passages, ears, and lymph nodes in the neck is indicated. If there is a cough the chest should certainly be examined. Blood tests and X-rays are only necessary if there is a suspicion of more serious disease.

Temperature Often people attempt to bring the temperature down by the use of aspirin or paracetamol. Sometimes this makes them feel a little better, but whether it is doing any good is questionable. Some even suggest that the temperature is part of the way the body fights infection. If this is so, bringing the temperature down could actually be harmful. Certainly very high temperatures can be damaging to the sufferer, e.g. 40°C and higher, and these should be brought down, preferably by sponging with lukewarm but not icy water (i.e. tepid sponging). This does not apply to the common cold because the temperature does not rise to this level unless there is secondary infection.

3.6 Headache

Almost everybody would suffer from headache at some time or other, and for some it is a frequent problem. Those who are unaccustomed to headache and who suddenly develop one for no obvious reason, or those who experience a sequence of headaches, are often concerned that they are suffering from a brain tumour. Fortunately, such tumours are rare and most general practitioners will only encounter one or two in a practising lifetime. The headaches of cerebral tumour are seldom continuous and usually not as severe as a bad migraine.

Headaches most frequently fall into one of two categories, being either *tension headache*, or *migraine*.

Tension headaches

The exact way in which tension headaches are produced is uncertain, but they are probably related to a tightening of muscles in the scalp. Any muscle which is placed under prolonged strain is likely eventually to go into spasm. Usually a person can voluntarily relax most muscles. Spasm of a muscle is really an uncontrolled contraction and there is little or no voluntary control over it. Spasm will subside spontaneously in time and often this can be hastened by the application of heat. Cold, on the other hand, may accentuate it.

Muscle spasm It seems likely that many of the aches and pains in the limbs and elsewhere that people suffer are due to muscle spasm, because the tightening of the muscles is usually accompanied by irritation of nerve endings in the muscles and this is felt as pain.

Many of us have bad posture and this can have the effect of putting extra strain on muscles and ligaments which are expected to perform tasks for which they were not designed. In time, the strain tells and the muscle goes into spasm. This is often experienced as an ache. A lot of backache is caused in this way. Similarly, I have known people who experienced pain in their jaw muscles simply because they had developed the habit of clenching their teeth for a prolonged time when they were worried. The same phenomenon occurs in tension headaches.

People who get tension headaches probably tighten their scalp muscles unconsciously when they are worried and anxious. Sometimes, if they think about it, they are able to relax, particularly if they have learnt the techniques of muscle relaxation (see pp. 192–3). Aspirin or other pain-killers can break the sequence of muscle spasm and pain. Alcohol can have a similar effect.

Tension headaches are usually not present on awakening in the morning, but gradually develop as the day proceeds. Commonly the evening is the worst time. The pain is usually an ache rather than a throb and the patient otherwise feels quite well.

Neck problems In some cases there appears to be a curious connection between bony abnormalities of the neck and tension headaches, for it is found that many patients who get these headaches also have neck problems. In a few cases manipulation or other treatment of the neck results in an improvement in the headaches. However, for most people the real answer is to try to come to terms with the reasons for their tension and this is usually due to something disturbing them in their past or present life, or perhaps worry about the future.

Eyestrain Eyestrain caused by defects in focusing (short sight, long sight, and astigmatism) or even reading in a bad light or at a bad angle can lead to strain of the scalp muscles and also the muscles which control eye movements. When this is prolonged, it too can lead to headaches which are probably due to muscle spasm. This is the main consequence of reading in a poor light which, contrary to popular opinion, has no permanent, damaging effects on the eyesight.

Migraine

Whereas tension headaches tend to produce a constant ache, *migraines* usually cause a throbbing pain. Migraines seem to be more common in people who are prone to asthma, hayfever and eczema. In a few patients the migraine seems to be clearly of dietary origin. For such people, removal of the offending substance from the diet can lead to freedom from further headaches. Cream is a common offending agent; other substances implicated are cheese, chocolate, citrus fruit, red wine and eggs. Although it is probably only about five out of every 100 sufferers from migraine who are able to identify any definite precipitant, the relief is so great that it is always worthwhile considering the diet to see if there is an association with any particular item of food.

Migraine also seems to be due to spasm of muscles but in this instance the muscle contraction is completely involuntary. This is because it involves the muscles in the walls of the blood vessels which supply the brain with blood. The blood vessels of migraine sufferers appear to be exceptionally sensitive to changes in diameter as a result of this muscle contraction within their walls. Just what causes the contraction in the majority of cases remains uncertain but there are probably several factors, of which emotional stress is likely to be one.

The pain of migraine, however, is not due to muscle contraction; all that this causes is a reduced blood flow to the brain, often leading to bizarre symptoms. Usually these are predominantly visual in nature, but sometimes there may be numbness of the whole of one side of the body, or even a temporary paralysis. At other times there may be restlessness or anxiety. The visual symptoms of migraine commonly take the form of flashing lights, or palisades, or even a half or a quarter of the field of vision of the sufferer being occluded. The first time these are experienced can be very alarming.

After the contraction of the blood vessels comes a dilatation so that there is an increased flow of blood to the brain. This is the stage at which there is usually severe, throbbing pain, and treatment is often directed to trying to restore the diameter of the blood vessels to normal. Interestingly, compression of the carotid artery on the side of the headache reduces the flow of blood and relieves the headache. This is not a useful thing for the patient to do but may help the doctor in making a diagnosis.

Pain relief Many migraines seem to respond quite well to simple painkillers. Others seem to do best with ergotamine, which comes in many forms. It is best given very early in the course of the migraine attack and if given by mouth, should be taken with metoclopramide (Maxolon), which hastens the stomach emptying time and so ensures that the ergotamine does not merely sit unabsorbed in the stomach. Without this, migraine has the effect of delaying the uptake of medicines. Ergotamine should not be given to people with impaired blood supply to the heart (i.e. angina) and the amount given to normal people should be strictly controlled as there is a risk of damaging the blood supply to the extremities. Some people find that they get so many migraine attacks that they have to take preventive treatment. For women, this can sometimes be achieved by reducing the oestrogen and increasing the progestagen content of the contraceptive pill. (See pp. 261-6.)

Pizotifen (Sandomigran) is another agent which is used. This is an antihistamine which has some additional properties. The beta blockers (see p. 245) have a place in the management of some cases, but should not be used when asthma coexists. Methysergide (Deseril) is used in particularly difficult cases, but should not be used for more than a few months at a time as prolonged use can lead to dangerous side effects. Given under supervision, with adequate intervals between courses, it can be very helpful.

The tricyclic antidepressants (e.g. amitriptyline) seem to be very useful for some patients.

Differentiation

Here is a table that highlights some of the differences between migraine and tension headaches. It should be remembered, however, that sometimes the two can coexist.

Tension headache	Migraine
Usually both sides of head	Usually one side of head only
Usually constant pain	Usually throbbing pain
No visual symptoms	Often associated with visual symptoms
Often relieved by alcohol	May be worsened by alcohol
No nausea	Nausea common
No difficulty in finding words	Often difficulty in finding words

People who suffer from both migraine and high blood pressure often find that their headaches improve when their blood pressure is brought under control.

The evaluation of a headache should include the taking of the blood pressure, an opthalmoscope examination of the eyes and an examination of the neck. Other parts of the body may require examination if indicated.

3.7 Fatigue

See also Chapter 2.4, The emotions and disease, p. 77, and
Chapter 4.1, Emotional and mental problems, p. 190.

This is one of the most common symptoms presenting to general practitioners and one of the most difficult to evaluate. It can be an indication of serious disease, but more often than not it is a manifestation of anxiety or depression. Any assessment must be based on the patient's history and the presence of other evidence of disease processes. Among the many causes having a physical basis one must think of: thyroid deficiency, anaemia, diabetes, kidney failure, tuberculosis, heart failure, cancer — and so on. The list is almost endless, but in these situations there is usually other evidence to give the doctor a clue. Many medications are capable of causing tiredness. In those who are anxious, the situation can become a vicious circle, with the presence of fatigue engendering further anxiety, and that, in turn, producing more feelings of fatigue.

The original anxiety is often the product of interpersonal conflicts and pressures — a combination of life events such as those listed by Holmes and Rahe (p. 178). Usually doctors will attempt to pinpoint the problem at a first visit and if sufficiently confident of the diagnosis, may tell the patient immediately that they believe his or her symptoms have an emotional origin. Having done that, they will often confirm this original diagnosis by doing a full physical examination and some blood tests. When these are reported as normal, the patient is further reassured.

If, however, doctors fail to recognise the nature of the problem initially, they may embark on a fruitless search for a physical cause, at the end of which they may have to say, 'Since all the tests are negative, I think the problem must have a "nervous" origin', which tends to leave the patient wondering whether every avenue has been explored and thinking that perhaps the doctor has missed something.

Assessment The patient can expect a fairly comprehensive history and examination and a few simple tests such as a blood count and urine examination. If the history or examination raise alternative possible diagnoses, the investigations may have to be more specific and complex. Occasionally the diagnosis is so clearly of emotional origin that no tests are necessary.

With adequate reassurance, fatigue will often subside promptly when the origin is not physical.

Tonics In the past many patients would ask for a 'tonic'. This is seen as something to provide extra energy, to give a sense of 'get up and go'. Today doctors seldom give tonics, which are usually mixtures containing a wondrous array of substances like iron, and vitamins. I always think of it as 'grapeshot therapy'. With grapeshot, many small bullets are fired at a target with the idea that at least one may hit the bullseye. A tonic is much the same — multiple medicines are administered in the hope that one at least will do some good. Doctors are taught to be specific in their diagnoses and then to give specific remedies. Actually, most of the more successful tonics of former times contained significant amounts of anxiety-relieving medicines, the forerunners of our modern tranquillisers.

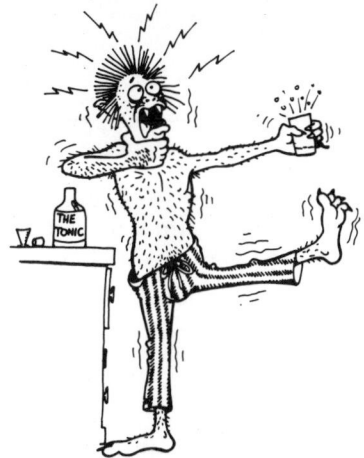

Many people suffering from fatigue will benefit from talking through their problems and learning relaxation techniques. Some merely need to slow up and not work themselves so hard. If the fatigue is due to depression, this may well need medication.

3.8 Pain in the chest

As with abdominal pain, there are many possible causes for chest pain. Most people realise that the heart is in the chest, so frequently there is anxiety about the possibility of the pain having its origins in the heart.

In medicine there are few absolutes, and one can only say that heart pain usually takes the form of a severe, tight, crushing feeling, most commonly in the centre of the chest, but often radiating to the neck or jaw and sometimes into one or both arms. The pain is a constant one, usually subsiding gradually. If the pain is severe enough to make the patient sweat, a doctor and ambulance should be called immediately. Even if the patient is not sweating, but clearly in considerable pain, unlike any that has been experienced before, it is probably wise to summon help.

Associated with the pain, a phenomenon known as *angor animi* is often encountered. This is really a Latin term for a sense of impending death or a fear for one's life.

Heart pain is caused when the heart is not receiving sufficient blood through the arteries which nourish the heart muscle. If the heart muscle is actually damaged, we say the patient is having a heart attack. A similar type of pain can be experienced by placing a tight tourniquet around the upper arm and continuing to exercise the lower arm. Quite soon a severe pain is felt in the muscles of the arm. This pain is promptly relieved when the tourniquet is released.

Angina
Some people experience a heart pain when they exert themselves or when they are upset. It tends to be worse in cold conditions. This is believed to be due to a reduced blood supply to the heart muscle rather than a complete blockage. This pain is known as *angina* and it is relatively common amongst the elderly. Anyone experiencing such pain for the first time

should get it assessed promptly by a doctor. It does not necessarily lead to heart damage.

Not all patients suffering from central chest pain have heart trouble and similarly not all people suffering heart attacks have central chest pain. In fact, sometimes the pain seems to be more in the upper abdomen and may be attributed to indigestion. Occasionally a person may suffer a 'heart attack' and have no pain at all.

Oesophageal spasms and other chest pains

One condition which often causes a similar pain is spasm of the *oesophagus* (gullet). This is a tightening of the muscles of the lower oesophagus, usually as a result of a regurgitation of acid from the stomach on to the less well-protected oesophagus.

In other cases chest pain like that produced by the heart can be due to wind in the abdomen or to trouble in the spine, such that there is pressure on the nerves which travel around the chest wall to the front of the body. Although in such cases there is actually nothing wrong in the front of the body, the brain interprets the messages that it receives from the nerves as coming from the front of the chest.

Many other conditions cause pain in the chest but it is worth remembering that the lungs which occupy so much of the chest do not cause pain. However, the outer lining of the lungs and the inner lining of the thoracic cage (i.e. ribcage) known as the *pleura*, is pain sensitive and the pain produced is known as *pleurisy*. This is described as a sharp, tearing pain and is made worse by deep breathing. Many people seem to experience lesser chest pains which are also affected by breathing, but these are seldom a true pleurisy.

Pleurisy

Pleurisy is due to an irritation of the pleura and usually it is caused by an infection in the lungs extending out to involve the pleural lining. In this situation there is likely to be a temperature. Sometimes other irritation is responsible, as when a rib is fractured. If fluid accumulates in the thoracic cage, it is likely to separate the two layers of the pleura, with consequent relief of symptoms.

Pericarditis

A similar but much rarer type of pain results from irritation of the lining membrane around the heart known as the *pericardium*. The resulting condition is called *pericarditis*. This can be due to a viral infection or be another manifestation of rheumatic fever, but probably it is seen most often as a consequence of damage to the heart muscle extending into the pericardium, after blockage of an artery to the heart (i.e. coronary artery).

In the investigation of chest pain, the patient's history is of the greatest importance: a full examination with a stethoscope may provide the answer. Sometimes a chest X-ray is helpful. If the heart is possibly involved, an electrocardiogram (ECG) is usually desirable, and certain blood tests may help to corroborate a diagnosis. If the pain is from the oesophagus, a barium swallow X-ray may help in the diagnosis.

3.9 Fever

See Chapter 3.5, The common cold (coryza), pp. 135-7.

3.10 Allergic rashes

Few people go through life without some form of skin allergy. The one which is usually easy to identify is the so-called 'contact dermatitis'. This means that the skin develops an allergy to something with which it is in direct contact. Common substances would include nickel, as in bangles, watches, bra buckles and costume jewellery; detergents; soaps where usually the perfume is responsible; dyestuffs in clothing materials; mascara; rubber, especially in gloves; together with many substances used in industry with which people come into contact when at work.

What needs to be remembered is that people do not develop an allergy the very first time they meet a substance. The first exposure may be responsible for making the sufferer sensitive to the offending agent, but the problem is not evident until a second or later exposure. Furthermore, people are often in contact with allergens (i.e. allergy-causing substances) for many years before they develop the sensitisation that results in an allergic condition.

A classic example would be a concrete worker who works with cement for many years and then suddenly finds that he cannot handle cement any more because an allergy has developed.

Of course, some chemicals have a much greater tendency to cause allergies than others. Some are so inclined to cause allergies (i.e. are allergenic) that most people can only handle them a few times before they develop an allergy. Penicillin on the skin is one such substance. People seem at times to become specially prone to develop allergies, so that a person who has recently developed an allergy to one substance is at greater than average risk of developing an allergy to some other substance at that time.

Urticaria

The allergic response takes many forms and in some instances can be very severe. One common form which often results from foods or medicines taken by mouth is known as *urticaria*. When this occurs, the patient, usually over the course of a very short time, develops irregular, reddened raised patches of very itchy skin. The patches vary in size from very small to those which are large enough to cover almost the whole of the body. These patches are described as *wheals* and they often disappear as rapidly as they developed.

Papular urticaria (hives) There is another form of urticaria known as *papular urticaria*, which is a fancy name for 'hives'. It is called 'papular' because the first sign of the condition is the development of tiny elevations of the skin (i.e. papules). Sometimes at the tip of these elevations is a small blister, but this is seldom as large or as colourless as the blisters (i.e. vesicles) which are seen in chickenpox. The papules in hives are very itchy and usually, sooner or later, the top is scratched off and a minute scab forms.

Some believe that hives are always caused by insect bites, but several cases I have encountered seem due to food allergies. One insect bite may be all that is required to stimulate the allergic response that results in multiple papules. The tiny papules that occur in scabies infestation are really yet another form of papular urticaria.

Angio-oedema The worst form of urticaria is that known as *giant urticaria* or *angio-oedema*. This condition usually develops most dramatically, sometimes only minutes or even seconds after the entry into the body of the offending agent. In many cases there is the same wheal formation but in addition there is a rapid outpouring of fluid into the tissues which become swollen (i.e. oedema accumulates). Notable among the tissues that may be affected are the lips, tongue and other structures in the back of the throat (pharynx). Usually the eyelids swell up too, and the patient may have difficulty in seeing as a result. The swelling of the mouth and throat is potentially very serious because it can compromise the airway and the patient could die from asphyxiation. Urgent medical attention is very important and the administration of adrenalin, followed by steroids, can be life saving. Although it is seldom so severe that the patient's life is in danger, there is no way of telling whether it will worsen or not, so it is important to get the patient to the doctor as quickly as possible. In bad cases a small surgical operation known as a *tracheotomy*, which involves making a hole in the windpipe (trachea) is necessary in order that the patient gets enough air to breathe.

Sometimes urticaria is chronic and by this we mean that it goes on for a prolonged period of time. This usually means that the patient is still taking the offending agent into the body, or else that something in the food is helping to make the allergic response worse.

Food additives

Certain chemical substances which commonly occur in our food have a particularly bad reputation for aggravating or even causing urticaria. Some of these chemicals occur naturally in raw fruit and vegetables; many others are added as part of the preservation process. These substances are *salicylates*, which of course are the principal constituents of aspirin (see p. 218), *benzoates* (see p. 95) and *tartrazines* (see also p. 95), which are food colouring agents, usually yellow or orange. The following lists indicate foods containing considerable amounts of these substances.

Foods containing tartrazine

Canned fish and canned shellfish
Fruit squash and cordial
Canned and bottled fruit juice, soft drinks
Syrups and toppings
Vinegar, pickles
Curry powder, mustard
Bottled sauces
Salad cream
Shop-bought cakes
Cake mix/instant puddings
Biscuits
Yellow pasta

Jam and marmalade
Packet and canned soups
Icecream, ice lollies
Jelly
Custard

Blancmange
Semolina
Coloured toothpaste
Coloured sweets and filled chocolates

Foods containing salicylate
Dried peas
Soups and mixtures containing dried peas
Blackcurrants, apples, bananas, grapes
Rhubarb
Beer
Wine

Cider
Apple drinks
Dried fruits, sultanas, raisins, currants, prunes
Vinegar
Bottled sauces containing vinegar
Pickles

Foods containing sodium benzoate
Bottled fruit squash and cordial
Tinned and bottled fruit juice
All carbonated drinks
Instant coffee and tea
Drinking chocolate
Chicory essence
Cider
Some beers
Jam, marmalade
Mustard
Curry powder
Horseradish sauce

Pickled foods
Bottled sauces
French dressing (i.e. oil and vinegar)
Tomato pulp and purée
Rennet
Cranberries
Prunes, plums and greengages
Cinnamon
Cloves
Tinned fruit
Shop-bought cakes and pastries
Artificial cream

The manifestations of these allergies do not necessarily occur on the skin. Some cases of irritable bowel are probably allergic in origin and there may be other unidentified disorders to which allergies may contribute. It is possible that food allergies play a part in some cases of asthma and in atopic eczema (see p. 164).

When doctors identify what appears to be an allergic rash, their first thought is that it might be caused by some medicine which the patient is taking, as this represents probably the commonest cause of allergic rashes in Western communities. Particularly high on the list are certain antibiotics, of which penicillin would be the worst offender. Occasionally the allergy to penicillin is so severe that people get it from drinking milk which contains minute traces of the penicillin which is used in treating mastitis — an infection of the teats and udder of the cow. Frequently an allergy persists for some weeks after the substance is taken into the body. In the case of penicillin, it usually lasts about ten days.

'Fixed drug rash' Some drugs (i.e. medicines) cause what is known as a *fixed drug rash*. This is usually a localised, rounded, reddened area of rash occurring after the intake of a particular medicine. After the medicine is discontinued, the rash fades, but should it be reintroduced, the rash returns again in the same place.

One needs to remember that not only the medicines which doctors prescribe, but also many over-the-counter medicines and even herbal remedies can cause allergic rashes.

Sensitivity to sunlight It is not only things which are taken by mouth which cause sensitisation (i.e. allergies). Sometimes people develop an undue sensitivity to sunlight. Thus there is a condition of *solar urticaria*, apparently induced by sunlight. This sensitivity is precipitated by some substance taken by the patient, or is associated with some disease such as the rare condition known as *porphyria*. Medicines which have a special tendency to produce sensitivity to the sun (i.e. photosensitivity) are the sulphonamides and certain medicines related to them, such as the thiazide diuretics and the anti-diabetic medicines known as sulphonylureas, which include tolbutamide and chlorpropamide; certain antibiotics such as some tetracyclines and griseofulvin; the phenothiazines such as chlorpromazine, promethazine and trimeprazine; chlordiazepoxide (Librium); chloroquin, an antimalarial, and occasionally others. These effects can be minimised by the use of sunscreening agents which absorb the ultraviolet rays.

Where an allergic response is brought about through involvement with a precipitating agent, the rash may not occur in the absence of the precipitant; otherwise allergies tend to last throughout life. Hence when there is an abnormal sensitivity to the sun produced by one of the medicines mentioned above, this usually disappears when the medicine is no longer present in the body.

3.11 Problems of the face and neck

See Chapter 3.28, Acne, p. 182; Chapter 3.10, Allergic rashes, p. 143; Chapter 3.19, Non-allergic rashes, p. 158; also Chapter 3.2, Back problems, p. 124.

3.12 Vision problems

People who consult the family practitioner with sight problems are usually having difficulties with focussing. As the body ages, the lens of the eye loses some of its flexibility, becoming more rigid and hence unable to adjust so readily to near and distant objects. It is usual for people to become long-sighted. In fact, a few people who in their youth are short-sighted, develop the ability to see close objects normally as a result of this phenomenon occurring as they grow older.

People with this complaint require correction with glasses and these may have to be modified quite frequently as time goes on. There is now available in some countries an operation which can be done on the lens of the eye, which is effective in eliminating the need for glasses in those who wish it. This operation was pioneered in the USSR.

Cataracts

Another common reason for difficulties with vision is the development of *cataracts*. These are blemishes in the lens of the eye which impede the passage of light and hence prevent visual images getting to the light and colour-sensitive area at the back of the eye known as the *retina*. Cataracts are more common in diabetics but can occur in anyone. There is some tendency for them to run in families. Occasionally they are the result of injury. These days it is common for eye surgeons to remove the affected lens from the eye and replace it with a plastic lens. The results are usually excellent.

'Floaters'

Another common complaint is of seeing spots, which apparently move about within the eye. Usually the observer, looking into the eye, can see nothing at all. This phenomenon is due to 'floaters'. These are small particles inside the eye which actually are remnants of structures which were important in the development of the eye before birth, but which while serving no present useful purpose, have now become dislodged and move about, producing the disquieting symptoms. They are not dangerous and the sight will not be otherwise impaired.

3.13 Weight gain

See Chapter 2.5, Diet, pp. 84–95, and Chapter 2.6, Special diets, pp. 96–101.

3.14 Vertigo

Vertigo (giddiness) is a condition in which sufferers have a sensation of movement or a feeling that everything is in motion around them. There is a feeling of unsteadiness, not unlike that associated with walking the decks of a rolling ship, and observers may suppose that the person is intoxicated. Sometimes the vertigo is so severe that the slightest movement of the head causes a loss of equilibrium and the patient is obliged to lie still with eyes closed. Usually the vertigo is associated with a feeling of nausea and vomiting may occur.

Semicircular canals

There are numerous conditions which can lead to vertigo, which must be carefully distinguished from a simple blurring of vision. Most cases are due to changes in the semicircular canals of the inner ear, which control balance. A large number appear to be due to *labyrinthitis* (otherwise known as *vestibular neuronitis*), a condition which is thought to be due usually to a virus infection involving the inner structures of the ear. It has a sudden onset, may last several days or weeks and then often settles down, never to occur again. Some people do have recurrent attacks over a period of 12 to 18 months, but there is no loss of hearing.

Another common cause would be a condition known as *Meniere's disease*. This condition usually starts with a severe attack of vertigo associated with nausea and vomiting. These attacks are briefer than those of labyrinthitis. Usually the patient also experiences noises in the ears (i.e. tinnitus). The condition tends to be recurrent and ultimately there is a loss of hearing, which initially fluctuates but finally becomes permanent.

Low blood pressure

Sometimes vertigo is the result of a sudden fall in blood pressure, as can occur when one abruptly arises from a recumbent position. This is particularly likely to occur in a hot environment, for example after a hot bath, or after a siesta in a tropical climate. The same phenomenon may occur in people who are on certain types of blood-pressure treatment. It is known as *postural hypotension*. The vertigo is a result of insufficient blood getting to the organs of balance.

Postural hypotension may occur spontaneously in the elderly who may learn that if they are to avoid falls, after arising from a lying position, they should sit on the side of the bed for 20 seconds or more before standing upright. Some diabetics, as a result of changes to the nerves which control the contraction of blood vessels, also have problems with postural hypotension.

Of course, the majority of people experiencing this drop in blood pressure on arising, do not suffer from vertigo but merely a dizziness, or in severe cases a fully developed faint.

Toxic substances which cause vertigo

Certain substances can cause vertigo and these include alcohol, streptomycin (an antibiotic which can affect the inner ear) and derivatives of opium. Some people believe caffeine and nicotine (e.g. in cigarettes) can also be implicated.

Aspirin can cause tinnitus (noises in the ears) but does not cause vertigo. Other medicines capable of causing tinnitus include quinine and streptomycin.

The examination

The doctor will seek to identify the cause of the vertigo and will examine the nervous system to determine if there is evidence of any nerve disorder in parts of the body other than the inner ear.

The ear itself will be examined as sometimes a virus infection of the nerve of hearing may be a cause. Occasionally wax in the ear is responsible, or even a blockage of the eustachian canal (see opposite). Hearing acuity will be checked. The inside of the eye will probably be examined with an ophthalmoscope, vision may be tested, and the blood pressure will be taken.

A blood test may be desirable to exclude anaemia or some other possible precipitating cause. If the condition does not settle or other symptoms suggest it might be a good idea, X-rays of the skull may be taken and the arteries in the neck may even be visualised to determine if there is a partial blockage. Other tests will be done as indicated, and if the symptoms persist, an ear, nose and throat specialist may be consulted.

Treatment
Fortunately, most cases of vertigo settle spontaneously and do not recur. In these cases, the doctor's task is principally to keep the patient as comfortable as possible until the condition resolves. Certain derivatives of the antihistamine medicines seem to be particularly helpful and even if they don't take the vertigo away, they are capable of reducing the nausea substantially. Medicines which are often used for this purpose include diphenhydramine (Benadryl), perphenazine (Trilafon) and meclizine (Antivert, Sea Legs). Diazepam (Valium) also seems to be very helpful in this condition. There is evidence that in Meniere's disease there is a buildup of fluid in the semicircular canals of the inner ear, and attempts have been made to alleviate the symptoms by giving a low-salt diet and sometimes by the administrations of diuretics (i.e. medicines designed to rid the body of excess fluid). Unfortunately there is no sure cure, but most cases settle with the passage of time, although sufferers are often left with a residual deafness.

3.15 Earache

There are two major causes of this very common problem. In childhood the most frequent cause would be the development of inflammation as a result of infection behind the drum. This is known as *otitis media* (otitis=inflammation of the ear, media=middle).

There is a small passage known as the *eustachian tube* which passes from an area at the back of the nose into the middle ear. When this is open it allows an equalisation of air pressure on either side of the eardrum. The eardrum is a semi-rigid membrane which is so called because it behaves like the membrane on the side of a drum. It vibrates in sympathy with the sounds from outside and these vibrations are transmitted from the drum via a series of small bones in the middle ear and then via the nerve of hearing (i.e. auditory nerve), to the brain.

When the drum is perforated it may continue to transmit sound vibrations but may do it less efficiently. Furthermore, when the drum is perforated it is sometimes possible, when blowing the nose, to blow air up the eustachian tube and then through the drum and out the ears — rather an alarming experience.

Eustachian blockage
It would appear that when the nose is blown very vigorously or perhaps even as a result of strenuous sniffing, nasal secretions and infected material can be blown up the eustachian tubes into the middle ear. If the eustachian tubes are well developed and not blocked, such material probably drains away quite promptly. However, if there is a blockage for one reason or another, including enlarged adenoids, the infected secretions may remain in the middle ear and form

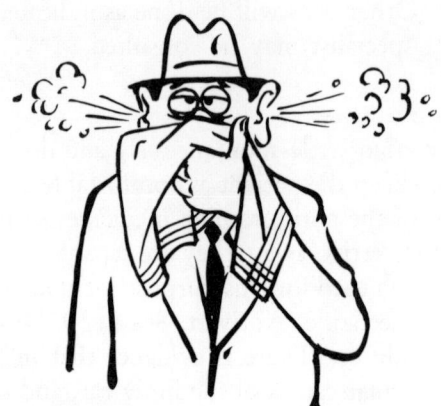

an abscess. If the drum is already perforated the pus will discharge into the outer ear. If the drum is not perforated, there is a good chance that the pressure will build up to such an extent that it will perforate and the patient becomes aware of a discharge on the pillow. This build-up of pressure produces a very painful throbbing until the drum breaks, the pressure is reduced and the pain immediately relieved. Unfortunately, because the pain has gone many people consider the problem has resolved.

Bacteria Several bacteria can be responsible for this infection and often it settles well with antibiotics, provided they are started soon enough. Occasionally doctors actually make a small incision (cut) in the drum with a view to ensuring that the opening occurs in an area that will heal well, rather than simply in the weakest part of the drum.

Unfortunately, not all natural perforations do heal well and sometimes they may persist. A perforated drum can restrict career opportunities and is unacceptable in the armed forces, or for airline pilots and persons whose work involves diving. People who have discharging ears should not be involved in the preparation of food.

Fortunately there are delicate surgical procedures by which a perforated drum may be closed, using the techniques of plastic surgery. Sometimes an infection in the middle ear may become chronic and if unchecked, it can involve the bony tissues adjacent and develop into the dangerous condition of *mastoiditis*. Any discharging ear should be seen by a doctor as soon as possible.

'Glue' ear After an attack of otitis media, it is usual for some fluid to remain behind the eardrum. In some cases this becomes very thick and is unable to drain away. This is known as 'glue' ear because the fluid is so tacky. It is often associated with some deafness but no pain. Usually the condition settles by itself over a period of some weeks or months. If it does not, it may be cured by either removing the adenoids, which tend to obstruct the eustachian tubes, or alternatively by making an incision in the eardrum, which is then kept open for some months by the insertion of tiny plastic grommets. Once the air gets to the 'glue' it slowly loosens up and drains away. Later the grommets fall out and the eardrum heals up again.

Antibiotics are seldom helpful in the treatment of 'glue' ear.

Otitis externa

The other important cause of earache is an infected outer ear canal. This is known as *otitis externa* or inflammation of the external ear. Frequently this develops as a result of an eczema (a sort of skin inflammation) in the canal becoming infected. The infection is usually a mixed one, being a combination of bacterial and fungal organisms. The precipitant is often water in the ears, which makes the lining skin of the ear canal very soggy, just as washing the dishes makes the skin of the hands soggy. Such sogginess makes the skin very susceptible to infection. Occasionally people get a boil or a pimple in the ear canal. This can be very painful. Doctors see most cases in summer after people have been disporting themselves in the water. In fact, keeping water out of the ear canal, e.g. with blue-tack plugs, will go a long way towards preventing this complaint, which is more common in adults than in children.

Treatment of otitis externa usually involves regular ear cleaning provided by a nurse or doctor, together with the local application of antibiotic and antifungal drops, sometimes with steroid drops.

In summary, one can say that otitis media is almost always associated with a runny, congested nose and a temperature, whereas otitis externa does not usually cause a temperature, but commonly follows a few days after getting water in the ears; the ear canal is sometimes itchy and often there is a smelly discharge. Otitis media is usually a disorder of children and otitis externa is usually a disorder of adults.

I regard otitis media as a medical emergency warranting prompt attention, because early intervention can usually lead to an abatement of the condition without perforation. Furthermore, it is usually very painful, and can cause temporary and even occasionally permanent deafness. Mild cases sometimes settle without antibiotics, but the decision on whether or not treatment is given should be left to the doctor.

3.16 High blood pressure

When we talk about *high blood pressure* we mean that the heart is having to work against a greater resistance than normal. This puts a strain on both the heart and the blood vessels. The resistance usually seems to be due to a contraction of the blood vessels.

High blood pressure is an insidious disorder which affects about 15 per cent of people over the age of 30 years. Occasionally it commences much earlier. Very few of those who suffer from it have symptoms as a result. It is usually only when the patient develops complications that symptoms occur, and as a result there are in most populations considerable numbers of people who have high blood pressure (otherwise known as *hypertension* or *hyperpiesis*) who are quite unaware of it.

It would seem that the prolonged extra pressure applied to the walls of the blood vessels leads to the early development of atheroma, which in turn can lead to further blockage of the blood vessels. These matters are dealt with in some detail in Chapter 2.1, p. 46, and the treatment is discussed in Chapter 4.6, pp. 243–8.

Patients on treatment for high blood pressure can expect their doctor to discuss regularly with them any untoward symptoms or problems with the treatment, e.g. side-effects of medicines; to measure the blood pressure; to make frequent examinations of the blood vessels in the back of the eyes (the one place where it is possible to examine the walls of the blood vessels directly); to check the heart sounds and listen to the lung bases for evidence of heart strain from time to time, and to assess the heart size, by X-ray, electrocardiogram, echocardiogram or physical examination at least once each year. In addition, an occasional blood and urine check on the workings of the kidneys is probably desirable, together with an evaluation of the peripheral circulation by examining the pulses in the legs and in the neck. There is thus more to the follow-up of a patient with high blood pressure than the mere taking of the blood pressure and most patients on treatment should be seen at least three-monthly. With very few exceptions, high blood pressure is not curable and most people who are started on treatment have to continue it for the rest of their lives if control is to be achieved. Often the dosage of the treatment used has to be varied, but this seldom means that the condition has worsened.

A high alcohol intake is an important reversible cause of hypertension. A few women develop an elevated blood pressure when taking certain contraceptive pills. Sometimes reducing the intake of salt is helpful in lowering the blood pressure but what part salt plays in causing the disorder remains uncertain.

3.17 Shortness of breath

Shortness of breath is a very alarming symptom and as discussed in the section on the emotions and disease (see pp. 79–80), is sometimes a response to anxiety. Probably the commonest cause is *bronchial asthma*, which must be differentiated from so-called 'cardiac asthma'.

Bronchial asthma

Bronchial asthma is the condition that occurs when there is a reversible obstruction to the free flow of air into and out of the lungs. This condition has much in common with the allergies of the nose described in the section on nasal congestion. There appear to be three principal factors at work in producing the obstruction:
1. A spasm (i.e. involuntary tightening) of the muscles in the bronchial tubes (i.e. the tubes leading to the recesses of the lungs).
2. An excessive production of thick secretions by the glands in the lining of the bronchial tubes.
3. A swelling of the lining membrane (i.e. mucosa) of the bronchial tubes.

Apart from the spasm of the bronchial muscles, the reaction is largely one of inflammation, and here again damage to the *mast cells* (see p. 222) seems to play a part.

Precipitants Many factors seem to participate in causing the wheezing which is so characteristic of an asthma attack. Frequently there appears to be an allergic basis; emotion can be a factor, as can infection, irritation and even cold or dry air. Exercise will often make the sufferer aware of a wheeziness which may not be apparent at rest.

Asthma attacks are always very distressing to the sufferer, whose apprehension will be heightened by sensing fear and anxiety in the faces or manner of onlookers.

Prompt treatment Most asthma attacks are readily controlled and usually they settle best if treatment is started early. The treatments available today are much superior to those used even ten or 15 years ago. Furthermore, by regularly using a *peak flow meter*, a small instrument designed to measure the flow rate of air breathed out from the lung, asthma sufferers can detect early deviations from the level which is normal for them, and modify their treatment accordingly. Asthmatics should obtain such a device and check themselves morning and night and perhaps even more often. It is a good idea to keep a diary of the results, together with the dosage of tablets or other treatment used.

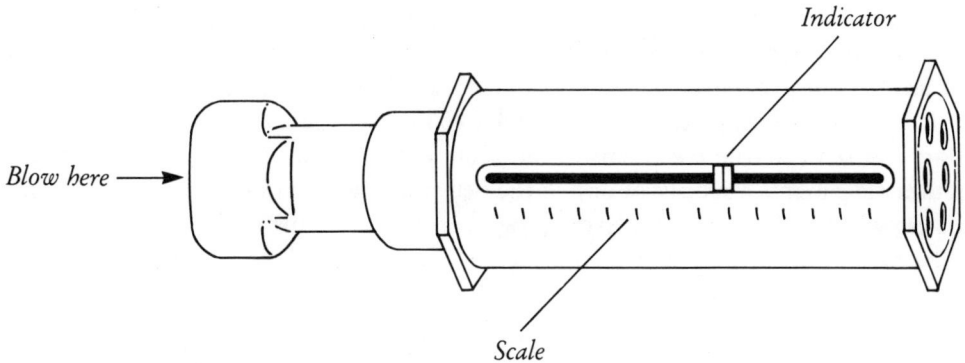

Peak flow meter

The aim of treatment in asthma is to relax the contraction of the muscles in the walls of the bronchial tubes, prevent or remove the excessive secretions and shrink up the swollen lining mucosa of the bronchial tubes. For many years the most widely used agents were adrenalin (i.e. epinephrine) and aminophylline.

As has been mentioned elsewhere, adrenalin has a powerful action in relaxing the muscles in the bronchial tubes. Unfortunately it is a stimulant to the heart, causing it to beat more rapidly. It is also very inclined to give patients tremors of their limbs. As a result, efforts have been made to develop medicines which will dilate the bronchi without adding to the strain on the heart and also produce less tremulousness.

Modern agents The agent, derived from adrenalin, which has probably proved most popular is salbutamol (Ventolin, Volmax). Also popular is terbutaline sulphate (Bricanyl), fenoterol hydrobromide (Berotec) and rimiterol hydrobromide (Pulmadil). Other medicines which are sometimes used are ephedrine and isoprenaline. The latter can be taken as a tablet which may be sucked under the tongue, as well as by aerosol. Orciprenaline sulphate (Alupent) is also widely used.

Aminophylline has a similar effect on the muscles of the bronchial tubes, but is rather inclined to irritate the stomach. It was falling into disuse until the introduction of some long-acting preparations (i.e. sustained release) which largely avoid this side-effect.

Long-acting preparations of theophylline, which is the active ingredient of aminophylline, include Nuelin, Theodur and Theograd and these are usually used in preventing attacks of asthma rather than in treating an acute episode. They can also be used as a supplement to the adrenalin-like preparations in an acute attack, as the effects seem to be additive. For people on long-term treatment with theophylline-type preparations, it is desirable to have regular blood tests to monitor the concentration of theophylline in the blood.

Steroids In severe attacks of asthma the steroids are among the most effective agents. (See section on anti-inflammatory medicines.) These are derivatives of hydrocortisone and they seem to be capable of suppressing inflammatory reactions, particularly those of an allergic nature. Steroids are usually given by mouth, by aerosol directly into the lungs, or by injection. As with most treatments, the earlier in the attack one starts, the better. In fact it is usually several hours after administration before the steroids have a significant effect.

There are, of course, hazards associated with the use of steroids, not least of which is stomach irritation. Many of the dangers, however, are due to long-term use and the risk to most people of a short course of steroid treatment for an acute exacerbation is small. Some doctors give their asthmatic patients a supply of one of the better-known steroids such as prednisone, for prompt use when an attack is anticipated, together with clear instructions about how many should be taken immediately and in the succeeding few days before starting a fairly rapid tailing-off process. Often developing attacks of asthma can be circumvented in this way.

Prevention A few people find that the only way they can lead comfortable lives is to take steroid treatment by mouth continuously. Because of the long-term side effects of steroids, this dosage needs to be kept to the minimum needed for control of wheeze — ideally less than 7.5 mg of prednisone, or its equivalent, daily.

A fairly recent development has been the steroid aerosol spray, and some people who formerly had to take steroids by mouth are now able to take them by inhalation. This means that the steroid is delivered directly to the site of action (i.e. the lungs) and there is relatively little absorbed into the bloodstream. Side effects are then very few. This treatment is not useful in controlling a severe flare-up of asthma once established, but if already being used should be continued throughout.

Sodium cromoglycate Yet another agent for preventing asthma attacks is the substance known as sodium cromoglycate (Intal), discussed in connection with allergic nasal congestion on p. 157.

This works on the mast cells in the bronchial mucosa in the same way as it works on the cells in the nasal mucosa. Similarly, it takes several weeks before it is fully effective, and patients who do not persevere with the treatment may be disappointed with the results. Even then it does not work for all asthmatics.

When to call the doctor

As a general rule it can be said that any asthmatic attack that is not responding to treatment should lead to a call to the doctor. It is particularly urgent if the patient is exhausted, blue, has difficulty in speaking because of breathlessness or if the lung flow rate on breathing out is less than 150 litres per minute when measured on the peak flow meter mentioned on p. 153. Severe attacks usually require hospitalisation.

It is important that people who are experiencing an asthmatic attack should not take medication which tends to make them drowsy, unless under the careful direction of a doctor. Breathing is controlled by a special centre in the brain, which is sensitive to the level of carbon dioxide in the blood. (Carbon dioxide is the substance produced when the oxygen we breathe is utilised in the body. It is usually expelled when we breathe out.) Drugs which cause drowsiness reduce the activity and sensitivity of that centre with the result that the lungs may not respond appropriately to a situation which requires more rapid breathing. This can lead to depression of respiration and even death.

Antibiotics Most asthmatic attacks appear to be unrelated to infection and as a result antibiotics should not be taken routinely. Although asthma is often associated with allergy, the antihistamines are of no value in asthma; ketotifen (Zasten) may be an exception. Probably the commonest mistake that asthmatics make is to ignore the existence of the earliest indications of an exacerbation of wheeze, thus not taking the steps which might abort an attack.

Many young people who suffer from asthma seem to lose the problem in adolescence.

Sufferers from asthma should try to lead lives which are as normal as possible. They must learn to cope with the disorder rather than pretending that it does not exist.

Swimming seems to be particularly good exercise for asthmatics.

The so-called beta-blocking medicines (see p. 245) which counteract the action of adrenalin and adrenalin-like medications may precipitate asthma and hinder the effective treatment of it, and so should not be used by asthmatics. A few people get asthma as a result of taking aspirin.

A patient who has a persistent cough which will not seem to resolve is occasionally found to be suffering from asthma.

Other causes of breathlessness

Cardiac asthma Cardiac asthma is an entirely different condition. It occurs in people whose heart is under strain — usually after experiencing prolonged high blood pressure or subsequent to a heart attack. Sometimes it occurs as a result of damage to the heart following rheumatic fever, or as a result of abnormal development of the heart before birth (i.e. congenital heart disease).

The breathlessness associated with strain of the left side of the heart is eased by sitting up.

Many attacks occur at night and the patient finds that it helps to sit on the bed with the feet on the floor. Often the sufferer experiences a sense of stuffiness in the room and opens all the windows. (See also section on cough, pp. 128–9 and medicines for the heart, p. 254.)

Pneumonia Sometimes breathlessness is due to a severe chest infection, as in pneumonia. This is a condition where one or more sectors of the lung are not working normally as a result of the presence of inflammation and infected secretions. Pneumonia is particularly serious in the elderly, and in anyone whose resistance is impaired for whatever reason. Pneumonia has sometimes been called 'the old man's friend' because it often occurs as a final incident in debilitating illnesses, and can lead to a quick, easy and painless demise, sparing the patient further suffering or indignity.

Emphysema A particularly unpleasant form of breathlessness is that associated with emphysema. In this condition many of the tiny saccules which form the terminations of the bronchial tree have been destroyed. This means that the area of the lung available for the exchange of oxygen and carbon dioxide is greatly reduced and more air has to be breathed in and out to enable sufficient oxygen to be obtained to meet the body's needs. Such people are often breathless all the time and although administration of medicines and oxygen may help relieve the symptoms, there is no cure. Many cases seem to follow upon a long history of smoking, but exposure to certain other air pollutants can also play a part.

3.18 Nasal congestion

See also Chapter 3.5, The common cold, p. 135–7.

The lining of the cavity of the nose is known as the 'mucosa'. It has been given this name because it contains many mucus-producing glands. *Mucus* is the clear, slightly viscous liquid which is produced by the nose in the early stages of a cold, or when it is irritated or inflamed for some other reason and the mucosa swells up and produces more mucus than normal. The usual causes of irritation are viral and bacterial infections, allergies and certain dusts. If the secretion of mucus and the swelling of the mucosa is sufficiently marked, the nasal passages will be blocked and the patient is obliged to breathe through the mouth.

Certain irritants (e.g. pepper) and most allergies (e.g. hayfever) stimulate a reflex which leads to vigorous and prolonged sneezing.

Blockage

When the nasal passages are blocked, the mucous secretions are often unable to drain away satisfactorily. In the resonating chambers adjacent to the nose (the sinuses, the antra) this accumulation of secretions may be subject to a secondary invasion of bacteria. At this stage the secretions from the nose become thicker and cease to be clear, becoming yellow, brown or green. (See section on common cold, pp. 135–7.)

Between the back of the nose and the middle ear there is a tube known as the *eustachian tube*. Secretions from the nose may get into the eustachian tubes, particularly when the nose is blown very vigorously against resistance. The result can be pain and a sensation of blockage in the ear. These symptoms are essentially the same as occurs in many air travellers when their plane descends and there is a delay in equalising the air pressure in the middle ear and the atmosphere. If the secretions are infected, an inflammation of the middle ear known as otitis media can occur. If this is not treated, the pressure in the inner ear may rise to the extent that the eardrum bursts, leading to a discharge from the outer ear. When the drum bursts the pain is relieved and any temperature which was present usually falls.

Sinusitis

Sometimes the pressure within the nasal cavities due to the infected discharge reaches a stage where there is acute pain and tenderness over the face on either side of the nose and sometimes over the forehead just above the eyes. Associated with this there is usually a high temperature and the patient may feel very ill. This condition is then known as *sinusitis*. Although strictly speaking any inflammation of the lining of the nose and sinus cavities could be regarded as sinusitis, the term is usually reserved for those acute situations where there is severe pain and fever.

Drainage From all this it should be clear that sinusitis is chiefly a drainage problem. Treatment is aimed at trying to shrink the mucosa of the nose, trying to reduce the secretions and, if present, trying to cope with secondary bacterial infection. Often it is important to establish whether the congestion is related to some nasal allergy. Usually allergies are characterised by recurrent sneezing. Many people who complain that they are always getting colds are really suffering from an allergy.

In those cases where allergy plays a prominent part, it is usually desirable to treat this. Sometimes the cause of the allergy can be identified. Common allergy-producing substances (allergens) include certain pollens and dusts, animal dander and certain mites which make their home in house dust. Here again nasal decongestants — sprays and drops — can improve the airway and the drainage of secretions. Local sprays of steroids, e.g. beclomethasone (Becotide, Aldecin, Becloforte, Beconase) may help, as may inhalations of various vapours, of which the best known are friar's balsam and Vicks. Antihistamines by mouth are often used but frequently cause a measure of drowsiness. Mebhydrolin (Fabahistin) and azatadine (Zadine) are said to be amongst the least likely to do this, and terfenadine (Teldane) and astemizole (Hismanal) are two new antihistamines claiming to avoid drowsiness altogether.

Another substance which is often used prophylactically (i.e. for prevention) is sodium cromoglycate (Intal, Lomusol, Nalcrom, Rynacrom). This is available in several forms, including a nasal spray.

Inflammation The reason for the inflammatory reactions seen in association with allergies is believed to be the rupture and discharge into surrounding tissues of certain substances found in those white blood corpuscles known as *mast cells*. Sodium cromoglycate is thought to interfere in this allergic response and so prevent the mast cells from rupturing. Regular use of sodium cromoglycate seems to be effective for many people in preventing hayfever. It needs to be remembered, however, that one has to persevere with the use of it for some time before protection is apparent.

Some noses become so blocked by the over-developed mucosa that this has to be burnt away before nose breathing is possible again. The situation is sometimes made worse when the central partition of the nose (i.e. the septum) is deviated to one or other side, as it sometimes is at birth or after injury.

3.19 Non-allergic rashes

There are many possible causes of skin irritation. Perhaps the best known are those due to local infection, usually either bacterial, viral or fungal and occasionally parasitic; those due to the infectious diseases, e.g. chickenpox and measles; those due to unknown causes such as atopic eczema and psoriasis; and those due to chronic irritation such as hyperkeratoses and industrial dermatitis. This section will take a broad view of irritation and will include a brief account of the features of the common infectious diseases which have skin involvement.

BACTERIAL INFECTIONS

Impetigo

Most children sooner or later experience the skin infection known as *impetigo* ('school sores'). Adults are not immune. The problem is characterised by a yellowish scab and sometimes there is oozing from under the scab or from surrounding broken skin areas. Infection is likely to occur whenever the skin is damaged and many attacks follow vigorous scratching as a result of insect bites or scabies infestation. Often grazes become infected before they have healed.

Many people do not seem to realise that whenever the skin surface is damaged, contact from clothing, however clean, will almost always lead to infection. I constantly see children who have suffered grazes on their limbs going about with them uncovered and rubbing on their sleeves, skirts or trousers. Many severe infections would be avoided if, when these injuries occur, the affected area was suitably bandaged and the dressings changed regularly. Exposure to the air and the light is excellent, but only if one is certain that the wound will not be in contact with anything which is likely to result in infection. Our everyday activities make this very difficult to achieve.

Impetigo is dangerous because it can occasionally lead to a very unpleasant kidney disorder known as nephritis (see p. 123). Impetigo is apparently caused by two bacterial families working in concert — the streptococci and the staphylococci. Fortunately, if the streptococci are controlled, the staphylococci seem to disappear also. Even more fortunately, the streptococci remain very sensitive to penicillin. As a result, most attacks of impetigo can be eradicated with a short course of penicillin. If the patient — usually a child — has a temperature, or if there is much reddening around the area of impetigo and perhaps extending in a line up a limb or elsewhere, or if there is a swollen lymph gland somewhere adjacent to the impetigo, it is usually best to have a course of penicillin (or some other antibiotic if the patient is allergic to penicillin).

Local treatment   Smaller areas of impetigo which do not have these features will often disappear with suitable local treatment. I usually apply an antibiotic ointment (not penicillin, which should never be used on the skin because of allergies) and cover the whole area with a piece of sticking plaster without gauze beneath it. With an uninfected wound I would always first apply gauze, which encourages a free flow of air in and around the wound and so promotes the development of a healthy scab. The scabs of impetigo, on the other hand, are unhealthy and form an impediment to healing. Excluding the air will prevent the formation of such a scab and healing will occur in a few days from below. Such treatment saves the patient from being exposed to the potential hazards of penicillin.

Boils

Boils are another form of bacterial infection producing skin irritation. They are caused by infection with the staphylococcus. Sometimes, if they are treated early, they will settle down after treatment with antibiotics. Flucloxacillin, a form of penicillin, is among the most effective antibiotics for most staphylococcal infections. Erythromycin can be used when there is an allergy to penicillin, as can a variety of other antibiotics. Some boils, however, are remarkably resistant to almost all antibiotics. Once a certain amount of pus has formed, it is usually necessary for this to be discharged before healing commences. There is an old surgical saying which states 'Where there is pus, let it out.'

It is my impression that the incidence of boils is often related to a diet over-rich in sugars. Certainly boils are sometimes the first evidence that a patient has diabetes. I usually advise patients to reduce their intake of foods rich in easily available carbohydrate, e.g. sweets, cakes, biscuits, soft drinks and sugar in tea and coffee.

People with skin infections are well advised to shower rather than use a bath. They should not share towels or clothes, and if they do have to use a basin or bath, these should be thoroughly cleaned afterwards with Dettol or some other good antiseptic. These measures are designed to prevent spread to other people.

VIRAL INFECTIONS

The best known of these are *herpes zoster* (shingles) and *herpes simplex* (cold sores).

Herpes zoster (shingles)

The interesting thing about herpes zoster is that the virus is the same one as causes chickenpox in children. Zoster is usually a disease of old people but occasionally it develops in children instead of chickenpox.

The suggestion is made that when people have chickenpox in childhood, they develop a resistance to the virus, but that as the years pass that resistance diminishes. Probably the virus remains dormant in the body and in later years, if resistance diminishes, it reappears. However, sufficient resistance remains to result in the infection taking a different form. In this case it actually invades the nerves and involves the pain fibres rather than the fibres which conduct the impulses which control movement. (These movement fibres are the ones which are infected and destroyed in poliomyelitis.)

This is the reason why herpes zoster is such a painful condition and why its distribution on the body is confined to the distribution of usually one, but occasionally two or more, nerve fibres. The site of the infection is usually marked by a linear red rash which later becomes blistered. Not only do patients have a painful time while the rash is present, but sometimes the nerves are permanently damaged so that after the infection is gone, they continue to send pain impulses to the brain. Sometimes this pain is very persistent and severe. It is known as 'post-herpetic neuralgia'. This pain sometimes seems to improve on carbamazepine (Tegretol) which is used in epilepsy, and, curiously, cimetidine (Tagamet), which is used to reduce acid production in peptic ulcers, is said by some to be useful in the acute stage as a means of preventing neuralgia.

Herpes simplex

An even better-known virus infection is herpes simplex. This is a much more localised infection and it is seen characteristically around the mouth. It is believed that, once acquired, this infection is a permanent inhabitant of the body. The viruses seem to multiply and cause symptoms when conditions are suitable. Heat seems to be attractive to these viruses and so they are likely to appear if the patient is experiencing a temperature. (Hence the term 'cold' sore, as they come out when the sufferer has a cold.) They will also appear sometimes after exposure to the sun.

There are now antiviral substances which, if taken by mouth or applied at the very earliest sign of the development of a cold sore, will often prevent it developing fully. Acyclovir (Zovirax) is one such substance, and idoxuridine (Herplex, Stoxil) is another. The latter can be applied locally but cannot be taken by mouth. Acyclovir can be used both locally and by mouth. These same agents are believed to have some benefit in herpes zoster, but the quantities used have to be much greater and their cost is still considerable.

Although herpes simplex usually occurs on the face and particularly about the mouth, it can occur elsewhere. Probably it is spread by kissing and people who have active herpes sores should avoid this practice. Particularly serious are herpes infections of the eye which can lead to permanent damage and even blindness.

Genital herpes Another form of herpes which has received a lot of publicity recently is genital herpes. This is essentially the same condition as herpes elsewhere, but usually it is spread by sexual contact. The sores, when they occur on the genital organs can be most painful and may interfere with sexual intercourse. There is some evidence that the presence of genital herpes may increase slightly the risk of women developing cancer of the cervix. Such women should have annual cervical smears. The treatment of genital herpes is the same as for herpes elsewhere. Patients are probably only infectious at the time when the sores are present.

FUNGAL INFECTIONS

Very few people do not experience a fungal infection at some time in their lives. Such infections often develop where two skin surfaces come together, as between the toes, the buttocks or the crutch. Usually these are situations which tend to be moist, either because of perspiration or else because they are difficult to dry after bathing. This is discussed at some length in the section on pruritus ani (see p. 167). Another site where fungal infections are common is in the ear and these frequently flare up in summer when people are more involved in water sports. Measures which encourage dryness of the skin are almost always helpful in dealing with fungal infections.

Curiously, this does not seem to apply to infections in the mouth, which are popularly known as *thrush*. These infections seem to occur most readily in mouths which are abnormally dry — particularly the elderly — but they also occur in small babies, apparently as a result of abrasions from sucking.

Ringworm Some fungal infections seem to develop on the skin irrespective of whether there is moisture present or not. An example would be the common ringworm. This infection is carried by animals, particularly cats and dogs, and hedgehogs are especially notorious. It is questionable whether ringworm ever passes from one human being to another.

Fungal infections tend to spread from their edges, which are usually curved, and as a result, patches which are more or less circular develop. There is usually some flaking of the skin and this is most obvious at the perimeter. The doctor can arrange for scrapings of the skin to be taken and if there are fungi present, these can be identified either directly with the microscope, or after being grown under laboratory conditions (i.e. cultured).

Treatments In some situations ringworm can be very difficult to treat by local applications (e.g. in the hair of the scalp) and there is now a substance called griseofulvin (Fulcin, Grisovin, Fulvicin) which can be taken by mouth. Usually the response is very slow, so the course is a long one and some people find the side-effects, which can include headaches and digestive disturbances, troublesome. Another problem is that after the consumption of alcohol, griseofulvin sometimes causes flushing and rapid beating of the heart.

Fungal infections of the finger and toe nails Many people develop very unpleasant fungal infections under the finger and toe nails. On the hands these are often the consequence of exposure to moisture when gardening in wet soil, or frequent dishwashing. Sometimes the only way these infections can be eradicated is by the use of griseofulvin. Without this the nails are often destroyed and the nail bed damaged in such a way that the developing nail is deformed.

PARASITIC INFECTIONS

Scabies

Probably the most intense itch is that due to scabies. This is caused by a minute parasite which burrows into the skin in order to lay its eggs. Strictly speaking, this irritation should be listed under those which are due to allergies. This is because the itch and the small pimples on the skin which develop are due to an allergic reaction to either the presence of the parasite or some waste product from its body. The spots are most noticeable in skin folds such as between the fingers, the wrists and under the armpits. Eventually the sufferer scratches the tops off the tiny pimples and crops of pinhead-sized scabs result. Often infection ensues, which usually takes the form of impetigo (q.v.).

The condition does not occur on the face of adults and this is thought to be because it flourishes in a warm atmosphere and the face is often cooler than the rest of the body, particularly in bed at night.

Scabies is very infectious and passes from person to person by close body contact. A variety of lotions and ointments are available for its treatment. All require application to the whole body, although the face can be omitted. This is usually best done after a hot bath or shower, followed by a brisk rub down with a coarse towel. The lotion is then applied with a shaving brush or else the palm of the hand. If the centre of the back is to be satisfactorily covered, most people will have to enlist the assistance of another. Usually the treatment is repeated after a few days. It is considered desirable that the whole household be treated. Sufferers should not be surprised if the itch continues for ten days to two weeks after the treatment, because this is due to the allergic reaction and the offending substances may remain active in the body for this length of time.

As the scabies organism can survive for some days on clothing, it is important that all garments should be boiled or otherwise thoroughly sterilised.

Lice

Like scabies, these too pass from person to person by close body contact. In the hair of the head, it is believed that the lice pass only when the hair of one person comes into contact with that of another, e.g. children playing together.

There are three types of lice: those that live on the hair of the head, those in body hair and those in the hair of the genital region (i.e. pubic hair).

The itchiness is again apparently an allergic reaction, this time to the bite of the louse. Sometimes the adult louse can be seen in the hair, but more often all that is found are the white spots attached to the shafts of the hairs, which are the eggs. Sometimes they are mistaken for dandruff. Usually there is considerable matting of the hair and often bacterial infection of the skin. Treatment is usually with a shampoo containing an insecticide. This is applied after the hair has been thoroughly washed and is allowed to remain in contact for 15 minutes or so, before rinsing off. Merely washing the hair does not drown or otherwise destroy the lice. It simply results in clean lice, as one authority puts it!

Lice in other sites can sometimes be eradicated by DDT powder. Patients were once recommended to follow the application of a shampoo by combing, using a special fine comb designed to slide the eggs along the shafts of the hairs, so removing them. With the newer insecticides this seems to be unnecessary.

Hair combing has some use, however, for it is likely to damage any adult lice in the hair, and once damaged, these lice invariably die — even if only a leg is injured.

THE INFECTIOUS DISEASES

The skin changes produced by the common infectious diseases are one of their main means of diagnosis. The following infectious diseases produce rashes on the skin (ie. exanthemata):
chickenpox
measles (morbilli, rubeola)
German measles (rubella)

There are also rashes which accompany a number of trivial viral infections, seen most often in children, e.g. hand, foot and mouth disease, and roseola infantum. Sometimes a rash may occur in glandular fever (infectious mononucleosis).

Chickenpox

The rash of chickenpox appears in crops. Often the first spots occur on the scalp, face or trunk. Later they tend to develop on the limbs. Initially the spots are just faint red areas on the skin, but these are quickly followed by blistering. At its height each spot looks like a drop of water sitting on the skin surrounded by a little redness. The spots are very itchy and often the blisters are damaged. The contents are very infectious. Eventually scabbing occurs, and in time the scabs come off, sometimes leaving a small white scar. The patient is usually considered to be no longer infectious when the scabs separate. Most patients will have some blisters in the mouth and these can be very painful. (See also Appendix 2, p. 288.)

Measles (morbilli)

The measles rash is quite different from that of chickenpox and several things occur before it becomes evident. Usually for 3–4 days prior to the rash appearing the patient will be clearly unwell, with a high temperature, cough, sore red eyes and congested nose. Sometimes small spots looking like grains of salt may be seen at the back and side of the throat (i.e. Koplik's spots). On the fourth day a blotchy red rash appears. This is usually first evident on the face and later comes to involve the rest of the body, lasting in all some 7–10 days. As the rash fades, the skin where it was tends to flake off in small scales like severe dandruff. (See Appendix 2, p. 288.)

German measles (rubella)

Rubella (or German measles) is different again. The condition is much milder than morbilli. The rash, which usually starts on the face, consists of pale pink spots which are smaller than those of morbilli and have less tendency to join together. Of special note in rubella are the enlarged lymph nodes almost always present just behind the ears.

The disorder would be of little consequence were it not for the fact that when women in the first three months of pregnancy get this infection there is a considerable risk of damage to the unborn child. A variety of very severe developmental defects may result, such that women who are known to have been infected are usually offered the opportunity of having an abortion. Among the better known problems which may occur in the unborn child are disorders of the heart, eye (even blindness) and hearing.

There are injections available which are capable of preventing this infection. (See p. 57.)

OTHER SKIN CONDITIONS

Atopic eczema (atopic dermatitis)

This very common condition is of unknown origin, but shows up particularly in families where there is a history of asthma and hayfever. So-called 'infantile eczema' is often the earliest evidence of this condition, which usually involves the face and trunk and may spread to the limbs and even the napkin area. In fact it is one of many causes of napkin rash.

There is no known cure for atopic eczema, but usually the condition can be controlled. Unless this is fully explained to patients at the outset, many are disappointed with the results of treatment and feel that their doctor is less than satisfactory.

In adolescence it is often confined almost entirely to the skin flexures, particularly the front of the elbows and wrists and the back of the knees. In later life patches may occur almost anywhere. The affected areas tend to be very itchy and the skin is dry. Often considerable relief can be obtained by the use of moisturising agents such as Alpha Keri or Aquacare. Most cases require the use of steroid creams or ointments in acute exacerbations. The weakest agent which gives relief of symptoms should be used. (See section on steroid applications, p. 220.)

Patients with atopic eczema should be at pains to avoid anything which irritates the skin. Soaps and harsh shampoos should not be used, nor should any irritating fabric or wool. Hot water is sometimes soothing.

Seborrhoeic dermatitis

Seborrhoeic dermatitis appears to be an entirely different condition which is associated with an excessive production by the skin of a fatty substance known as sebum. It is not clear whether the scaly rash that ensues is due to the excess sebum or whether this is simply a by-product of the disorder. Certainly the condition is most prevalent at the ages at which sebum production is at a maximum, viz the newborn and adolescence. The rash is usually seen particularly along the hairline of the scalp, behind the ears, in the eyebrows and the fold of skin between the nostrils and the outer margins of the lips. Seborrhoeic dermatitis also seems to settle well with steroid applications, but again there is no permanent cure.

When it occurs on the scalp in babies it is known as *cradle cap*. Some people believe that dandruff is a mild form of seborrhoeic dermatitis. The latter condition seems to respond best to shampoos containing selenium sulphide such as Selsun.

Psoriasis

This is yet another scaling skin condition which is very frequently seen. It usually takes the form of well defined scaly plaques. The cause is not known but the condition tends to run in families. A few cases appear to follow infection with the streptococcus but such cases usually clear up after a few months. In general the condition tends to be chronic and although remissions are common, there is no known treatment which will effect a cure.

Various preparations of coal tar seem to be helpful and usually steroid applications will settle an acute flare-up. The condition is particularly common on the scalp, but can occur anywhere on the body. Severe scalp involvement is often mistaken for gross dandruff because of the massive scaling of the skin from the affected area.

Sometimes the finger nails are involved and this may simply take the form of pitting, or may be very severe and hard to distinguish from a fungal infection.

Exposure to the sun is helpful in treatment.

Intertrigo

This is considered by some to be a form of seborrhoeic dermatitis. It is really skin damage occurring as a result of the apposition and rubbing of two skin surfaces. The problem is compounded by the presence of moisture, particularly perspiration. It is seen most frequently under the breasts of overweight women. Usually a fungal infection ensues and the result can be a very unpleasant odour and much discomfort.

This condition can usually be prevented by careful hygiene, meticulous drying of the area and, provided the skin is unbroken, the application of talc to facilitate the movement of the skin surfaces over each other.

CHRONIC IRRITATION

The last group of skin problems included in this section are those related to chronic irritation.

Hyperkeratosis

In those countries where there is frequent exposure to bright sunlight such as Australia and New Zealand, the presence of *hyperkeratosis* on exposed skin surfaces is common, particularly on the forehead and the back of the hands. This is an overdevelopment and heaping up of the outer horny layers of the skin. When they are small, hyperkeratoses can usually be picked off, leaving a painful break in the skin. This is not helpful, for within a few days a new roughening of the skin has appeared. Occasionally they become large and almost horn-like, although seldom more than a centimetre in diameter.

Hyperkeratoses tend to be unslightly and often get damaged and so most people prefer to be without them. Furthermore, after many years they can become cancerous. Fortunately even at the cancerous stage they are still easily cured unless left untreated for an inordinately long time. Skin cancers of this type are slow to spread and the good result obtained with treatment is one of the things which help make the figures for cancer cure look so encouraging. Hyperkeratoses are usually readily removed with treatment by liquid nitrogen or else burned away by a process known as diathermy. They can also be treated with fluorouracil (Efudix), a potent preparation which should only be used under strict medical supervision.

'Rodent ulcers'

Another skin condition seen in elderly people and probably related to exposure to the sun, is the so called 'rodent ulcer'. Doctors know these as basal cell carcinomas (B.C.C.) and usually they start as small elevations of the skin surface which subsequently develop a pearl-like appearance. Later still they tend to ulcerate in the centre, forming craters with a pearly perimeter. This is a form of cancer which invades tissues locally but does not spread to other parts of the body. Rodent ulcers are usually readily cured by surgical removal or deep X-ray. Very occasionally they are fatal, but only when neglected and allowed to invade deeper and deeper into the body structures. They are seen most commonly on the face and ears and other exposed areas.

Changes in moles

Those cancers of the skin which can supervene on hyperkeratosis and which are very amenable to treatment should not be confused with the pigmented cancers which can arise in the skin either spontaneously or as a result of changes in a mole. These spread very rapidly and if not caught early, tend to be very dangerous. Anyone who observes an increase in the size of a mole, a change in colour — particularly a darkening of colour — a thickening or bleeding, should see a doctor as promptly as possible. Complete surgical removal may be necessary. There is a special risk from moles which are subject to frequent irritation, as on the palms of the hands or the soles of the feet.

Changes in moles also seem to be related to exposure to bright sunlight and as a result it is clearly wise to avoid too prolonged exposure to the sun, and in particular, severe sunburn.

Age changes in the skin

As we age, a variety of changes occur in the skin and one of the most frequent is the development of pigmented spots of one kind or another. Most of these are of no consequence, but if in doubt it is wise to have them looked at by a doctor.

Few older people escape without so-called 'liver spots' on their hands. These are not related to the liver and are quite harmless. Another blemish is unkindly known as a 'senile wart' or 'seborrhoeic wart'. In fact I have occasionally found them in quite young people. These are greasy, slightly elevated patches, the tops of which can often be picked away, leaving an area oozing blood. Often they are pigmented. Although unsightly, they are quite harmless, but may cause anxiety if confused with an enlarging mole. They can be cut away but unless the appearance is particularly distressing, they are usually best left alone.

3.20 Anal and rectal problems

The most common problems in this region patients bring for treatment by the general practitioner would be either *haemorrhoids*, *perianal haematoma* or *pruritus ani*.

Haemorrhoids (piles)

The reasons why some people develop hemorrhoids and others do not, remain unclear. There does seem to be some relationship to constipation and straining to have a bowel motion. It is my impression that they are more likely to occur in people with varicose veins, so perhaps they reflect an inherent weakness in the walls of the veins.

In reality, haemorrhoids represent dilated, engorged veins and any obstruction to the free drainage of blood from the veins around the anus can help to produce them. Thus women in pregnancy, where the unborn baby may be pressing on a variety of abdominal structures, are particularly prone to this problem.

People who have disorders of the liver (i.e. cirrhosis) impeding the free return of blood from the anal region also often experience haemorrhoids.

In all cases engorged veins swell up and sometimes extend outside the anus after the passage of a bowel motion. They are also liable to injury from the motion and as a consequence often bleed. Note that bleeding from the bowel should always be investigated by a doctor and should never be assumed to be due to haemorrhoids until investigations have demonstrated unequivocally that they are present.

Small haemorrhoids sometimes respond to a diet which encourages regular, easy bowel motions so that straining becomes unnecessary. This may be facilitated by softening agents such as bisacodyl (Dulcolax) and certainly is aided by an adequate intake of fluid and fibre and regular exercise.

Suppositories (q.v.), inserted into the lower bowel and containing astringents (which cause contraction of tissues) and decongestants (which help to empty the blood vessels), are sometimes helpful. Mild haemorrhoids may disappear after injection into them of substances designed to cause a clot to form and later promote the development of fibrous tissue. These are called 'sclerosants' and a similar treatment is sometimes used for early varicose veins.

If all else fails, the hemorrhoids may be removed completely and this is done either by banding them (rather similar to the rubber-band method of removing the tails of lambs) or else complete surgical removal, stitching up the base afterwards.

External piles

The so-called 'perianal haematoma' is sometimes referred to as an *external pile*. Unlike haemorrhoids, this condition occurs suddenly and is very painful. It too is related to the veins in the region of the anus. It appears to be caused by a blow-out in one of the veins around the outer edge of the anus and subsequent clotting. It is not clear what causes this to occur, but patients with this problem suddenly become aware of a very tender lump near the anus. After a few days the pain settles, but the patient is left with an annoying tag of skin which may get injured by toilet paper and clothing and makes it rather difficult to maintain good anal hygiene. Some doctors will open the vein when the clot occurs, and remove it, something which is possible if the patient presents soon after it develops. More often than not, it is left to settle and later, if the tag is a nuisance, it is removed surgically at a convenient time.

Pruritus ani

'Pruritus ani' simply means 'itch of the anus' and this is a very common condition which has many causes.

In children itchiness of the anus brings to mind the possibility of worms. It should not be treated as this, however, unless the worms are actually seen. It is amazing how many mothers dose their children with over-the-counter worm medicines simply because their children are irritable or have been scratching the anal area.

A very common cause of itch in this region is a fungal infection and such infections may develop in any area of the body which fulfils three conditions:
1. It is moist.
2. It is warm.
3. It is out of the light.

In order to eradicate such infections, it is desirable as far as possible to reverse these conditions. Thus loose-fitting clothes will help to prevent sweating and will enable the air to circulate, so helping to maintain coolness and dryness. In babies, exposure of the bottom to the daylight by leaving the napkins off is often very helpful. This exposure is not really practicable in adults unless they attend a nudist colony! Careful attention to anal hygiene and adequate drying after bathing is always desirable.

Many itches seem to be self perpetuating, as constant scratching of the skin seems to make the skin more irritable and induce a vicious cycle. Scratching of the anal area, once established, seems sometimes to come into this category and many people suffer from chronic perianal itch long after the initial precipitant has apparently disappeared. Such people sometimes benefit from the use of steroid applications (q.v.) but run the risk that if these are overused, the skin will lose its texture and become thinner and more liable to injury.

See also commentary on cancer of the bowel, pp. 75–6.

3.21 Joint problems

Many of the patients who come to the general practitioner with apparent joint problems actually have trouble related to the muscles and ligaments around the joint rather than in the joint itself. Most problems in the shoulder region are of this nature. Sometimes the trouble seems to start when muscles or ligaments are put to unaccustomed use. e.g. a game of golf or tennis by someone who does not usually play such sport. Sometimes muscles are strained because they are put to strenuous use too abruptly. Seasoned athletes always 'warm up' with muscle stretching exercises before they undertake vigorous activity. (See p. 105.)

Repeated minor damage can also have detrimental effects and lately much as been heard of R.S.I. which stands for 'repetitive strain injury'. This can occur in any muscle which is being overused, but has been seen particularly in typists using modern electric typewriters or computers for prolonged periods. It is now clear that such people require frequent breaks from their work throughout the day.

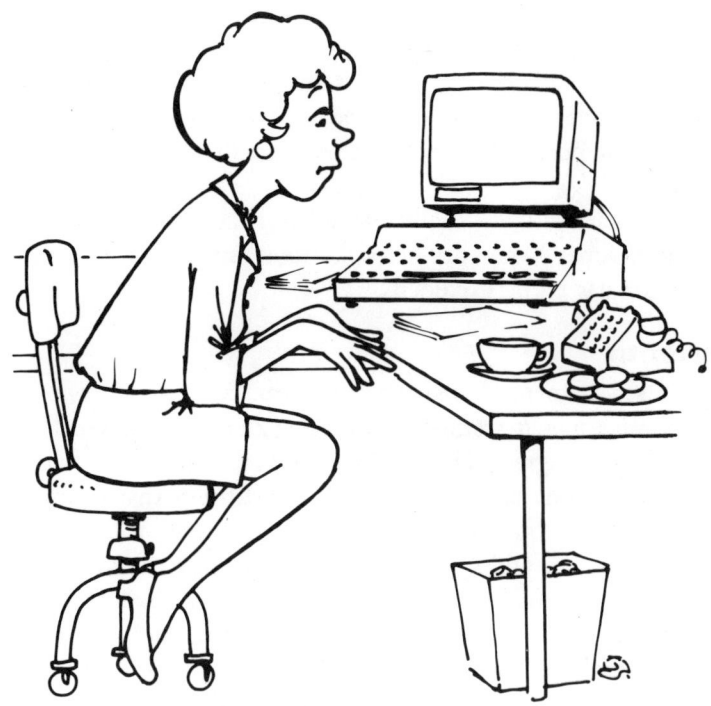

A variety of treatments are available for these muscle and ligament problems. Often they benefit from various forms of physiotherapy and sometimes an injection of hydrocortisone into the affected area is beneficial.

Osteoarthritis

Where the problem involves damage to the joint itself, it is usually given the label *arthritis*. It is very important to realise that there are many different types of arthritis. The most common would be that which is called *osteo-arthritis* (or *osteo-arthrosis*). This condition has every appearance of being due to wear and tear and tends to be most common in the elderly. There is probably more to it than this, because surprisingly, a few people achieve a great age with very little evidence of osteoarthritis while others develop it quite early in life. A joint that has been subject to injury of some sort is at special risk. Thus people who have torn a cartilage in the knee or who have had a dislocated hip often develop osteoarthritis in the joint in later years.

Overuse of the joint Excessive use would be the most usual cause of an attack of pain in the early stages of osteoarthritis. Rest, on the other hand, frequently leads to a regression of symptoms. On the whole the condition tends to be progressive and as age advances, the pain on movement of the joint may well become chronic. In general, pain tends to be least obvious at the onset of activity and gets worse with continued use. There is no known cure but relief may be obtained with non-steroidal anti-inflammatory medicines (NSAIDS, see p. 222), rest, physiotherapy and sometimes an injection of a steroid into or around the joint. The latter has the disadvantage that, because it may relieve the pain, the sufferer may be encouraged to continue overusing the joint and so exacerbate the damage.

In some cases it is now possible to replace the joint, in whole or part, with a prosthesis (i.e. artificial joint).

The diagnosis of osteoarthritis is usually made from the patient's history and an examination of the joint. Sometimes X-rays are helpful; blood tests are of no assistance unless some other cause of arthritis has to be excluded.

Rheumatoid arthritis

This is a particularly severe form of arthritis which can occur at any age. Usually the condition is chronic but sometimes it seems to burn itself out. A variety of treatments are used in an endeavour to halt its progress. The condition mostly starts in the fingers or wrists, tends to affect both sides of the body and is notable for the stiffness that is present in the affected joints after rest. This is very obvious in the morning, tending to wear off with use.

The joints are apt to be hot and swollen and the skin over them becomes quite smooth. In a surprisingly short time considerable deformity may develop. Although initially the condition tends to affect the hands and wrists, later the knees, ankles, elbows and shoulders are often involved. On the whole, the best treatment for the joints seems to be rest, but they should nevertheless be put through their full range of movement several times each day. Without this they seize up and become immobile.

Exercise The improvement in stiffness that occurs with exercise is misleading as it often makes patients suppose that strenuous exercise is the best treatment. Attempts at this are usually rewarded with increased pain and stiffness the following day. Soluble aspirin in high dosage or other NSAIDS are still the first line of treatment, but care must be taken that they do not irritate the stomach.

Some cases require steroids (e.g. prednisolone) in order to get relief, but because of the dangers associated with long-term use of these agents, the dosage is kept as low as possible, attempting to achieve a working compromise between pain relief and side-effects.

A remission sometimes seems to be hastened by injections of minute amounts of a gold salt. A series of injections at weekly intervals over several months seems to be helpful to some sufferers. Patients on this treatment require regular tests of urine and blood to ensure that no side-effects involving the blood or kidneys are occurring.

Another agent which helps some people is a substance known as D-penicillamine. This is taken by mouth and like gold, can sometimes affect the blood or kidneys, so frequent blood and urine tests are necessary here also.

Curiously, chloroquine, which is better known as an antimalarial, is beneficial to some patients. This has the disadvantage that it can damage the eye. This damage is reversible so long as it is recognised early and patients on this treatment should have regular eye examinations.

There are numerous other substances which have proved helpful in particular cases, which leads one to feel that it may not be too long before a really satisfactory answer to this disease is found.

Almost all patients with rheumatoid arthritis suffer from an associated anaemia which often requires treatment by injections of iron. This is because iron taken by mouth is not well absorbed in this condition.

Surgery Where joint problems are very severe, surgery can play a part either by rendering the joint immobile or else by replacing the damaged joint with an artificial one. Removal of the lining membrane of the joint (i.e. synovial membrane) may be helpful as this is where most of the inflammation seems to be.

Diagnosis The doctor will suspect the diagnosis of rheumatoid arthritis from the patient's history and the appearance of the affected joints, which are also notable for their tenderness. The diagnosis is confirmed by blood tests, which usually show evidence of anaemia and a raised sedimentation rate (p. 284). There are a number of fairly specific tests for rheumatoid arthritis which are also helpful. Throughout the course of the illness, progress is checked by following the sedimentation rate and looking for evidence of anaemia. Most sufferers benefit from regular physiotherapy designed to maintain muscle strength and prevent deformity from occurring.

Gout

This condition occurs most commonly in men, but is not unknown in women. It usually affects a single joint and has a special predilection for the great toe, although it can strike anywhere.

Attacks often follow an infection, or an injury including a surgical operation, but may develop for no obvious reason. There is some association with the taking of alcohol, but not every sufferer is a drinker. The use of diuretics is a common precipitant.

The pain is described as being comparable to having 'barbed wire pulled through the joint'. Sufferers usually have an excess of uric acid in their bloodstream and the tendency to accumulate this substance is commonly due to an inherited disorder of the body's metabolism, although in a few instances it is due to a deterioration in kidney function. An excess of uric acid in the urine is one cause of kidney stones, which can lead to the very painful condition of renal colic (see p. 130).

The doctor will make the diagnosis from the appearance of the joint, which is usually hot, red and tender, together with a blood test for uric acid. Treatment is usually with a non-steroidal anti-inflammatory agent or else a medicine called colchicine which is a very old remedy derived from a plant. Those cases that do not respond to these medicines will usually improve on the steroids.

In persons whose uric acid reading is consistently high, certain medicines may be taken regularly to improve the kidney's ability to remove it from the bloodstream. Probenecid (Benemid) or sulfinpyrazone (Anturan, SP2) are two such. Aspirin interferes with their action. There is another substance called allopurinol (Zyloprim) which, when taken regularly, reduces the production of uric acid by the body. This is the medicine which is most frequently used by people whose excess of uric acid is likely to lead to kidney stones or kidney damage.

Patients are encouraged to drink plenty of fluids and careful dieting can play some part in keeping the uric acid of the body within normal limits.

Here is a list of substances which enthusiasts for dietary restriction say are best avoided by people with a tendency to gout:

Asparagus	Onions	Sweetbreads	Sardines
Cauliflower	Garlic	Liver	Anchovies
Brussel sprouts	Rhubarb	Kidneys	Fish roe
Cabbage	Strawberries	Tongue	Meat extracts
Broccoli	Heart	Brains	

— plus spices, beer, ales and red wine.

However, it would seem that most of the uric acid in the body does not come from the food which we eat, but from the metabolic processes of the body.

3.22 Nervousness

See Chapter 2.4, The emotions and disease, pp. 77–83, and Chapter 4.1, Emotional and mental problems, pp. 190–203.

3.23 Depression and reactions to loss

The problems of depression are dealt with in much more detail in another section of this book. (See p. 195.) It should be noted, however, that depression is a common reaction to loss.

The reactions to serious loss are essentially the same, no matter what its nature. Elizabeth Kubler-Ross, who has done so much to help in the understanding and care of the dying, first categorised the reactions to loss amongst the bereaved, but the same reactions can be observed in those who are suffering from illness (loss of health), the menopause (loss of fertility, loss of youth), amputation (loss of limb), children leaving home (loss of dependants), paraplegia (loss of the use of the lower half of the body), and so on.

Where the loss is anticipated, some of the emotions may be experienced prior to the event, but this does not usually make the grief much easier to bear, because until a loss actually happens, there is usually the hope that it might not occur.

It is sometimes helpful to those who are suffering serious loss to have explained to them the feelings they are likely to experience. The order of events varies considerably and not everyone experiences all the emotions. There is also a great variation in the time spent by different people in each of the emotional stages. Occasionally someone may seem to become stuck for a prolonged time with one emotion, such as anger or depression. However, this is rare if a person is allowed to express emotions in the way that is right for him or her.

Denial Almost always there is *denial*. The patient, the family, or both, deny that the loss has occurred. In the case of bereavement, this situation is often relieved if those who are denying the loss are shown the body of the person who has died. Relatives who refuse to see the body or who for some reason are unable to do so, may have much more difficulty in accepting the death.

Anger Anger is common in grief. 'Why should this happen to me?' is a common reponse. Anger can arise at any time during grief, sometimes when quite unexpected. This can be quite disconcerting and may bring with it feelings of guilt.

Bargaining Some people make an irrational attempt to bargain with God. 'If You give me more time' or 'if You restore my health, I will dedicate myself to good works' etc. Often such people have had no previous association with religion.

Depression Depression is often associated with grief and may be particularly difficult to master. Anti-depressant medicines are only likely to be helpful if the depression lasts a long time and interferes with a person's ability to function.

Acceptance Finally most people accept their loss. They become resigned to the facts of the situation. Where feasible, this may be the platform upon which a new life is established, as in the case of a paraplegic who finds a new vocation and makes the best of remaining faculties.

Throughout any reaction to serious loss, the sufferers require support and empathy; caring concern. The doctor and the family have an important role in this. Unwanted information should not be forced upon the patient, but doctors can help by being available to answer questions honestly when these are presented. In this situation you soon come to know who you can trust and who is genuinely concerned for your welfare. Doctors cannot be distant and detached and some measure of emotional involvement is inevitable if the best care is to be given. Some doctors have difficulty in knowing how much of themselves to give in these circumstances and occasionally err on the side of giving too little. Serious loss can be a draining experience for all concerned.

3.24 Vaginal discharge

This problem is a very distressing and embarrassing one when the discharge is excessive or irritating. A certain amount of clear, non-irritating discharge is perfectly normal and this may increase a little just before the menstrual period; midway in the cycle at the time when the ovary is producing the ovum (egg), i.e. at ovulation (see also pp. 268-9); in pregnancy, and at times of sexual excitement. Abnormal discharges are usually associated with itchiness, irritation or soreness and/or an unpleasant odour.

The commonest form of abnormal discharge is due to infection, but other factors such as injury from surgery or childbirth, or even the insertion of an intra-uterine device (IUD) for contraception, can play a part. Irritating douches and occasionally forgotten tampons can also contribute. Rarely a discharge may be the first evidence of the presence of a tumour involving the uterus (womb) or the vagina.

The infections which can occur may involve either the cervix (neck of the womb) or the vagina itself.

Infections of the cervix

These are relatively uncommon, but usually spread by sexual intercourse. The principal infecting agent is the chlamydia organism which is the same one as causes a condition known as non-specific urethritis or NSU (an infection of the tube known as the urethra, which leads from the bladder to the exterior). Non-specific urethritis, which is identified most frequently in males, has symptoms not unlike those of gonorrhoea (see also p. 185). In fact, gonorrhoea itself is another cause of infection of the cervix.

Yet another infective agent is the virus responsible for herpes simplex (i.e. cold sores). These infections are more common on the outer genital structures than the cervix, but sometimes they do lodge here.

Finally, there are occasionally other infections which develop in the cervix after local injury, as may occur in association with IUD insertion or surgery in this region. A variety of bacteria may then be responsible for the infection.

Infections of the vagina

These are more common and there are three organisms which account for almost all of them. The most frequent are caused by the ubiquitous candida albicans, which causes vaginal 'thrush'; others are the bacteria gardnerella vaginalis and certain organisms, larger than bacteria, known as *protozoa*, viz. trichomonas vaginalis.

With candida the most disturbing symptom is usually itch. There is often a curdy discharge and there is much redness of the involved tissues. The condition seldom occurs in young women before the onset of their periods or in older women after the periods cease.

Gardnerella infections are most notable for their odour, which is described as 'fishy'. There is usually considerable soreness and the discharge tends to be grey-white in colour but is not purulent (i.e. does not contain pus).

Trichomonas infections also produce an odour which in this case is said to be 'musty'. The discharge usually contains pus and is frothy. Sometimes it is greenish in colour. There is soreness and redness of the vagina and often considerable itch.

Sometimes these symptoms are mistaken for a urine infection. Trichomonas infection, gonorrhoea and chlamydia can all involve the urethra and cause a burning pain throughout the time that the bladder is being emptied. Candida infections may involve the urethral opening, and so may herpes. In these cases the pain associated with the passage of water is noticed particularly at the beginning and the end of the process of passing urine (micturition).

Whatever the cause of the infection or irritation, it is usually important that the doctor should inspect the area of soreness and look into the vagina. Examination of the vagina is done with a metal or plastic instrument called a *speculum*. Most doctors will warm the speculum before inserting it. The examination is accomplished readily and usually with little or no pain if the patient is properly relaxed, and the doctor is gentle. If the patient is unable to relax and holds herself tight, or the doctor is ham-fisted, the examination can be uncomfortable and even painful. Usually a swab is taken during this examination for sending to the laboratory.

After the speculum is removed the doctor may wish to examine the internal organs manually and this is done by inserting two fingers, encased in a glove, into the vagina. This is particularly important if pain has been associated with the discharge or an abnormality of the tubes, uterus or cervix is suspected.

Finally, the doctor may ask the patient to supply a sample of urine so that this can be checked to make sure there is no infection present.

Treatment

Candida albicans infections are treated with antifungals and there are many of these. A dye obtained from the gentian plant known as gentian violet is very effective, but is not often used these days as it is rather messy and stains any clothing with which it comes into contact. (See also pp. 241–2.)

Here are some of the commonly used antifungal preparations:
Miconazole (Daktarin, Gyno-Daktarin)
Clotrimazole (Canesten)
Econazole (Ecostatin, Gyno-Pevaryl)

Ketoconazole (Nizoral)
Nystatin (Mycostatin, Nilstat)
Ticonazole (Gyno-Trosyd)

These are usually administered by pessary and a course of seven days is frequently prescribed. Many people recommend the use of two pessaries, inserted together, in the evening on retiring to bed. To obtain good coverage of the vaginal walls, the pessary should be inserted, in the applicator provided, as far up the vagina as possible. Ideally the patient should do this in bed and should not arise for some hours subsequently. This is to prevent the pessary slipping down in the vagina and so denying some of the vaginal wall adequate coverage.

It is said that about one case in five will recur soon after the end of the first treatment. If a menstrual period occurs during the course of treatment, it is recommended that the treatment should be continued regardless.

Thrush infections of the vagina often occur for the first time after a course of antibiotics. It is normal to have a balance of organisms in the vagina, consisting of certain bacteria and candida albicans. This balance is self-sustaining and causes no problems. The same may occur in the lower bowel. When antibiotics are given, the balance may be disturbed by the destruction of the bacteria, and the candida, having no opposition, overgrows and produces symptoms — irritation in the vagina or diarrhoea in the bowel. This is yet another reason why only necessary antibiotics should be prescribed.

If the patient is known to react in this way to the administration of antibiotics, doctors sometimes prescribe antifungal treatment as a precautionary measure to combat the candida albicans at the same time as they give the antibiotic. Males also suffer from candida infections of the genitals, particularly if uncircumcised (i.e. foreskin of penis retained). For this reason it is common for both partners to be treated simultaneously. If this is not done, the complaint may pass to and fro, from one to the other.

Trichomonas infection is thought to be sexually transmitted and this is another condition where it is common to treat both partners. The treatment of infection is simple, as this protozoa responds well to metronidazole (Flagyl) taken by mouth. A few days on this treatment usually eradicates the causative agent and relieves symptoms.

Happily, gardnerella infections also respond well to a short course of metronidazole or similar agents such as ornidazole or tinidazole.

Chlamydia infections, on the other hand, usually settle after treatment with either tetracycline or erythromycin. In this instance also the patient's sexual partner should be treated if there is any likelihood of infection.

Prevention

Some general advice on preventing vaginal discharge and irritation:
1. Always wear clean, properly washed underwear, preferably cotton. Avoid tight clothing. Nylon panties may retain moisture and encourage the growth of organisms. Cotton panties should be worn under pantyhose.
2. Personal hygiene is important. Regular washing is desirable, particularly at the time of menstruation when the risk of infection is higher.

3. Avoid vaginal deodorants and sprays as these often cause irritation.

4. It is often helpful if, after the passage of a bowel motion, the toilet paper is passed from the front to the back, thus avoiding the spread of organisms from the back passage (anus) to the vagina.

5. The use of condoms may help in preventing the spread of those organisms which are transmitted sexually.

6. Women who have inadequate secretions at intercourse — often due to unsatisfactory or too hasty foreplay — may prevent irritation by using an artificial lubricant. Some lubricants are themselves irritating (e.g. vaseline) but others such as KY jelly and another known as Silk, can be strongly recommended.

Note that after the menopause some vaginal irritation can be due to a dryness and atrophy of the vaginal lining. Hormone replacement treatment can, if necessary, often restore the lining to its normal state.

3.25 Nausea, vomiting and diarrhoea

Nausea is a feeling of sickness and there are many causes of this very unpleasant symptom, but the commonest would probably be what is known as *gastro-enteritis*. This is the situation in which viruses and bacteria infect the stomach and the intestines. Occasionally it is caused by some irritating substance which has been taken. 'Gastro' refers to the stomach and 'entero' relates to the large and small bowel. If the stomach only is involved it is called *gastritis* and if just the bowel is involved it is called *enteritis*. Thus the combination of the two comes to be known as gastro-enteritis and this is usually accompanied by both vomiting and diarrhoea.

Most attacks of 'food poisoning' are due to eating food which contains bacteria — usually staphylococci — as a result of imperfect cooking, being handled by someone with an infected sore, or being reheated after standing for a prolonged time. At other times the attack is due to a viral infection, probably passed from one person to another by the use of eating or drinking utensils which have not been adequately washed, by kissing, or even possibly through breathing the same air! Sometimes the water we drink is infected. Occasionally the gastro-enteritis is simply a symptom of some other condition which may start that way, as in some cases of hepatitis.

Gastro-enteritis treatment Most people with gastro-enteritis will find that their stomach settles spontaneously and all that is required is to ensure that the patient does not become dehydrated and is receiving adequate nutrition. Sometimes medicines can be used to reduce the misery of the complaint. Many medicines in the phenothiazine group (see p. 227) are capable of relieving nausea and probably the most widely used would be prochlorperazine (Stemetil). Another is cyclizine (Marzine), which is used extensively for motion sickness. Metoclopramide (Maxolon) is capable of relieving nausea also. Its principal action is to hasten the emptying of the stomach. This is particularly important for those suffering from migraine, a condition in which stomach-emptying time is very slow. Since tablets are not absorbed in the stomach, it is important that their passage to the small intestine should not be delayed or they will be ineffective. Therefore metoclopramide is given at the same time as other agents specific for migraine.

Another type of medicine altogether is scopolamine (Hyoscine, Kwells). This slows down the activity of the intestines. It is used particularly in motion (i.e. travel) sickness. Recently a preparation has been produced which is absorbed from a patch applied to the skin behind the ear. Provided it is commenced well before the journey begins, it seems to be very helpful to those so afflicted. It should not be used if there is a risk of glaucoma (an eye disorder).

Most current treatments for gastro-enteritis aim to rest the gastro-intestinal canal. This means that only foods which are known to be non-irritant and easily digested are given. Some people advocate fluids alone, initially. Milk is best avoided, as are fluids which themselves are known to increase the activity of the bowel, e.g. orange juice. If there is vomiting, any fluid is probably best given in frequent sips rather than a glassful at a time. This is less likely to induce the stomach spasms which cause vomiting. Everybody has their own favourite, but I usually suggest just water, or else ginger ale from which all the fizz has been allowed to disperse. Plenty of fluid is very important as much will be lost from the bowel as diarrhoea or from the stomach as vomit.

There are commercial preparations (e.g. Plasmalyte-O or Gastrolyte) which the doctor can prescribe if that seems desirable. These have the advantage that they provide nourishment, and also replace some of the minerals lost.

When the problem seems to be resolving, it may be desirable to introduce some solids. These should be bland, easily digested foods and I usually suggest starting with boiled rice or banana, cold, dry toast, cracker biscuits, boiled fish or boiled chicken. Later, when further improvement occurs, dairy products and other fruits may be contemplated.

Diarrhoea treatment There is debate about the treatment of diarrhoea. Some believe that artificially reducing the activity of the bowel gives an opportunity for toxic materials to be absorbed into the body. Certainly if the diarrhoea is mild it may be as well to let nature take its course. Nevertheless, the diarrhoea is often so severe that any relief is greatly welcomed.

A number of agents very powerfully slow the bowel. These include diphenoxylate (Lomotil, Diastop), which is related to opium, and loperamide (Imodium). Also sometimes used is kaolin which is a powder — a sort of pulverised clay — which has the property of absorbing toxic substances and increasing the bulk of the bowel motion. It can be helpful in the control of diarrhoea.

All these agents must be used with discretion. If the dosage is excessive, the patient may swing from diarrhoea to very stubborn constipation.

Remember that it is very seldom necessary for antibiotics to be used in the management of diarrhoea. The most important treatment is the replacement of lost fluid. This is particularly important in young children who become dangerously dehydrated very quickly. The dehydration is advanced and needs urgent treatment if the skin seems loose on the body, the eyes are sunken, there are few or no tears, the mouth and tongue are dry and there is very little urine, which appears particularly dark. It is always wise to obtain the advice of a doctor before the condition advances to this stage.

If diarrhoea persists longer than expected, causes other than infection will be sought by the doctor. Sometimes an X-ray of the lower bowel, called a barium enema, is necessary. Examination with a telescope-like instrument, known as a sigmoidoscope, can give the user a chance to view the bowel wall closely and perhaps identify the nature of the irritant.

3.26 Pain and irritation of the eye

The commonest cause of irritation would be an inflammation of the conjunctiva, the lining membrane of the eye. This is *conjunctivitis* and it is usually due to either a bacterial or viral infection. Sometimes it is caused by an allergy, e.g. from pollens. The eye is red and sticky — so sticky that when the sufferer wakes, the lids are often stuck together and have to be prised open. Often this is best done after the application of warm water.

Provided the choice of antibiotic drops or ointment is correct, the infection responds rapidly to treatment. In fact, if there is not a substantial improvement, perhaps even cure, in 48 hours, it is probable the bacteria are insensitive to the antibiotic or the diagnosis is wrong. The doctor should be notified and will probably wish to re-examine the eyes. Drops in the eye need to be applied frequently. Ointments work for a little longer (see section on use of eye drops, p. 211).

Another cause of irritation of the eyes is injury. The source of this may vary from a foreign body such as birdseed, dust or a flying splinter, to irritation from minute and often invisible eyelashes, or even just vigorous rubbing. It is important that the cause should be identified and measures taken to remove the irritant.

Other causes of painful eyes include *glaucoma* and *iritis*, serious disorders which are beyond the scope of this book and which require specialist advice.

3.27 Menstrual disorders

There is still a lot of misunderstanding about menstruation. This is often perceived as the removal of poisons from the body, and women whose periods cease often fear that somehow there will be an accumulation of harmful toxic substances. In fact, under the influence of hormones (i.e. messenger substances), the lining of the uterus (womb) is prepared to receive a fertilised ovum (egg) each month. If this does not occur, this specially prepared surface is shed and discharged. In the process of shedding the lining, which is known as the *endometrium*, there is some bleeding. The combination of blood and shed endometrium is what constitutes the menstrual flow.

These changes in the endometrium are brought about by hormones from the ovary. These, in turn, like the thyroid gland, are under the influence of the *pituitary gland*, which is situated at the base of the brain.

Contraceptive pills contain a combination of hormones which simulate those which are produced by the ovary. In simple terms, the *oestrogen* causes development of the endometrium and *progesterone* (and its derivatives, known collectively as *progestagens*) causes its shedding.

Changes in the character of the menstrual flow may indicate many conditions. These may vary from absent periods in pregnancy, at the menopause and in anorexia nervosa; scanty periods in association with hormone treatment (e.g. the contraceptive pill), increased thyroid activity and numerous other conditions.

Unless the cause is obvious, (e.g. pregnancy), menstrual changes should not be ignored and medical help should be sought promptly.

The pituitary gland is influenced by the emotions and this seems to be why some menstrual abnormalities are produced by stress. The pituitary gland is also affected by starvation and this is the principal reason for the cessation of periods in anorexia nervosa.

The thyroid gland, which also produces hormones, is itself under the control of the pituitary, although occasionally it acts independently. The thyroid, too, has an action on menstruation, with scanty periods occurring when it is overactive and heavy periods when it is underactive. Most women, after they have an IUCD (intra-uterine contraceptive device) inserted, find that their periods are heavier than before. Those on the contraceptive pill usually find their periods diminish (see section on the pill, pp. 261–9).

Other causes Certain abnormalities of the uterus and the neck of the uterus (cervix) are also capable of causing changes in menstruation. One of the most common would be the presence of fibrous lumps in the muscle of the uterus. These are known as *fibroids*. They are not cancerous but can at times become very large. They are most common in women who have never borne children.

Occasionally abnormal periods are due to cancer of the uterus or cervix, and it is important that sufferers get very rapid attention.

Examination procedures

The doctor will take a detailed history, look for possible hormone abnormalities and do an internal examination. If this does not provide an indication of the cause of the problem, it may be necessary for an examination of the endometrium to be done. This usually involves an anaesthetic, under which the cervix is dilated and a long scraper, known as a *curette*, is inserted into the uterus. With this instrument the endometrial lining of the uterus is removed and the scrapings sent to the laboratory for microscopic examination. This examination can often give useful information about the cause of the menstrual abnormality and the hormonal status of the patient. The procedure is known as a *dilatation and curettage* or D & C.

Heavy periods

Heavy menstrual periods (known as *menorrhagia*) can lead to a significant loss of blood and subsequent anaemia. This may become a vicious circle as anaemia itself can cause the periods to be heavy. Because the blood lost contains iron, the anaemia is usually of the iron-deficiency type and women with this problem often need to have their iron intake supplemented.

Blood tests to evaluate any anaemia and to further elucidate the menstrual abnormality may be required. (See p. 282.)

Dysmenorrhoea

Cramping pains in the lower abdomen and backaches at the time of the period and for some time before, is known as *dysmenorrhoea*. It is most common in women under 25 years of age and often disappears after childbirth.

The first few menstrual cycles experienced by an adolescent girl are usually pain free. In these cycles there is usually no ovum (i.e. egg) produced. Once ovulation (i.e. the production of an ovum or egg) commences, dysmenorrhea is common and sometimes very severe. Treatment with a contraceptive pill, which has the effect of suppressing ovulation, may give temporary relief. Many women can cope reasonably well once they have a proper understanding of the condition and are assured that nothing serious is wrong. Others will require pain relief. Sometimes a non-steroidal anti-inflammatory drug is helpful. (See p. 219.) The development of dysmenorrhea later in life raises the possibility of infection in the pelvic organs or perhaps a condition known as *endometriosis*.

Endometriosis

The latter is due to some of the cells which normally line the inner surface of the uterus (womb) establishing themselves on structures in the pelvis. Thus the outer walls of the uterus, the ovaries, the fallopian tubes (which convey the ovum to the uterus) and even the lower bowel may be involved. These cells are subject to the same cyclic changes, as a result of hormonal influence, as are the cells of the lining of the uterus. About the time of the menstrual period they become more prominent and often very painful. Sometimes the pain is so great that an operation has to be performed to remove the misplaced tissue. In other cases, hormone treatment will control the symptoms. If the patient can tolerate the symptoms for that long, they disappear after the menopause.

Pre-menstrual tension

Yet another very troublesome problem is that of pre-menstrual tension (PMT). Most women suffer some measure of this, but for a few it can be quite incapacitating. Women who suffer severely experience a sensation of bloating and often there is evidence of retention of fluid, usually shown by ankle swelling. The legs, the abdomen and the breasts may all feel unpleasantly heavy. Frequently there is headache and almost always there is depression and irritability. Some women find that they are unable to control their tears and weep copiously. Uncharacteristic outbursts of temper can be frequent, leaving husband and children bewildered and upset. Women seldom become involved in violent crime, but those who do are quite often found to be suffering from pre-menstrual tension at the time. As a result of all this, the few days leading up to the menstrual period can be a time of much anguish for some women.

There is now evidence that a hormone (i.e. messenger substance) called prostaglandin plays a part in this problem. If the output of prostaglandin can be reduced, the symptoms may be alleviated. Those medicines referred to as NSAIDS (non-steroidal anti-inflammatory drugs) seem to help to do this and one, mefenamic acid, known as Ponstan, seems to have a particularly good reputation in this respect. There is also evidence that a folk remedy — oil of the evening primrose — may be effective.

3.28 Acne

Acne is a condition which causes many young people much distress and embarrassment. It is usually at its worst in adolescence, but advice to the patient to 'wait and you'll grow out of it' is small consolation and sometimes not true. A few sufferers continue to have problems into their 30s or even 40s.

Apparently the cause is partly due to hormones in the body. We all have many of these chemical messenger substances, produced naturally in glands called the *endocrine glands*. The word 'endocrine' indicates that their products are secreted directly into the bloodstream, in contrast to 'exocrine' glands which secrete into a hollow organ or on to the skin. The glands in the skin which produce the sweat and oily substances which protect our skin are sometimes referred to as *holocrine glands* because their secretion includes some of the gland's own cellular material, and this plays a part in acne. Probably largely as a result of the influence of the secretions of certain of the endocrine glands, these holocrine glands seem to be exceptionally active so that sufferers produce more secretions than normal.

In addition there is an abnormal production by the skin of a substance called *keratin*. This material is constantly lost from the body in the form of minute, scale-like collections of cells. The keratin has the ability to block the opening of glands in the skin (sometimes visible as what is known as a *comedone* or *blackhead*), which rather than causing the glands to cease their secretion, leads to an accumulation of secretions in the gland, which consequently swells up. Bacteria on the skin play a part and lead to an inflammatory reaction (p. 218) in the secretions and surrounding tissues, resulting in the production of the typical acne pimple.

Treatment

Acne treatment attempts to remove the keratin from the skin, reduce the greasiness which causes the keratin to be more prone to block the gland openings, and to destroy the bacteria which play a part in producing the inflammation.

There are many things which are used to achieve these objectives. Benzoyl peroxide (Benoxyl) has the ability to both remove the keratin and to kill bacteria. Retinoic acid (Retina A) and its products also appear to help remove keratin, but additionally have an action on the initial production of keratin. Both agents need to be applied very cautiously in the first instance, as some people have skins which are so sensitive that they do not tolerate them well.

As might be expected, antibiotics to kill bacteria have a role in this condition and several of them seem helpful. The tetraclines, erythromycin and cotrimoxazole have all been used successfully when taken by mouth. Curiously, the action seems to go further than just killing the bacteria and it is thought by some that in these circumstances these substances may have a secondary, anti-inflammatory action.

Local antibiotics are sometimes used and clindamycin (Dalacin T) is the one which seems to be most effective.

As with so many common conditions, we still do not know as much about acne as we should. As a result there is a conflict of opinion on what advice should be given. Most would agree that efforts to reduce the oily substances on the skin are worthwhile and some people find that wiping cotton wool soaked in alcohol over the affected area once each day is helpful. Others find that this is too drying.

In a similar way, some people maintain that diet is of no value and that advice to avoid foods which are rich in sugar, and in particular, chocolate, is unnecessary. My own experience, and that of many patients that I have interviewed, suggests that this is helpful in some cases at least. In fact, in earlier years, after a few pieces of chocolate I could almost guarantee to produce a new acne spot on my own face within 48 hours.

Some people seem to get their spots predominantly on their forehead and others on the chin. It has been my observation that these sites often relate to the way that a patient sits, with either forehead or chin resting on the hands. It would seem reasonable, therefore, to recommend that people keep their hands right away from their faces. It is also unhelpful to pick or squeeze the spots. Such practices invite further infection and seem to encourage scars and permanent blemishes of the skin. Women should avoid cosmetics which have a greasy base.

Sometimes the skin is improved when the contraceptive pill is commenced, apparently as a result of the changes in the hormone balance which ensues. (See p. 262.)

Any treatment should be given at least a four- or six-weeks trial before being abandoned as unsuccessful.

3.29 Painful urination (dysuria)

Pain on passing urine is usually an indication that there is infection in the urinary tract or urine itself. Sometimes it is due to irritation around the opening of the urinary passages to the exterior (i.e. urethra). Thus a fungal or even a bacterial infection in this area may lead to pain. Injury in this region can also give rise to discomfort.

Females are more prone to urine infections than males and this is attributed to the shorter distance from the exterior to the bladder. In fact, males seldom get urinary infections unless there is some anatomical abnormality of the urine-collecting system. In older men this is usually an enlarged prostate. Unless there is an obvious cause for the infection, any male patient should have an X-ray of the kidneys, the ureter and bladder.

Many women experience their first urinary infection (*cystitis*) at the time of commencing an active sexual life. The act of intercourse seems to precipitate the infection. Where this association seems certain, an X-ray is probably unnecessary. All other females should have an X-ray, as should the males.

Fortunately urine infections do not seem to cause much permanent damage except in children and in pregnancy. (See bacteriuria, p. 69.)

The bacteria which cause the infection are usually those found in the bowel. In consequence, meticulous toilet hygiene is advocated. It is also suggested that it may be helpful to pass the toilet paper from in front, backwards, after a bowel motion. Clothing should be loose fitting. Women who get infections as a result of sexual intercourse are encouraged to empty the bladder immediately afterwards. This should have the effect of flushing bacteria out of the urinary system. Sometimes they are also given an antibiotic to take at such times. It is believed that concentrated urine is more likely to become infected than dilute urine, so an adequate fluid intake is desirable.

Diabetics are particularly prone to urine infections because sugar in the urine is very attractive to bacteria.

Symptoms The most notable symptom of urinary tract infection is pain or burning on passing urine. There is usually a feeling of urgency to pass urine. Sometimes there is pain in the lower abdomen or in the loins or back. Usually the urine is cloudy, sometimes blood stained, and there may be a noticeable odour.

In children, bedwetting can be a symptom of urinary infection. Occasionally there are no symptoms at all, or perhaps just a temperature and a vague sense of being unwell (i.e. malaise). Some doctors will test the urine in the office, but more often the patient is asked to go to the laboratory, where a sample is passed into a special sterile container. This will be examined under the microscope and any bacteria causing the infection may be identified and an appropriate antibiotic prescribed.

At times the symptoms are so severe that the doctor will prescribe an antibiotic on a 'best guess' principle, i.e. the doctor will give an antibiotic which is successful in the majority of patients. Even in these circumstances it is wise to have a urine sample cultured before starting the antibiotic, so that if the treatment should be unsuccessful, knowledge of the best antibiotic to substitute will be available.

If the treatment is going to be successful, the patient will usually be free of symptoms within about 36 hours, but even so, the full course should be taken. Inadequate treatment sometimes allows an infection to smoulder on without any indication of its presence. Some treatments depend on a single large dose of antibiotic.

About 2–3 weeks after completion of the treatment, I like to have a further urine test done, just to check that there has not been a recurrence of the infection.

It is probably unwise to rely on home remedies for a urinary infection, for although these may allay the symptoms, it is unlikely that they will eradicate the bacteria altogether. A few patients have recurrent or chronic infections and sometimes the only way to control these is to take antibiotics all the time.

Urethritis

Sometimes the same symptoms may be caused by an inflammation of the bladder neck without infection of the urine. This is known as a *urethritis*.

The gonococcus (which causes gonorrhea) is one micro-organism which is capable of causing urethritis; chlamydia is another. These two, but not all infections, are the result of sexual intercourse.

In men the urethritis may be associated with an infection of the prostate gland (i.e. prostatitis). The doctor may insert a gloved finger into the anus (back passage) as a means of feeling the prostate gland to ascertain whether it is enlarged and tender. Tenderness is usual in a prostatitis. Sometimes a sample of the infected material can be obtained by massaging the prostate until some discharge appears at the end of the penis. This can then be examined in the laboratory and any micro-organisms grown on culture plates.

3.30 Diarrhoea

See Chapter 3.25, Nausea, vomiting and diarrhoea, pp. 177–9.

3.31 The menopause

This is the term given to the time when a woman's periods cease, usually between 45 and 52 years of age. The situation is occasioned by the ovaries ceasing to respond to the hormones produced by the pituitary gland at the base of the brain.

The menopause signifies the end of reproductive life for a woman and can be a time of emotional turmoil, sometimes leading to depression. On the other hand, many women have few, if any, symptoms, and rejoice in the extra freedom that not having monthly periods and anxiety about pregnancy gives them.

When symptoms do occur, some of them are emotional in nature, e.g. headaches, indigestion, back pain and chest pain may be of this origin. Careful examination by the doctor to exclude physical disease is important and thereafter appropriate reassurance is helpful. This is a time when much skill is required on the part of the doctor and the benefits of a sound, long-term relationship between doctor and patient can pay great dividends. Many patients require much understanding and support.

At menopause some women experience a sudden cessation of periods; others find that the periods slowly diminish in volume until they stop completely, while yet others find that the interval between periods increases from two to three or even six months before stopping altogether. It is important to remember that it is abnormal:
1. If the bleeding occurs more frequently than once monthly.
2. If the menstrual volume increases rather than diminishes.
3. If the menstrual period ceases for more than six months and then returns.

Oestrogen deficiency

There are a number of symptoms which are believed due to a deficiency of oestrogens. These can often be reversed by the administration of oestrogen replacement, but there is debate about the safety of long-term treatment with oestrogens in the necessary dosage, and some doctors prefer not to give them or else give them in short courses only. Certainly, giving oestrogens for this purpose is likely to cause renewed development of the endometrium (the lining of the uterus), leading to further uterine bleeding. This then leads to problems about the nature of the 'post-menopausal bleeding' and whether it really is due to the administered oestrogen or whether it is caused by some abnormality of the uterus. The use of a repeated cycle of oestrogen and progesterone, as in the contraceptive pill, can help overcome this problem. Furthermore, since cancer of the endometrium is a possible complication of oestrogen treatment given alone, women requiring such treatment who have not had their womb removed at hysterectomy, should always be prescribed cyclical progestagen to counteract this problem.

Oestrogens in high dosages also tend to alter the clotting characteristics of the blood, increasing the possibility of clots (deep vein thrombosis) in the veins of the legs or elsewhere.

Oestrogen deficiency can lead to the following:

Hot flushes These are probably the commonest of the menopausal symptoms. Their frequency and severity varies greatly from one person to another. They may be accompanied by sweating. Most women are concerned that their flushes will be obvious to others and are embarrassed because of this. In fact it is uncommon for flushes to be apparent to an observer, so the fear is usually unfounded. Most flushes occur spontaneously, but some women find that anxiety, excitement or certain items of their diet, such as alcohol or coffee, precipitate them. If necessary, flushes can be controlled by oestrogens, although some people believe this is just postponing the time when they cease spontaneously. Clonidine, which has been mentioned in connection with migraine and hypertension, has an action on the blood vessels and can also be used to control flushing.

Changes in the lining of the vagina and diminished vaginal secretions Despite popular belief, sexual interest and activity can continue into old age. For women, sometimes this is impeded or made painful by menopausal changes, but usually they can be reversed by local treatment with creams which contain oestrogen.

Osteoporosis

This is probably the most serious and least understood of the problems of the menopause. It is a condition in which the bone loses some of its density, predominantly as a result of the loss of calcium. The process seems to be almost universal from middle age on, but is more marked in women.

After the ovaries cease to function at the menopause, women have less oestrogen present in the body and this seems to be the important factor. Women who have their ovaries removed early in life develop osteoporosis prematurely unless they are given oestrogen supplements. Other factors which work to increase osteoporosis are inactivity — particularly long periods in bed — the use of steroids (see p. 220), smoking, and certain disorders of the thyroid gland resulting in excessive production of thyroid hormone. Interestingly, it is a major problem in space travel when there is weightlessness.

The problem is more common in some families than others. Those people who start life with well calcified, large bones appear to have some protection from the disorder, as even if they lose some of the calcium from their skeleton, there is still sufficient bone substance to provide the necessary support. This is a reason why an adequate calcium and vitamin D intake in both pregnancy and childhood is so important.

A well constructed diet plus adequate sunlight should be capable of providing both these essentials without resort to medicines. (See list of foods high in calcium, p. 100.) It is thought that the Pritikin Diet may lead to calcium deficiency if persevered with for too long.

How effective late measures are in preventing osteoporosis remains uncertain. Certainly, when oestrogen levels are low, less calcium loss does seem to occur after these are administered. Unfortunately the effective levels of oestrogen are prone to cause complications, of which the most important is probably the already mentioned increased tendency to clotting in blood vessels. Some authorities advocate the use of calcium supplements to prevent osteoporosis, but the evidence that these are able to stem the tide of calcium loss is conflicting. In fact most say that there is no way that the lost calcium can be replaced, but that oestrogen supplements will halt further loss.

As a result of the reduction of bone density, there tends to be a collapse of the vertebrae in the spine, usually precipitated by lifting. This has the effect of reducing a person's height. Most people do not notice this themselves, but one of the best ways of achieving an early diagnosis is regular measurement of height. Later the patient may become stooped. Symptoms are usually caused by the resulting pressure on the nerve roots as they pass through the vertebrae to the rest of the body. Sometimes the pain is not felt in the back but in the area of the body which the nerves supply.

Another place where osteoporosis causes trouble is the hip and many fractures of the hip occur as a consequence of comparatively trivial injury because of the presence of this condition.

The diagnosis of osteoporosis is usually made on the appearance of the bone on X-ray. Sometimes it is necessary to check out other possible causes of changes in the bones. Some of these show up as an abnormality of the blood test for alkaline phosphatase (see p. 284). The blood tests in osteoporosis are normal. The worst feature of osteoporosis is the pain and it is important that sufferers get adequate relief when this is severe. Because the pain is likely to be chronic, those agents capable of causing dependence are usually best avoided.

SECTION FOUR
Treatment

4.1 Emotional and mental problems

> 'Canst thou not minister to a mind diseased,
> Pluck from the memory a rooted sorrow,
> Raze out the written troubles of the brain,
> And with some sweet oblivious antidote,
> Cleanse the stuff'd bosom of that perilous stuff,
> Which weighs upon the heart?'
> — Shakespeare: *Macbeth* 5, iii

Some doctors devote all their time to patients whose problems are psychological. If they have passed through a special training course and are deemed to have had suitable experience, they are designated as *psychiatrists*. All psychiatrists are fully qualified medically before they commence their specialised training.

Many doctors have to deal with people who have emotional problems or disordered thought processes, but few more than the general practitioner. Some general practitioners find this a very interesting and fruitful area to work in and their skills may fall little short of the psychiatrist's. Others feel that their basic training has left them ill-prepared for this work and either ignore psychological problems or else refer them to people who they feel are able to provide the necessary skills. Such problems tend to be very time-consuming and, apart from obtaining the help of psychiatrists, the aid of psychologists, counsellors and practice nurses may be enlisted.

Physical symptoms only? Unfortunately there seem to be many people who feel that general practitioners are only interested in physical symptoms. They are reluctant to come to the doctor with emotional problems and some people even engineer a physical symptom as a sort of ticket to get them into the doctor's office. General practitioners soon learn that many of the symptoms patients present to them have a basis in emotional problems. Thus a lot of headaches and many abdominal pains have their origin in anxiety. In these circumstances doctors who simply provide immediate relief for symptoms and do not explore the background to them are failing in their duty, and patients are getting second-rate care.

Anxiety and depression In the psychological area, the two most common problems seen by general practitioners are anxiety and depression. Each can be either the cause or the result of symptoms. Obviously anybody who has a serious complaint is going to experience anxiety about it, and if the outcome is in doubt, a likely result is often depression. Here are some of the symptoms of anxiety:

tremulousness	frequent urination	rapid breathing
sweating	lack of interest in self	muscle tension
looseness of the bowels	thumping of the heart	headache

Unexplained surges of anxiety are sometimes described as *panic attacks*.

What can the doctor do? Probably the most important thing that the doctor can do is to identify the nature of the complaint. You as the patient are likely to be most reassured if this can be done positively rather than as a result of excluding physical problems. It isn't always very reassuring to be told that 'every possible physical cause for your complaint has been explored and has proved negative, so I have to assume that the problem is psychological (or emotional).' You are likely to be more convinced if the doctor is in a position to say in the first instance, 'Your symptoms suggest to me very strongly that they have a psychological basis, but before we accept that totally, I would like to satisfy myself that this diagnosis is correct by excluding one or two physical possibilities.' Alternatively, your doctor may occasionally be so sure of the diagnosis that no tests at all are necessary.

The patient's medical history In order to be able to make a positive diagnosis the doctor usually has to make the time to take a comprehensive *medical history* of the patient. Some doctors have adopted a schedule such that a prolonged consultation would throw the rest of their day out of kilter. These are the doctors who, sometimes out of necessity, but more often by design, see large numbers of patients in the minimum of time. Often they are very popular because usually patients don't have to wait long for the consultation. Patients get a bottle of tranquillisers or the like, and they often feel better, but the underlying problem remains.

However, even the doctor who accurately identifies the nature of a problem does not always get results, but often patients who feel they have had a thorough assessment, and that the doctor really understands their problem, are greatly reassured, and this may go a long way towards alleviating their anxiety.

Maintaining perspective People who have serious anxieties often have difficulty in seeing them in perspective. Their problems appear excessive because they lack dimensions. Their thoughts are in turmoil and ideas and worries keep on reappearing in their consciousness. Curiously, putting these anxieties into words often seems to help give them perspective and the problems then seem more manageable. What at first seemed infinite in its enormity, becomes finite. To achieve this, one needs an interested and concerned listener, be that doctor, psychologist or the next-door neighbour.

Interest and concern Most people will respond favourably to anyone who shows interest and concern for their welfare. There is a well-worn adage that 'a problem shared is a problem halved'. This sharing of concerns is the chief ingredient of what is known as 'empathy'. A listener who can truly share the feelings of a sufferer is said to show empathy. Usually it is necessary for the listener to make it apparent to the sufferer that the feelings are shared and this is often best achieved when the listener paraphrases the words of the patient. That is to say, rephrases the expressions of feeling in such a way that the sufferer comes to realise that he or she is not alone with those feelings.

Relaxation techniques

If reassurance alone is not enough to alleviate anxiety, many doctors will spend time explaining to their patients techniques that may be used to aid in achieving relaxation. Such *relaxation techniques* require perseverance and continuing practice. Time must be set aside each day from the hustle of home and workplace in order to refine the process and achieve competence. Even when the techniques are mastered, it is important to cultivate them in an appropriate quiet environment and relaxed frame of mind. Many methods rely on a measure of self-hypnosis, and breath control can help to achieve added benefits.

Probably the commonest symptom of emotional tension is muscular tension. The muscles most frequently involved are those of the scalp. Muscles which are subject to prolonged tension which has a voluntary component are prone to go into involuntary spasm and it seems that this spasm is the cause of pain such as that of the tension headache. Some other muscle aches and pains probably occur on this basis and bad posture can play a part, perhaps aggravating the situation. Actively moving each muscle group and then deliberately relaxing it so that the limb or other part of the body concerned comes to feel heavy is a method that is often used.

A relaxation routine Here is a typical routine adapted with permission from a 'wellness workbook' produced by Pierre Beautrais (unpublished). He says, 'Practise relaxing in a quiet, warm, comfortable place, free from interruption. Lie down on a reasonably firm surface. Close your eyes and breathe in, slowly, as deeply as you can. Hold your breath a few seconds, then let it go, saying "Calm" to yourself as you breathe out. Keep saying "Calm" every time you breathe out.

'Now concentrate on your hands. When you breathe in, grip the hands quite firmly and notice the sensations. The knuckles turn white, the muscles feel hard and tense. As you breathe out, and again say the word "Calm", let the tension go. The hands will return to their normal colour and feel heavy, warm and tingly as the blood flows freely. Savour that sensation, let it increase. Release a little more tension. When your hands feel quite relaxed, move on through the other major muscle groups in your body, following the same procedure. Remember to say the word "Calm" to yourself each time you breathe out.

'Lightly flex the muscles to identify them. Begin with the forearms and upper arms, then focus on your shoulders, which can appear as if the weight of the world is on them. Let them flop. With your feet, wiggle your toes to get them comfortable, then relax them and your arches and ankles. With your calf muscles, let them become soft, long and smooth. Thighs and buttocks: release the big muscles until you feel as if you are sinking into the floor. Stomach muscles: check that you are allowing them to gently rise and fall with every breath. Allow the oxygen to seemingly nourish and cleanse every cell. Back muscles: focus on the back muscles all the way up your spine. Let your neck muscles come into focus. Gently move your head from side to side. Let these muscles relax completely. Become aware of your jaw and chin. As you breathe out, let your teeth be about 25 mm (1/4 in.) apart, and your mouth open if that is comfortable for you. Eyes and forehead: clench your eyes and wrinkle your forehead as you breathe in. Then as you breathe out, smooth out the wrinkles. Let your eyelids hang slightly closed. Relax your forehead until your whole head feels calm and your body peaceful.

'Now check to see if you have missed any tension spots. If you find some, concentrate on them individually. If tension is particularly hard to shift, clench that muscle lightly and then relax. Repeat this as often as it takes to move the tension. Be conscious of the weight of your body and of your limbs. When you feel completely relaxed, just lie there for a few minutes and enjoy the sensation and allow a picture of peace to form in a favourite setting. When you are ready, slowly open your eyes. Don't get up immediately, but wait until you are ready, and then imagine your body filled with fresh energy, entering each part of the body from the toes to the head. Now, refreshed, slowly sit up.'

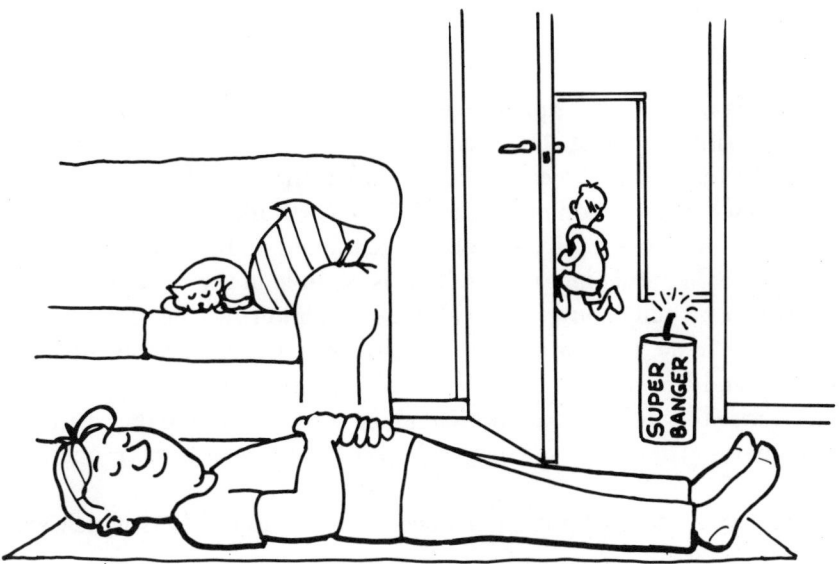

Breathing

Controlled breathing, alone, can be useful and patients are often told to practise *diaphragmatic breathing*. This is breathing in which the muscular partition between the abdomen and the chest (the diaphragm) does most of the work. It may be that the extra attention to muscle movement which this engenders is as important as the relaxation which is produced. Getting your mind off your anxieties can be very helpful.

Exercise

Exercise also helps in relaxation. A person who is physically weary seems to have less nervous energy to put into muscle tightening and the other manifestations of tension. It is also possible that the exercise leads to the production of certain substances, called *endorphins*, from the pituitary and these appear to give a sense of wellbeing sometimes referred to as a 'natural high'. This seems to be incompatible with anxiety. For some, the best answer is a change of environment and occasionally this means a change of occupation, something which should never be recommended without very good reason, as some people find that they cannot get another job, or alternatively the stress of adapting to a new position is as great as that of continuing in the old. For the few, it can make all the difference.

Indecision

A frequent stress-promoting situation is that of *indecision*. Individuals who come to a crossroads in their lives often experience serious anxiety until such time as they can make up their mind one way or another. Usually once they have decided and embarked upon a course of action, the anxiety disappears. A few will continue to worry for a time as to whether they have taken the right course of action.

Action-taking

A major part of counselling is devoted to helping people who are in a situation of stress to identify for themselves the possible lines of action available and then to encourage them to choose the one which is right for them. The counsellor often has the task of motivating the patient or client to persevere with that action once chosen. It is worth mentioning as an aside that these days doctors are trained in simple counselling techniques and are encouraged to make the patient part of the decision-making process. This is possible in the medical context provided the doctor makes patients fully conversant with their condition and the various treatment options available. In medicine, there are many occasions when there are decisions to be made about management and frequently there are several treatments possible. In the past some doctors have been criticised for being too authoritarian, i.e. always ordering their patients about, regardless of how they — the patients — have felt about their treatment. Hopefully that is changing.

This book is designed partly as a way of putting patients in possession of facts which will help in their decision-making.

Tranquillisers

The last resort of patients with symptoms of anxiety should be the tranquilliser bottle. Paradoxically, this easy answer to their problem is also often the hardest in the end. Although the relief provided is often immediate and profound, patients develop dependence so that when the medicine is withdrawn, anxiety symptoms much worse than those with which they started manifest themselves. It is usually safe to take tranquillisers for a few days, but if given for more than a couple of weeks the risk of dependence increases very markedly. Patients who have experienced the relief from anxiety that the tablets can provide are naturally often reluctant to discontinue the treatment.

Unfortunately many people seem to feel that if they are paying the doctor, they are not getting value for money if they only get a discussion about relaxation techniques and do not come away with a prescription for a bottle of medicine. Doctors in turn may be concerned that their patients should not feel short-changed, and so may be tempted to prescribe unnecessarily, thus establishing a sort of vicious circle.

Depression

Depression is a different matter. Sometimes depression seems to occur as a result of chronic anxiety and once the latter is relieved, the depression lifts. Unfortunately this is the exception.

Some depression seems to be a reaction to external events, e.g. a response to bereavement. Usually it is relatively short lived and the patient is aware of the background to it. (See Chapter 3.23, Depression and reactions to loss, pp. 173–4.) Others develop depression for no apparent reason and many explanations have been offered. There seems to be some tendency for it to occur in certain families. Some authorities have even suggested that it is a learnt behaviour, a way of coping with stressful situations, while others attribute it to suppressed anger. Some depression follows clear-cut cycles. This may be *manic-depression*, also known as 'bipolar affective disorder', the sufferers from which often respond well to treatment with lithium.

Diagnosis of depression A person is considered to be suffering from depression if four of the following conditions are present:
1. Change of appetite (diminished or increased).
2. Change in sleep patterns (inability to sleep or tendency to sleep all the time).
3. Excessive tiredness or loss of energy.
4. Loss of interest in activities which have usually given pleasure, e.g. sex or reading.
5. Thoughts of self-reproach or guilt.
6. Reduced mental and physical activity, or else agitation.
7. Reduced ability to think or concentrate.
8. Thoughts of death or suicide.

With the passage of time, most depressions lift spontaneously, but until that occurs the patient may suffer very acutely and if it is severe enough, there is a real danger of suicide. Provided patients persevere with treatment, most will ultimately obtain relief of their symptoms, but sometimes several medicines, even from among the same group, have to be tried before the most effective is found. Patients should not hesitate to see their doctor if there is no improvement after a fair trial. This may take several weeks.

Medication As described in Chapter 4.4, there are two families of medicines which have been shown to be particularly useful in treating depression. Probably the most widely used, but slowest to start working, are the *tricyclics* (and now the *tetracyclics*), while the others are the *mono-amine oxidase inhibitors* (MAOIs). The latter have the disadvantage that they interact adversely with certain foodstuffs, leading to symptoms of headache and palpitations, together with serious elevations of blood pressure. The foods to be avoided with MAOIs are listed in Chapter 4.4 on p. 230.

ECT ('shock treatment')   A few people will not respond to any medication and with some reluctance the psychiatrist may advise *'shock treatment'* (i.e. *electro-convulsive therapy* or *ECT*). This involves the passage of a brief electric current through the brain between the terminals of shock-producing equipment applied to the skin of the scalp. Some people regard this as barbaric, but provided the patient is well prepared it is not nearly as bad as is often thought. The disadvantage is that after the electric shock which is given to the anaesthetised patient, there is commonly a loss of memory of what went on for some time before. This loss of memory is distressing to some people. Shock treatment is not universally popular, but for those who have been through the peculiar hell that is deep depression, it may bring a blissful relief of their symptoms and one might argue that it is cruel not to make it available in such circumstances, when other treatments are ineffective.

Psychosis

There is another area of psychiatric work which deals with people who appear to have lost touch with reality. These patients are said to suffer from a *psychosis*. Some types of depression can be caused by a psychosis.

Patients who are psychotic may show this in many ways. Thus people may have quite unrealistic fears and may suppose that they are receiving personal and terrifying messages through the television or radio. They may have the impression that they have seen or heard things which were not seen or heard by others (i.e. *hallucinations*), or they may have an unwarranted sense of their own importance and capabilities. Others will believe themselves to be personalities from the past. Often the presentations are very bizarre and the lay public label the sufferer as 'mad' or 'insane'. Sometimes such episodes are the result of another disease process and the classic example is syphilis, which in some cases ends up as GPI, which stands for *general paralysis of the insane*. Van Gogh, the artist, is believed to have suffered from this condition and it has been claimed by some that it was the principal factor in his favouring the use of the very bright colours that characterised his now famous impressionistic style. In an exacerbation of his psychosis, he cut off his ear.

Schizophrenia

Many of the people who suffer from psychosis in the community today are suffering from *schizophrenia*, a mental disorder which can take a variety of forms. The cause of this condition remains unknown, although there are many theories and there is some tendency for it to run in families. The majority of schizophrenics, with or without specialised help, manage to function in the community without being institutionalised.

Usually the condition is manifest first in adolescence, although sometimes there is evidence of it in childhood. In the early phases, such people find it difficult to make deep friendships, tend to distance themselves from others, and often appear very shy, sensitive and solitary.

Others live a very stormy life, oscillating from aggressiveness to submissiveness so that they move from one crisis to another. Others again are of a very suspicious turn of mind and do not trust others. They frequently have feelings of inferiority and harbour many grievances.

William Goldfarb, a psychiatrist, has listed nine diagnostic points for the established condition:
1. Severe and continued impairment of emotional relationships with others. This is a further development of the aloofness referred to above as an early manifestation.
2. A lack of awareness of personal identity. There may be abnormal behaviour towards oneself; examining parts of the body as though they belonged to another. There may be acts of self-inflicted injury.
3. An abnormal preoccupation with certain objects, unrelated to their normal uses.
4. Continued resistance to environmental changes, often promoting what for others would seem to be monotony and boredom.
5. Abnormal perceptions. This may take the form of increased or reduced or unexpected responses to the various senses, e.g. hallucinations of hearing or sight, lack of sensation to pain or temperature, etc.
6. Acute and abnormal anxiety without reasonable basis. Circumstances or even objects which under ordinary conditions would cause little or no anxiety, become the source of irrational fear.
7. Speech abnormalities. Words may be uttered which do not make sense. Speech may show a variety of mannerisms and the patient may become confused about personal pronouns. Patients may automatically repeat back many times words and phrases used in their presence.
8. Abnormalities of movement. There may be excessive movements, or a reduction of movement. Sometimes patients will adopt unusual and inappropriate postures, or may maintain rigidly any position into which they are put.
9. An apparent diminished intellect with occasional evidence of normality or even flashes of brilliance.

Treatment The response to treatment of schizophrenia is variable. Some treatments are founded on the view that there is an underlying disorder of the chemistry of the cells, while others are based on the idea that the thought processes of the patient need examining and reorientating. Some theories of causation are based on the belief that the sufferer has in earlier life been subjected to contradictory messages, e.g. a mother who constantly avows that she loves a child but never shows this in any physical way, and in fact yells at the child every time it enters the room. In other words, there is a verbal expression of love, but both verbal and non-verbal messages suggest disapproval or even dislike. The result is confusion in the mind of the child. It would appear that sometimes discussion and analysis by and with the patient can help to a better adjustment. It is said that the therapist's role in this situation is 'to help patients to understand themselves better'.

Most treatments depend heavily on the use of the phenothiazine group of medicines (see p. 227) which seem to have an almost specific effect. A close relative to these, known as haloperidol, has fewer side-effects for many people and may also be used. Those who seem to do best on treatment appear to be (a) those who are better off financially; (b) persons who before they developed severe symptoms, appeared to have good social, marital and sexual adjustment; (c) those who are married; (d) those with outgoing personalities; (e) those where there are obvious precipitating factors, with a marked emotional response, e.g. depressed, anxious or confused; (f) those with disorders of movement.

It is very important that persons who are started on phenothiazines or haloperidol should continue with this treatment. There is a great temptation for people who perceive themselves to be well again to discontinue medication. Often within a few days they are back where they began.

A brief review of some theories of psychotherapy

Treatment using psychological methods which is designed to help people emotionally is often described by the rather grandiose term *psychotherapy*. In fact we all perform a little psychotherapy from time to time, as for example giving somebody a few words of praise, or a pat on the back, to indicate approval and support. Psychotherapy of one sort or another is used in almost all psychological disorders and there are various opinions about which approach is best in particular circumstances. It seldom seems to play a very important part in the management of psychoses. Some basic concepts are outlined here as these techniques are sometimes used by general practitioners.

Psychoanalysis Sigmund Freud was one of the first to popularise the concept of *psychotherapeutic analysis*. He believed that in any personality there were three principal subconscious conflicting forces:
1) the 'Super-ego', which in simple terms might be thought of as being similar to the conscience;
2) the 'Id', which represents essentially instinctive drives like hunger and sex;
3) the 'Ego', which was seen as a sort of referee acting out of self-interest.

Free association In order to identify and help the patient analyse these forces, Freud popularised the concept of *free association* where patients are encouraged to let their mind wander and express thoughts aloud. This may allow previously suppressed material to come to the surface of consciousness.

Abreaction *Abreaction* is a technique used to help people re-live past damaging experiences. Often this is facilitated by the use of a sedating drug which helps to lower inhibitions and so enable previously repressed emotions to be expressed.

Insight Freud aimed to give patients *insight* so that they could understand the reasons for the conflicts in their psychological makeup. However, he did not accept that simply understanding the dynamics of the situation was sufficient. He also believed that the patient had to *feel* emotion and *grow* emotionally.

Transference Freud also alerted people to the phenomenon of *transference* — something which probably is present in almost every interpersonal transaction but is seen most vividly in the psychotherapeutic situation. In its simplest form this may occur where the patient sees in the therapist many of the qualities of a parent and may in consequence react and respond to the therapist as if to a parent. *Counter-transference* may occur when the therapist sees in patients the characteristics of their own children, or others close to them, and come to treat them accordingly. Sometimes transference can lead to bizarre and unexpected reactions. To a lesser degree, whenever we meet someone, we see in that person some of the characteristics of other people that we have known, and probably we either like them or not, according to the way that we reacted to those others. Usually this would seem to occur at a subconscious level.

After Freud, many others sought to develop techniques of analytical psychotherapy, but most psychotherapists do not confine their approach to just one school of thought. Most are eclectic, which means that they pick out what they regard as the best parts from a variety of psychotherapeutic techniques.

Rational emotive therapy (RET)

Albert Ellis was one who thought that most emotional problems could be dealt with on an intellectual level. He tended to the view that if the patient had a proper understanding of the basis upon which they responded emotionally to any situation, then they would be able to reason their way out of it. He developed *rational emotive therapy* (RET) and propounded the *ABC theory*, which could be simplified as follows:

Let us suppose the patient, a student, feels that his happiness is dependent upon maintaining his self-esteem by achieving the goals that his parents have set him.

A stands for the *activating event*, which in the above example might be considered to be the qualifying exams for a professional career.

B stands for the *belief system* held by the patient relating to the foundation on which he thinks his happiness depends.

C stands for the *consequences*, emotionally, of A, i.e. happiess or unhappiness, depending upon whether he passes the examinations or fails.

Ellis took the view that most of us have some irrational beliefs and that as a result we often 'catastrophise' a situation and so exaggerate in our minds its 'awfulness'. The aim of the therapy is to help people to deal with their irrational beliefs. The patient must be convinced that even if the exams are not passed, it is still possible to please the parents and so maintain self-esteem, or else that it is not necessary to satisfy the parents' needs, and so on. Clearly this is a rather trivial example, but the principles apply in much more complex situations. This approach is at a thinking rather than a feeling level and many therapists reject RET on that account.

Carl Rogers

Carl Rogers is another psychologist turned psychotherapist who has had a wide following. He pioneered the idea that each of us, given the opportunity, can find our own solution to our particular problems. The therapist's task is to provide a warm, supportive, encouraging environment within which this can be achieved.

Self-worth Like most such therapy, Rogers' basic aim is to build up a patient's sense of *self-worth*. The patient is encouraged to talk and to ventilate negative feelings such as anger, jealousy and hate. The therapist avoids making judgements but helps the patient clarify the feelings. As far as possible, the discussion relates to the present and tries to avoid relating problems to past events. The therapist tries to be non-directive so that the patient achieves his or her own insights and ultimately an interpretation of what is happening emotionally. The aim is to achieve a change in feelings and attitudes.

Most therapists would take the view that a truly non-directive approach is probably an unattainable ideal, and that even non-verbal signals, however subtle, give the patient an inkling of the therapist's preferences. There is a great temptation in any counselling situation for the therapist to try and impose his or her views and ideas on the patient. The traditional medical model (where the doctor is seen as the all-wise advisor) in which most present-day doctors were reared, runs directly counter to this concept. Nevertheless, modern medical schools are now emphasising that with adequate information, the patient can and should play a significant part in the decision-making process. Of course, some patients feel uncomfortable with this —as do some doctors — but the principle is one that should be encouraged.

Transactional analysis

Transactional analysis (TA) was devised by E. Berne, the author of *Games People Play*. He presented a simple method whereby people could analyse their own behaviour. Berne believed, like Freud, that the personality of each of us had three components. He said that one part of us represented *the parent*. Berne said that the messages represented by the parent were mostly learnt in the first five years of life, and that for the majority they were predominantly negative messages, usually 'Don't do' instructions, but sometimes positive, as when the child does something which pleases or impresses the parent — 'you clever little person'.

The second component was described as *the child*, and this represents the *responses* of the child to what is seen and heard in the first five years of life. These, then, are mostly *feelings*. Again, as the messages are mostly negative, so are the *feelings* mostly negative. This leads the child to feel that 'I'm not OK', in the jargon of transactional analysis. In later life, when situations arise which are analogous to those which caused problems in childhood, the patient reverts to the same responses as in earlier life. Thus a frustrating situation is often dealt with by anger rather than reason.

The third component is *the adult*. Once developing children reach about ten months of age, Berne believed they achieve some ability to interpret the messages which they receive. Later these powers increase. The 'adult' can be thought of as the response of the person to the 'parent' and the 'child'. It is therefore the intellectual interpretation of the learnt responses and feelings of early life.

Life positions Berne described four life positions relating to oneself and one's relationship with other people. They are:
1. I'm not OK — you're OK
2. I'm not OK — you're not OK
3. I'm OK — you're not OK
4. I'm OK — you're OK

The latter life situation is considered the ideal and this is what transactional analysis hopes to achieve.

Reality therapy

Yet another approach is that of William Glasser. It is called *reality therapy*. Once again, it apparently has special value for those who have low self esteem, a major problem with a large number of people who seek counselling and/or psychotherapy. These are the people who see themselves as failures.

Glasser emphasised two major concepts:
1. The need for everybody to love and be loved. ('Everybody needs somebody' as the song goes).
2. The need for everybody to feel that they are worthwhile to themselves and to others.

Few could argue with these principles, but in order to achieve success, it requires great commitment on the part of the therapist, and real involvement. It belies the old idea that the doctor or therapist should not become involved with the patient. There was a time when one of the virtues extolled by medical teachers was the concept of 'clinical detachment', and probably this idea has had a lot to do with the distant, impersonal attitude of some doctors who strive hard not to get close to their patients emotionally.

Obviously there are limitations to the extent that medical workers can become involved with their patients. If such people fully shared the emotions of all their patients all the time, they would not get through the day. There has to be a compromise, and after a patient or client leaves the consultation, the worker has to put the worries of that person out of his or her mind as far as possible. Glasser was particularly aware of this and as part of the contract with patients he made it quite clear that during the course of the interview his full attention and all his concerns were for that patient, but once the interview was over, he was essentially unavailable. This would also help to prevent the creation of too great a dependence by the patient on the therapist.

In the course of treatment the patient is given small tasks to do and when these are successfully completed, the success is praised. If the patient fails, there is no punishment. As time passes the patient is encouraged to attempt more and so achieve even greater success. In such a way the self-image of the patient is slowly built up. The emphasis in this therapy is more on behaviour than feelings.

The patients are encouraged to examine their behaviour in terms of whether what they do is good for them and the people they care about and whether what they do is acceptable to the wider community. The therapist is neutral and non-judgemental.

Behavioural therapy

The reinforcement of those things which are positive has much in common with *behavioural therapy*. The latter is more mechanistic in its approach and insight on the part of the patient is not seen as important. Several techniques are used, but underlying all is the concept of *facilitation*. This term relates to research which shows that a nerve impulse following a particular track within the nervous system will pass along the pathway more readily, the more often it occurs. This phenomenon is seen in the many things which we do automatically, such as tying a tie. Most of us can do it quite well, but if asked exactly what we do, we are hard put to explain. The nerve pathways from the brain to the arms have been facilitated and we are said to have been *conditioned* to perform these actions. In a similar way, the dogs of the Russian researcher, Ivan Pavlov, were taught to expect a meal and produce saliva when bells were rung. The sound of the bells came to be associated in their minds with the arrival of food so that eventually they salivated when bells rang, regardless of whether food was forthcoming.

Conditioning

Conditioning is a psychological term used in certain situations where the patient is rewarded for desired behaviour and so encouraged to repeat the behaviour. Conditioning techniques are sometimes successful with people who have phobias such as a fear of spiders or a fear of open spaces. This process is sometimes called *desensitisation*. In desensitisation, a patient is gradually brought to accept an anxiety-producing stimulus. Thus a person with a fear of heights might be encouraged to take a few steps up a ladder and so become accustomed to that. As time goes by, further steps are taken, and so on until ultimately the patient has the confidence to go to the very top of a high ladder.

Many men suffering from impotence — a failure to complete the sexual act — have nothing physically wrong with them, but their efforts to have intercourse are impeded by their fear of failure, and the more often they fail, the more they are conditioned to fail in the future. Often the best treatment for them is to be encouraged to lie with their partners, to pleasure them, but to avoid intercourse for a time. The pressure to perform is removed, and frequently after a relatively short period of time their normal sexual reactions return and intercourse resumes. This too is a form of desensitisation.

Flooding Another behavioural technique is called *flooding*. Using this method, anxious patients may be overwhelmed with the things which create the anxiety. Patients are taught to cope, because they know that the treatment is being given in a safe, supervised setting. Most techniques of desensitisation as described above use a gradual introduction of things which produce anxiety, moving from the least to the greatest. In flooding there is no such gradation — the aim is to maximise the anxiety. Thus it is conceivable that a patient who was abnormally afraid of water might be suddenly plunged into the sea. This type of treatment, which is usually more subtle than this, is also known as *implosive therapy*. More often the exposure is not to the real thing but in the patient's mind, so that patients who have a fear of water are called upon to imagine themselves in the sea. This treatment is often successful in people suffering from phobias.

In some medical schools it used to be common to show medical students a series of sexually explicit films in order to condition them to aspects of sexual activity. It was considered that after this exposure they would be able to discuss sexual matters with their patients with much less embarrassment. This is another form of flooding.

Aversive conditioning

Aversive conditioning is another technique. This requires the use of an unpleasant stimulus to alter a person's attitude. Most people believe it is most successful when it is used in association with positive conditioning.

This technique has been used in attempts to help homosexuals who were dissatisfied with their sexual orientation. I have not heard of any real success. The approach was to provide some unpleasant stimulus, such as taking a drink to induce vomiting, every time a picture which evoked homosexual feelings was shown. The hope was that the homosexual would be conditioned to experience nausea and perhaps vomit even in the absence of the vomit-producing drink, every time he or she felt stimulated in a homosexual way.

Aversive conditioning has also been suggested as a treatment for alcoholics. Based on the observation that alcoholics seem to sip their drinks more frequently than non-alcoholics, some workers have set up bars where the alcoholics are connected to an electrical apparatus which gives them a shock if they sip their drinks at a rate that is greater than acceptable. It was hoped that these heavy drinkers might be converted into social drinkers in this way, but again I have not heard of any successes.

Operant conditioning is a technique whereby the patient is given some reward for successful cooperation. A simple example would be bed-wetting children who are given gold stars for a dry night. When several gold stars are accumulated they can be exchanged for a small toy, or some other appropriate reward.

Other approaches to psychotherapy

There are many other approaches to psychotherapy — *gestalt*, *encounter therapy*, *psychodrama*, and so on. Latterly there has been renewed interest in *hypnotherapy* and some workers report success with this in helping patients over the early and most severe stages of tobacco withdrawal. Hypnosis can have profound effects, but has the disadvantage that the suggestion is of limited duration. This problem can be overcome to some extent by frequent sessions until a new pattern of behaviour becomes second nature.

Family therapy is also popular. This is based on the idea that many emotional problems in individuals are merely the symptom of a family that is not functioning well as a unit (i.e. dysfunctional). In family therapy, the therapist meets with the whole family and observes the patterns of behaviour. Thus it may be that one member of the family is always dominant, another excessively passive; yet another may be the scapegoat, and so on. A skilled therapist, who must be objective, can draw the attention of the family members to the effects their attitudes and actions are having on each other and so help them to interact in positive and constructive ways. Often real communication between family members occurs for the first time. In recent times, with so much pressure on the family unit, family therapy assumes a special importance. It is a very powerful tool which has special relevance for family practice.

4.2 About your medication and reading your prescription

'The quack has a considerable advantage over the regular practitioner. If any of his promises become realised, he is applauded to the skies; and if the patient finds himself deceived, he is obliged in honour to be silent, that he may not expose himself to blame for having confided himself to a wretch who has the more right to deceive, as the number of simple people is always the greatest. Besides, this daring man risks no loss of reputation; because as it exists only among ignorant people, the blame will always incline towards those who have listened to him. Men are so fond of the marvellous that the quack has above all others the power of making the vulgar relish novelty. The more absurd his promises are, the more he is attended to. He applies a barbarous name to a plant he has just gathered at the entrance of the village and then, giving the details of his miracles, this plant is adopted for the cure of every infirmity.'

— Dr Zimmermann,
A treatise on experience in Physic, 1782

A great deal of the treatment provided by general practitioners centres around the use of medicines.* Throughout history Man has sought substances which will relieve symptoms or even cure illness when the occasion demands. In the animal world some animals seem to have an instinct which enables them to identify certain plants which will be helpful to them if unwell. A cat, for example, will sometimes seek out certain grasses to eat if it is feeling ill.

Over the years mankind has developed a knowledge of many substances, most of which are of vegetable origin, and a listing of these, together with their uses and dangers, is known as a *pharmacopoeia*.

Herbal remedies Even today many of the refined substances administered for medicinal purposes are derived from herbal remedies. Thus the herbal physician who prescribes extract or tincture of foxglove (*digitalis* spp.) is merely prescribing an unrefined form of digoxin. Digoxin is the chemical name of a pure substance derived from digitalis leaf. It has the

---

*It should be noted that throughout this book the word 'drug' has been used as little as possible. In fact, it is a term which has been used widely for many years for medicines. In some countries pharmacists are referred to as 'druggists'. Latterly, much has been heard about drug abuse and the word has been debased, coming to be associated with dependency and illicit activities. To avoid confusion, alternative terms have been used whenever possible in this book.

advantage that the dose is known precisely and other contaminating substances are eliminated. To this extent the modern doctor and the herbalist are not far apart. Many people who advocate returning to nature and herbal remedies would be surprised to learn how many of the medicines currently in use are merely purified chemical variations of the naturally occurring substances.

Had digitalis been discovered in the twentieth century, there is little doubt that it would have been hailed as a 'wonder drug', quite as remarkable in its own way as penicillin or any other medicine.

Individual differences One thing that many people find hard to understand is the fact that individuals differ in the way their bodies deal with medicines. The same thing applies to food, of course, for while one person may be able to eat any quantity of certain foods, another may find that one mouthful causes uncomfortable symptoms. If everybody was the same in this respect, the doctor's lot would be much easier. It would also mean that it would be quite acceptable for one person to give their medicine to another. In fact, this is a very dangerous thing to do, as will be reiterated elsewhere in this book.

Side-effects

A careful doctor will use a knowledge of the patient, together with a knowledge of the side-effects of medication, to find the best and safest preparation to recommend for any particular patient. Often information about side-effects caused by other medicines in the same person is helpful in this connection.

The doctor having a knowledge of possible complications from a medicine will also advise the patient about these, so that the patient will know what action to take should they occur. Even the common aspirin can be very dangerous to some people, having the ability to cause or precipitate a stomach ulcer or occasionally a stomach haemorrhage. It can also bring on very severe asthma and other allergic reactions in susceptible people.

It is probably fair to say that there is no medicine known which is completely free of unwanted effects — usually referred to as 'side-effects' or 'adverse drug reactions'. The same can also be said for everything we eat or drink. Water, if taken to excess, can be dangerous.

In a sense, the administration of any medicine to any patient (or any herbal remedy for that matter) is an individual experiment. The doctor will make sure that as far as possible the benefits of the medicine outweigh the possible disadvantages. The doctor will also know that there is a small but definite risk of the patient experiencing unwanted side-effects. The level of acceptability of the risk will depend very much on the severity of the condition being treated. In other words, very serious disease may justify much more heroic (i.e. risky) treatment than minor disease. Such decisions often require great skill on the part of the doctor, and whenever possible informed cooperation from the patient.

An example of this would be the use of chloramphenicol. This is an excellent agent for the killing of bacteria. Unfortunately it has a side-effect which, when it occurs, can be quite devastating. It can lead to a disorder of the bone marrow so that certain types of cells necessary for the normal functioning of the body are no longer produced. When this occurs (and fortunately it is quite rare), the patient often dies. Because of this, chloramphenicol is not used unless the patient is in dire straits and there is no alternative. Thus, sometimes a patient may be suffering from a severe infection which does not seem to respond to other bacteria-killing medicines (i.e. antibacterials), or alternatively the patient may have developed an allergy to the other possible agents. Happily this problem does not occur when chloramphenicol is used locally in the eye or on the skin.

Allergic reactions

Allergies to medicines represent one of the possible side-effects that can occur. Some people seem to have a special predisposition to allergies and some medicines seem to have a greater than average tendency to cause them.

This tendency to allergic reactions is another reason why medicines should not be administered indiscriminately without a really good indication. It is common for people to go to their doctor with complaints such as influenza and sometimes they are disappointed when they are not given an antibiotic. In fact they should be glad that the doctor does not consider it necessary for them to have such treatment because they will not be exposed to the risk of developing an allergic reaction to the antibiotic. The more often one is exposed to an antibiotic, the more likely one is to develop an allergy.

Penicillin, which in its various forms is the most widely used antibiotic, has a particularly high incidence of allergic reactions. The difficulty is that, once an allergic tendency to a particular medicine is discovered, it becomes very hazardous to give that medicine again. Even if the allergy when first detected only took the form of a skin rash, there is a fair chance that when given again, the reaction will be more severe and sometimes even life threatening. Most doctors, before they prescribe a medicine, will enquire whether the patient has had it before and if he or she has, whether it caused any problems.

Follow instructions

It is very important that medicines should be taken according to instructions. Some medicines are only properly absorbed if there is no food in the stomach. It is useful in this connection to remember that *after a meal it usually takes about two hours for the stomach to empty.*

If it is recommended that a medicine be taken *before meals*, that usually means that it should be taken on an empty stomach, i.e. *any time greater than two hours after the last meal.*

Other medicines are prescribed to be taken *with food* or *after food*. This usually means that the medicine is better absorbed into the bloodstream when mixed with food, or that the medicine is irritating to the stomach. In the latter case, the food in the stomach will act as a buffer to protect the lining of the stomach from damage from the medication.

In doctor jargon

  ac (ante cibum) means 'before food' pc (post cibum) means 'after food'

Sometimes the order is to take medicine twice daily, or more often.

   bds or bid means 'twice a day' qid means '4 times daily'
   tds or tid means 'three times a day' q4h means '4 hourly'

(See also the section on reading your own prescription, p. 214.)

If the doctor feels that an even concentration of a medicine is of considerable importance, the prescription can be written with the recommendation that it be taken six hourly or even four hourly. In general, this means that the dose should be spread out as evenly as possible. In this way one can keep the concentration of the medicine in the body at a satisfactory level. If the dose is taken less frequently, there is a likelihood of wide fluctuations in the concentration of the medicine in the body and sometimes this can mean a 'stop-start' sort of treatment which is seldom in the patient's best interests.

In these cases it may be desirable to take all necessary steps to ensure that the treatment is taken around the clock, even going to the extent of setting the alarm to wake oneself up in order to take the medication throughout the night. More often the timing is not so critical and it is reasonable to take the medicine first thing in the morning, about noon and then again last thing at night. Sometimes a good night's rest is almost as important as the medicine, and the even concentration of the substance in the bloodstream is a lesser consideration.

Complete the course

A common mistake that many people make is to assume that once they are feeling better, they can discontinue a course of antibiotics or other medicine. What is not always realised is that many infections can smoulder on, sometimes without symptoms. An example of this would be a urine infection. If the infection is severe, the patient may be aware of *pain* on passing urine and also often an *urgent* desire to pass urine, usually coupled with a *frequent need* to pass urine. With appropriate treatment the concentration of bacteria is reduced and the patient loses these symptoms. This does not necessarily mean that the infection has been cleared. At such times patients sometimes stop the treatment and shortly afterwards often regret the decision because the symptoms return. What is worse, the short course of antibiotic may have killed off the weaker bacteria while the stronger ones have survived to reproduce and repopulate the urine with a more resistant strain which is hard to eradicate.

Hence, unless a medicine is causing undesirable side-effects, it is best to complete the prescribed course of treatment. To overcome this problem, some newer treatments consist of one single large dose of antibiotic designed to kill all the bacteria at once.

The right dose and duration of the treatment

Yet another reason for not taking medicines without a doctor's approval is the fact that people differ in the quantity of medicine that is appropriate for them. A heavily-built person will probably require a bigger dose than a small, frail person. Children, not surprisingly, usually require smaller doses than middle-aged patients, and so on. Thus it can be said that the type of treatment and the dosage must be tailored to the condition and to the patient. Modern medicines are so potent and the potential for harm (and good, of course) is so great that this is not a place for amateurs.

Another problem not recognised by everybody is the way in which different medicines interact. In some instances two medicines taken together will cancel out each other, whereas others will have an additive effect, i.e. potentiate each other. For example, when the tricyclic medicines which are administered for depression are taken at the same time as certain medicines which reduce the blood pressure, the latter are likely to be rendered ineffective.

The same tricyclic medicines usually have a tendency to cause drowsiness and if given in association with certain tranquillisers, may make the patient very sleepy indeed. The doctor needs to use much skill in deciding whether a particular combination of medicines is likely to be effective and tolerable. Since each person's responses to medication seem to be different, it is almost inevitable that difficulties will sometimes arise. For this reason it is not surprising that medications often have to be changed and that most doctors try to be very conservative in their prescribing. The more medications the patient is on, the more likely it is that untoward, unwanted reactions will occur. It is a fortunate patient whose doctor can say, 'Your problem is going to clear up by itself. There is no need for any medicines'.

Scepticism

The body has most remarkable powers of healing and human nature being what it is, it is understandable that any medicine which is being administered when improvement occurs will be credited with producing that improvement. Most doctors have long since learnt to be very sceptical about the efficacy of apparent cures, despite being constantly assailed by patients who declare that they have received great benefit from all sorts of unlikely remedies.

Many supposed 'cures' appear to be based on false premises. For example, there are those who believe that 'arthritis' is due to too much 'acid' in the blood. This possibly derives from the fact that one form of arthritis — gout — is associated with too much uric acid in the bloodstream. The proponents of the acid theory of arthritis strongly recommend that all acid foods should be avoided in arthritis, regardless of its cause. On the other hand, one can find others who earnestly believe that taking large quantities of acetic acid is the best way to treat arthritis and will recommend it to all who will listen. Orthodox medicine believes that arthritis is not just one disease, but several, and can be caused by many factors.

Similarly, there is a condition of *parathyroid deficiency* (parathyroids are small glands in the neck within the thyroid gland) which can cause cataracts. If this condition is found early and the missing parathyroid hormone administered, the cataracts will regress. As a result, some non-medical enthusiasts have advocated such treatment for all cataracts. It would be wonderful if this medical approach to the common cataract were effective, but of course it almost always fails.

One has to realise that there are many disorders which at first appear similar in their manifestations, but which have very different origins. This is yet another reason why it is so very unwise for one person to take another's medicines. 'My doctor gave me these tablets for my arthritis. They've made all the difference to me. Here are some for you to try. I'm sure they will help your joints, too', says a concerned friend. Such a friend might unknowingly do incalculable harm.

The evaluation of medicine

Any new medications have to be very thoroughly evaluated before they are made available to the public. This is a process that takes years, first to establish efficacy and secondly to establish safety.

One of the best ways to do this is by the 'double blind' trial. In such a trial the researcher administers, with the permission of a 'guinea pig' patient, a prepared medication. The person who has done the preparation fills a series of coded containers with the medicine. Half of the containers will contain the new medicine under trial and the other half will contain either an inert substance or a known active ingredient made up to look exactly like the medicine under trial. Thus the researcher does not know whether any individual patient is getting the new medicine under trial or the other agent similarly packed.

The idea is that when the researchers are evaluating whether the patient has benefited from the treatment, they will not be biassed toward one preparation or the other and a completely objective assessment can be made. Similarly, the patients will not know whether they are getting an active ingredient or whether an inert substance has been administered. The patient will judge the medicine given entirely on its merits. It is surprising how often strange side-effects are described for something which is known to be as innocuous as water. At the end of the experiment, after many patients have been treated and assessed, the code will be broken and the researchers can determine whether the new medicine is better than the other agent which has been administered.

Usually hundreds and sometimes thousands of people have to be treated in this way before the researchers can say with confidence that a new preparation is satisfactorily free of significant side-effects and useful for the purpose for which it was intended. Such is the power of the mind over the body — the power of suggestion — that it is often hard to determine whether the medicine has really made a difference to the patient or if the very fact of taking a medicine has helped. Doctors refer to this as the 'placebo' effect and in the past, knowing this, some have prescribed rose-coloured water or similar preparations for those patients who have demanded medication but who on investigation have been found to have little or nothing wrong with them.

The word *placebo* takes its origin from a Latin word which means 'to please' and the word 'placate' comes from the same root. Many patients still come to the doctor in the belief that all they need is a bottle of medicine. Doctors, too, often form the opinion that the patient will not be 'pleased' if they go home with lots of good advice and reassurance but no medicine. This is a major reason why some decide to placate the patient with a placebo.

Some people feel that too much time in the early years of medical training are spent learning about scientific method. On the other hand, medical leaders often express disquiet about some members of the profession becoming caught up in treatments which have not been proven to be of any value. Some will respond by saying that all their patients who have had the unproven treatment seem to be getting benefit from it, often forgetting what is known about the 'placebo effect'. They usually go on to say that the patients are no worse off, so what is the harm?

Doctors who dabble in the unproven or the unorthodox usually attract quite a following because there are always some patients on the lookout for something new and different, particularly for stubborn, hard-to-treat complaints. These patients often feel a need to justify the fact that they have sought an unorthodox treatment and will as a result, hail any slight change for the better as a major breakthrough, thus adding to the number of those claiming significant benefit. (See also my quotation by Dr Zimmermann at the beginning of this chapter.)

Sometimes we forget that most disorders have a fluctuating course; the majority are self-limiting and will ultimately disappear spontaneously, while those which do not, usually have remissions and exacerbations.

Alternative ways of giving medicines

Most medicines are taken by mouth and come in the form of tablets or mixtures.

Tablets have the advantage that the dosage can be accurately determined. Usually adults soon learn how to swallow tablets with the aid of water and sometimes people learn how to swallow them without. Tablets are particularly useful for unpleasant medicines because they go down so rapidly that there is seldom any sensation of taste. Children often have trouble with tablets and so their medication may be prescribed in the form of a *mixture*. Unfortunately such mixtures are frequently very syrupy and it is probably a good idea for them to brush their teeth before and after each dose lest the syrup encourage dental caries.

Usually the trick when swallowing tablets is to place the pills as far back on the tongue as possible and then to swallow some water so that they are washed down into the gullet. Many make the mistake of not placing the tablet far enough back on the tongue. Some people find that swallowing the tablet is facilitated if, instead of placing the tablet on the surface of the tongue, it is placed under the tongue, immediately behind the front teeth, again a mouthful of water is swallowed and somehow the tablet goes with it. I find that this will usually work for me.

Unpleasant tastes can sometimes be prevented by placing a block of ice on the tongue for a short time before taking the medicine. This seems to prevent the taste buds from functioning normally.

Other types of tablet In addition to tablets taken by mouth, there are some which are designed for use in other body orifices.

Suppositories are a type of tablet designed to be absorbed from the rectum (lower bowel). These need to be pushed well into the anus (back passage). Remember it is important that their protective covering be removed before insertion, otherwise they will not be effective. Such suppositories are usually designed to melt at body temperatures and hence if they have to be kept for any time should be stored in the refrigerator. Wearing a disposable plastic glove, which can usually be bought at the pharmacy, is often helpful when inserting such suppositories.

A similar tablet for vaginal use is usually referred to as a *pessary*. These are best inserted after the patient is in bed as otherwise they have a tendency to slip down the vagina. This can mean that when they dissolve, some parts of the vaginal wall will not be covered and the treatment will be rendered relatively ineffective. Most manufacturers supply a special applicator for pessaries to assist in the insertion process.

Other routes of administration

Injections are another way of adminstering medicines, but usually these are given by the doctor or a nurse. Sometimes patients are required to do this themselves, as many diabetics will know.

Another method of giving treatment is by *nasal or oral inhalation*. If a substance is well absorbed by the nose or lung lining, this is a quick way of getting it into the bloodstream. Sometimes inhaled substances have a direct local effect on the muscles of the tubes to the lungs (i.e. bronchial tubes), or the lining of the nose, and do not enter the rest of the body. This can be a way of avoiding some of the side-effects of such substances which, if they are in the bloodstream, circulate all round the body.

Recently ways have been developed for facilitating the passage of medicines through the skin without injection and some agents seem to be well absorbed in this way. Glyceryl trinitrate, which is used in the prevention and treatment of heart pain (angina), is a typical example. A patch containing this substance is applied to a suitable area of the sufferer's skin. The patch is designed to release slowly the active substance and so provide some protection from the pain throughout the day.

Eye, ear and nose drops

Drops are frequently used, particularly in the eye, ear and nose. Quite often they are not as effective as they should be, because patients are not adequately instructed in their use.

Eye drops: Whenever possible, these should be administered by a second person. If no one is available to help, the patient should stand before a mirror. The lower lid of the eye is grasped between thumb and forefinger and pulled forward, away from the eyeball. This produces a small cup immediately in front of the eyeball and the drop or drops are placed in this area and then the lids are closed for a second or two. Eye ointments are applied in the same way and have the advantage that they remain longer in contact with the structures of the eye, but the vision is often blurred for a considerable time afterwards. They are particularly useful for application at night. Eye drops are washed away so rapidly that for best results they often have to be applied every one to two hours.

Ear drops: If possible, these should be warmed before use. Should they be very cold when placed in the ear, they may cause giddiness. The patient should lie on one side, the affected ear uppermost. The drops, usually four or five in number, are placed in the ear canal and then, while the patient remains on the side, pressure is applied with a finger to the outer ear, immediately in front of the ear canal. The finger is then wiggled a little and in this way the drops are brought into contact with the whole of the inner surface of the ear canal. The usual mistake with ear drops is to use too few drops.

Nose drops: If nose drops are going to be used the patient should lie flat on his or her back. The drops are put in one nostril and almost immediately afterwards the patient, remaining supine, should turn the head to the side involved and stay in that position for about half a minute. Thereafter the same routine is repeated with the other nostril. This procedure encourages the drops to enter the nasal cavities (sinuses) which lie on the outer side of each nasal passage (nares). If this is not done, it is likely that the drops will simply run down the back of the nose into the throat and the benefit will be minimal.

Preparations for skin conditions

There are numerous preparations designed specifically for the treatment of skin conditions. These usually come in the form of ointments, creams, pastes, powders and paints.

Ointments tend to be greasy, and help to prevent the loss of moisture from the skin. They also have a soothing and softening effect. They are usually used on dry and scaly skin surfaces.

Creams are usually more oily. They too have soothing and softening effects and may also act as moisturisers and even have a cooling action. They may be used on either dry or wet surfaces and are less messy than ointments.

Lotions are drying, soothing and cooling. They are particularly useful on broken, oozing skin surfaces.

Pastes can also be used on broken skin surfaces. They are protective and may have a drying effect on wet areas.

Dusting powders are usually used in areas where the skin bends or folds, as under the arms or the groin, particularly when they are sore and moist. They reduce the friction of two skin surfaces rubbing together and assist in drying moist areas.

Paints also tend to be used in areas where the skin bends or folds and their principal action is a drying one. Sometimes they have intrinsic antibacterial or antifungal properties.

Reading your prescription

Prescriptions are not confidential documents and there is no reason why they should not be read by patients if that is their wish. However, your doctor should explain to you what the medicine is and what it is expected to do. Feel free to ask about anything that you don't understand. Most of the symbols used are just convenient abbreviations — a hangover from the days when doctors demonstrated their erudition by writing in latin.

The symbol at the head of the prescription is usually an R with a cross through the descending tail — thus **R**. This stands for *recipe*, which is the latin word for 'prepare' or 'make up'.

Thereafter the doctor usually indicates the formulation that is to be used, e.g. tablet (usually abbreviated to 'tab').

Here are some other words which may be seen and their abbreviations, although most are seldom used today and they may have little more than curiosity value.

Ampoule = Amp. (a small glass container of liquid)
Auristillae = Aur. (ear drops)
Capsule = Caps. (a dissolvable container for a single measured dose of a medicine)
Collyrium = Col. (an eye wash)
Cremor = Crem. (a cream)
Elixir = Elix. (a sweet-tasting, alcohol-based mixture or suspension)
Expectorant = Expect. (an agent to assist in bringing up sputum from the lungs)
Gargarisma = Garg. (a gargle)
Guttae = Gutt. (drops, usually for the eye)
Haustra = Haus. (a draught)
Injection = Inj. (an injectable material)

Liniment = Lin. (a liniment)
Linctus = Linct. (a cough medicine)
Mistura = Mist. (a mixture)
Nebuliser = Neb. (apparatus for production of a fine mist)
Oculentum = Oculent. (an eye ointment)
Oleum = Ol. (an oil)
Pigmentum = Pig. (a colouring material)
Pulvis = Pulv. (a powder)
Suspension = Susp. (a suspension of active ingredient in a fluid)
Syrup = Syr. (a syrup)
Unguentum = Ung. (an ointment)

Usually following the name of the agent to be used is the size of a standard dose of the preparation to be prescribed. Thus some substances are produced in preparations of different strengths, e.g. amoxycillin is available in capsules of 250 mg or 500 mg. If the doctor wishes the patient to have the smaller size, 'Caps amoxycillin 250 mg' will be at the head of the prescription.

Almost all medicines have two or more names. One is the *generic* name, which is the official name, in this case amoxycillin, and the other is the *trade name* given by manufacturers to distinguish their product from other brands; in this case the developer, Beecham's Research Laboratories, has called their product Amoxil. *Throughout this book the generic name has been used and trade names, starting with a capital letter, have been inserted in brackets afterwards to aid identification*

The next line of the prescription will indicate how this dosage is to be given. Often this instruction is preceded by the abbreviation 'Sig.' or even just S. This stands for 'signatur' which means 'label'. The line below this is usually preceded by the word 'mitte' or an abbreviation for it. This is the latin word for 'send' and is followed by an indication of the amount of the substance which the doctor wishes to be supplied.

So our prescription for amoxycillin might look like this:

R
Caps amoxycillin 250 mg
S. Caps ī three times daily
M. 15

This means that the capsules are to be labelled so that the recipient knows to take them three times a day and that the total number to be supplied should be 15. The number of capsules in each dose is usually indicated by roman numerals, written with a line above.

Sometimes at the end of the first line is another abbreviation such as 'BNF' or 'BPC' or 'USP'. These are abbreviations for special, recognised pharmaceutical manuals and the inclusion of one means that the preparation requested should be made up in accordance with the directions in that book, e.g.

BNF refers to the *British National Formulary*;
BP is the *British Pharmacopoeia*;
BPC is the *British Pharmaceutical Codex*;
USP is an abbreviation for the *United States Pharmacopoeia*.

These abbreviations are used particularly for mixtures, as they save the doctor having to specify in detail the contents of the preparation required. The pharmacist will find that information upon consulting the relevant book. Here is a simple prescription for ear drops from the *British Pharmacopoeia* (BP)

℞
Sodium bicarbonate 5 g
Glycerol 30 ml
Purified water (freshly boiled and cooled) to 100 ml

The doctor will simply write on the prescription:

℞
Aur. Sod. Bicarb BP
S 3–4 drops to be put in affected ear tds
M. 10 ml

and the prescription from the *British Pharmacopoeia* will be given to the patient. In fact the doctor does not even need to write the instructions, except the frequency of use (in this case tds, which means 'three times daily'), as this too is indicated in the pharmacopoeia, together with the amount to be dispensed, unless otherwise advised by the doctor.

As you will have noticed, this prescription contained some other abbreviations. Here is a list of some of the most frequently used:

Abbreviation	Derivation	Meaning
aa	ana	of each
ac	ante cibum	before meals
aq	aqua	water
bd/bid	bis in die	twice daily
det	detur	give
e. aq.	ex aqua	with water
e. lact.	ex lacte	with milk
ft.	fiat	make
g		gram
hn	hac nocte	tonight
hs	hora somni	at bedtime
m	misce	mix
mane		morning
mdu	modo dictu utendus	use as directed
mitte		dispense
mg		milligram

Abbreviation	Derivation	Meaning
ml		millilitre
nnp	no name please	
np	name please	
nr	non repetatum	no repeats
nocte		at night
od	omni dei	every day
om	omni mane	every morning
on	omni nocte	every night
paa	part affectae applicandus	apply to affected part
pc	post cibum	after meal
po	per os	by mouth
ppa	philala prius agitata	shake bottle before taking
pr	per rectum	use rectally
prn	pro re nata	use as required
q3h	quaqua 3 hora	every 3 hours
q6h	quaqua 6 hora	every 6 hours
qd/qid/qds	quater in die sumendum	4 times a day
qh	quaqua hora	every hour
qqh	quaqua quater hora	every 4 hours
qs	quantum sufficit	as much as necessary
qos	quoties opus sit	as often as necessary
R	recipe	prepare
rep/rpt	repetatum	repeat
sig	signatur	label
stat	statim	at once
tds/tid	ter in die sumendum	3 times a day
ut dict	ut dictum	as directed

Some general rules for patients on medications

Try to remember or make a note of the medicines you are using or, better still, take the bottles to the surgery. Usually the doctor has a record, but this is not always quickly available. It is seldom helpful to say 'the little white tablets with the groove across them' as there are probably dozens of such tablets made, and the doctor possibly does not know what the tablets look like anyway. Tell the doctor about all the medicines you are taking — including those bought over the counter from the chemist or other stockist — in case any new medicines prescribed do not mix well with them.

Before the doctor prescribes for you, mention any allergies or other reactions which you have had to previous medicines. Take the opportunity to ask the doctor whether you can expect any side-effects from the medicines you are being given.

Never give your medicines to anyone else and never take medicines which have been prescribed for someone else.

Do not use old medicines which may have deteriorated. Your pharmacist may be able to tell you whether agents which he or she has dispensed are still safe to take.

The medicine container should be clearly labelled with the instructions for use. These instructions must be followed meticulously.

Never put medicines from one container into another unless you are certain that they are identical. Women who think there is a possibility that they might be pregnant should ask the doctor whether any medicine is safe to take in pregnancy.

Do not hoard medicines and always ensure that they are in a place where children cannot get hold of them.

Unless they are not agreeing with you, always complete a recommended course of antibiotics even if your symptoms seem to have disappeared. If in doubt, ask your doctor. If you do have medicines left over after a course of treatment, offer them back to the pharmacist or else flush them down the toilet.

If you have medicines which have to be taken regularly regardless of circumstances — such as insulin, or steroids — make sure that you have a card on your person indicating this and informing people of the usual dosage.

Always remember any instructions you are given such as those relating to food interactions with the mono-amine oxidase inhibitors (see p. 230) or to the possibility of feeling drowsy which would be dangerous if you are driving or working with dangerous machinery. Note too that alcohol usually adds to these risks.

Should you feel unwell or experience any untoward symptom shortly after commencing a new medication, remember that although this is not necessarily the cause, it must be considered a likely possibility. Discuss the matter with your general practitioner before discontinuing the treatment. Sometimes side-effects do not appear until quite a long time after starting treatment. Others cease to be a problem after a time.

Some people on sleeping tablets experience difficulty in remembering whether they have taken their tablets and are tempted to take a further dose during the night. As a consequence, it is wise to keep the tablets well away from the bedroom so that this temptation is reduced.

Some commonly used medications

4.3 Anti-inflammatory agents

Inflammation is a response of the body to injury, infection or other irritant resulting in the dilation of blood vessels, or the oozing of body fluids into the tissue, or the accumulation of white blood cells, or any combination of the three. Inflammation is usually accompanied by increased warmth in the affected part, increased redness, swelling and pain. There is frequently some reduction in function.

An *anti-inflammatory* agent is a substance which is designed to reduce some or all of these symptoms and signs. Most anti-inflammatory agents have, additionally, some painkilling (analgesic) properties and sometimes they are used for this purpose only. Usually the anti-inflammatory effect is only useful if they are taken on a regular basis. Anti-inflammatories are used most frequently in conditions associated with disorders of the back, the joints, the muscles and ligaments. Thus they are widely used in arthritic conditions and in strains and sprains.

Common anti-inflammatory agents

The most frequently used anti-inflammatory agent is undoubtedly aspirin. This is used in many situations for its painkilling properties, but needs to be taken in high dosage, 4-6 hourly, if it is going to be effective as an anti-inflammatory. Paracetamol and codeine, incidentally, are agents which give pain relief but which have little or no anti-inflammatory effect so they come into a different category.

As already mentioned, for most people aspirin is a very safe preparation, but for a few it is very irritating to the stomach and can actually cause ulcers, or make existing ulcers bleed. Some people also find that it aggravates allergic reactions and may even precipitate severe asthma. It should be avoided by people known to have a tendency to stomach ulcers or severe indigestion and also by people with kidney or liver problems. It should only be given on medical advice to children less than one year of age, women in late pregnancy or breast feeding and to anyone who is on anti-clotting tablets. In very high dosage it may cause noises in the ears.

Many preparations have been developed in an effort to achieve the same anti-inflammatory effect without stomach irritation. Unfortunately, they all share the same side-effects as aspirin, although in some stomach irritation is less marked. Naproxen (Naprosyn)* is a popular choice.

---

*Throughout this book generic names of all medicines are quoted, with the trade names given in parentheses afterwards. (See also p. 213.)

It has the advantage that it need be given only twice daily. Others include diflunisal (Dolobid), sulindac (Clinoril), fenoprofen calcium (Fenopron), flurbiprofen (Froben), ketoprofen (Alrheumat, Orudis, Oruvail), azapropazone (Rheumox), diclofenac sodium (Voltaren), fenbufen (Lederfen), piroxicam (Feldene) tiaprofenic acid (Surgam) and tolmetin (Tolectin), and these suit some people well but also often cause stomach irritation.

Ibuprofen (Brufen) has fewer side-effects than naproxen but is also a weaker anti-inflammatory. Some of these, e.g. piroxicam, need only be given once daily.

Mefenamic acid (Ponstan) is a painkiller with slight anti-inflammatory action. It seems to have a special place in the management of menstrual pain. Indomethacin (Indocid) is a powerful anti-inflammatory which, like most of the others, is also useful in the joint condition known as gout. It is usually best tolerated if it is started in small doses and gradually increased. Phenylbutazone (Butazolidin) is probably the strongest in this family of anti-inflammatory medications, but the incidence of stomach irritation and other side-effects from phenylbutazone is such that it is usually reserved for cases which fail to respond to all other anti-inflammatories. The most serious of the side-effects is a reduction in the ability of the bone marrow to make certain elements of the blood — a disorder which sometimes proves fatal.

Anti-inflammatories sometimes interfere with the action of medicines known as diuretics, which help the kidneys rid the body of retained fluid.

Cortisone

After aspirin, the best known anti-inflammatory agent is *cortisone*. This is usually administered as *hydrocortisone* as it is more rapidly utilised by the body in that form. This is a substance that is manufactured by the body in the adrenal gland. If the adrenal glands have ceased to work, as they do in Addison's disease, hydrocortisone or one of its derivatives is given as a replacement. When it is produced in excess by the body, as occurs in Cushing's syndrome,* a patient may experience all the consequences of over-dosage by cortisone without taking any medication. These side-effects can include increased weight gain, retention of fluid (oedema), raised blood pressure, loss of calcium from the bones, stomach ulcers and impaired healing of the skin. The patient may also show a tendency to diabetes and a greater susceptibility to infections.

Steroids Cortisone and the other medicines derived from it are often loosely spoken of as *corticosteroids* or simply *steroids*. There are other substances which share a steroid chemical structure, but for practical purposes when a doctor talks about treatment with steroids, the allusion is to cortisone or closely allied medicines. When cortisone was first isolated, it was soon recognised for its extraordinary anti-inflammatory properties. In fact some patients with rheumatoid arthritis lost so much of the inflammation in their joints that they were able to walk for the first time in years. It was hailed as a 'miracle drug', and not without reason. Then came the disappointment. In a short time many patients began to experience some or all of the side-effects noted above. The worst was the softening of the bones due to the loss of

---

*Syndrome — a collection of signs and symptoms.

calcium. In some people the spinal column collapsed, leading to pressure on the roots of nerves, with very severe pain resulting. This loss of calcium from the bones is called *osteoporosis* and it is very difficult, if not impossible, to reverse the process. Such a condition often occurs spontaneously in elderly people and is particularly common in women. (See pp. 186–7.) It can also occur in people who are obliged to spend long periods of time in a recumbent position as a result of a paralysis of their limbs or other enforced bed rest.

Derivatives Much effort has been devoted to developing derivatives of cortisone which are capable of providing the very important anti-inflammatory effect, yet minimising the side-effects. Unfortunately none has been entirely successful and these medicines must always be used with discretion and only for very clear reasons. Steroids have a great many uses and many lives have been saved as a result. However, they do not cure but simply halt the destructive process while the body marshals its own defences.

Skin disorders Hydrocortisone and its derivatives can actually be absorbed through the skin and are very helpful in the management of many different types of skin disorder. Even here the steroids must be administered carefully, for if they are used over a wide area of the body for a long time there is considerable absorption and the patient may experience the same side-effects as if the substance were taken by mouth. However, a more common problem is the local effect that the steroid has on the skin — usually a thinning, so that it can sustain injury less well. The skin may also develop a permanent unnatural pallor and sometimes there are minute blood vessels which become prominent and unsightly in the affected area.

These effects are almost never seen in patients who are treated with hydrocortisone, but are more likely to occur, the more powerful the steroid. Regrettably, some skin conditions can only be kept under control with regular use of the very powerful steroids, but whenever possible a doctor will bring a condition under control with a strong steroid and then change to a weaker form for maintenance.

Skin damage is particularly acute on the face, and if at all possible, steroids should be avoided here.

The least potent of the steroids for local application is hydrocortisone; somewhat stronger is clobetasone butyrate (Eumovate) followed by betamethasone valerate (Betnovate) and hydrocortisone 17-butyrate (Locoid). The strongest of all is probably clobetasol propionate (Dermovate).

Here is a list of some of the conditions of the skin where the steroids can be helpful:
Atopic eczema
Contact dermatitis and seborrhoeic dermatitis
Psoriasis
Allergic rashes and insect bites
Sunburn
Some forms of napkin rash

Steroid injections   Yet another way that steroids may be used is by injection directly into an inflamed joint or other tissue. Thus steroids are often injected into the joints, or the tissues surrounding the joints, of patients with rheumatoid arthritis; they are injected into the inflamed area of the elbow in so-called 'tennis elbow'; they may be injected into painful tissues in an inflamed shoulder, and so on. So long as the injections are not too large or too frequent, there is little need to worry about the side-effects associated with too much steroid in the body.

Many people with arthritis and other disorders of the musculo-skeletal system have every reason to be very grateful to the scientists who first isolated cortisone and who have subsequently refined it for specific purposes.

Other uses of steroids are in:

Acquired haemolytic anaemia	Nephrosis
Allergy (e.g. hayfever and hives)	Polyarteritis nodosa
Aphthous ulcers of the mouth	Rheumatic fever
Asthma	Shock
Chronic active hepatitis	Systemic lupus erythematosus
Crohn's disease	Thrombocytopaenic purpura
Some forms of leukaemia	Ulcerative colitis

Steroids, because of their anti-inflammatory action, can have the effect of encouraging the spread of infection insofar as some inflammation is helpful and represents part of the body's defence mechanisms. Consequently steroids are not given for infections (either viral or bacterial) unless something else is given simultaneously to control the infection. Interestingly, viral infections of the eye represent one of the greatest hazards. If steroid drops or ointment are put into the eye when it is infected with the 'cold sore' virus (herpes simplex) and no antiviral agent is used, the condition can be greatly worsened and blindness can occur.

It should be repeated that *steroids do not cure disease but suppress inflammation*. In effect, they buy time and enable the body's own defences to come to the rescue.

When corticosteroids are given in high dosage for a prolonged time they have the effect of reducing the production of natural steroids by the body. When the treatment is stopped it takes some time for the adrenal gland to start operating normally again and during this time the patient may suffer from an acute and dangerous deficiency of steroids. It is for this reason that doctors will reduce the dosage of administered steroids slowly (i.e. tailing off) so that the natural processes can gradually take over again.

For the same reason, when prolonged treatment is discontinued abruptly, there may be a dangerous exacerbation of the condition, often referred to as 'rebound'. Sometimes the dosage of steroid will be adjusted so that it is given on alternate days, or in some other similar way, in an effort to reduce the degree of suppression of the naturally occurring hydrocortisone.

Treatment card   Because of the dangers of long-term treatment with steroids, persons required to take them for a prolonged time are strongly recommended to carry in their wallet or handbag a card giving details of the dosage and possible complications should treatment be inadvertently stopped. A 'Medicalert' bracelet is also a good idea.

The usual card states: 'I am a patient on steroid treatment which must not be stopped abruptly and in the case of intercurrent illness, may have to be increased.' It then goes on to give the following instructions: 'Do not stop taking the steroid except on medical advice. Always have a supply in reserve. In case of feverish illness, accident, operation (emergency or otherwise), diarrhoea or vomiting, the steroid must be continued. Your doctor may wish you to have a larger dose or injection at such times. If the tablets cause indigestion, consult your doctor at once. Always carry this card while receiving steroid treatment and show it to any doctor, dentist, nurse or midwife whom you may consult. After your treatment has finished, you must still tell any new doctor, dentist, nurse or midwife that you have had steroid treatment.'

Because of the special properties (and dangers) of the steroidal anti-inflammatory medicines, it is common to refer to all other anti-inflammatory medicines as 'non-steroidal anti-inflammatory drugs' and this is frequently abbreviated to NSAID.

Allergies

The body has a number of protective mechanisms, and these include the ability to produce substances called *antibodies* in response to the presence of various foreign substances, particularly when they consist of protein. Thus, antibodies are produced as a means of coping with the invasion of the body by micro-organisms. The substances which produce the antibody response are called *antigens* (sometimes referred to as *allergens*).

Apart from micro-organisms, a wide variety of substances can act as antigens, but some are more likely to do so than others. Furthermore, some people differ in the way they respond to antigens. The first time a person comes into contact with an antigen, the production of antibodies is stimulated. This is a slow process and is usually associated with destruction of the foreign substance. When the body comes into contact with the same antigen on a later occasion, there is already some antibody present and the reaction between antigen and antibody is much more rapid. In some cases, the reaction is excessive and accompanied by symptoms. This is known as *hypersensitivity* and the body's responses are described as an *allergy* — really another form of inflammation. Antibodies are produced in the lymphatic tissues, principally by white blood cells known as *plasma cells*, which are a type of lymphocyte.

The reaction between antigen and antibody, when excessive, leads to damage to yet other cells, the *mast cells* and *basophils*. Their cell walls are injured and certain substances are released into the tissues. These include histamine, serotonin and kinins. These substances produce a localised inflammation and some contraction of certain muscles which are not under voluntary control. The result is usually an increase in the fluid in the tissues, causing swelling and congestion and often a tightening of the muscles.

Such changes play an important part in, for example, some cases of asthma, where the small tubes to the lungs may be narrowed by three things: the swelling of the tissues, the production of mucus and the contraction of the muscles in the bronchial walls. Hayfever, where there are changes in the lining of the nose, is another example of an allergic reaction.

In fact, there are many types of allergy and a great many parts of the body can be involved. Some people suffer allergies of the skin and many examples of contact dermatitis come into this category. Others have allergies of the gastro-intestinal passages (i.e. alimentary canal) to certain foodstuffs, while allergies to medicines, showing up in a variety of ways, are commonplace.

Usually the best way to deal with an allergic reaction is to avoid all contact with the agent causing it, if that is possible. Of course, it may be difficult to identify causative agents in the first place. Sometimes, as with foods, it is possible to do this by a process of elimination (see Chapter 2.6 on diets for allergy), while on other occasions skin tests may be helpful.

In skin testing, very dilute suspensions of likely causative agents are prepared. A small drop of each of these is then placed in rows on the patient's skin, usually on the forearm. A tiny prick is made into the skin through the drop so that a trace of each of the substances under investigation enters the tissues. Shortly afterwards the area is re-examined and a note made of any site where there is marked reddening, swelling and itching which would suggest that the substance placed there is the offending agent.

Many hayfever sufferers find that they are allergic to pollens in the atmosphere, and animal dander is another common cause. Ubiquitous mites which live in house dust create problems for many people. Unfortunately it is not always possible to eliminate substances which are acting as allergens (i.e., causing allergies) and the best that can be done is to try to minimise the effects. Sometimes the *antihistamines* are effective. These help to neutralise the action of histamine which is a principal cause of allergic inflammation. Most antihistamines cause drowsiness but recently two new ones, terfenadine (Teldane) and astemizole (Hismanal) have been developed which appear to be free of this side-effect. Unfortunately they are rather expensive. Antihistamines do not seem to be helpful in asthma.

Another substance, known as sodium cromoglycate, appears to act on the mast cells, helping to make the walls of these cells impervious to histamine, serotonin and the like, so that these substances do not escape and damage the tissues. Sodium cromoglycate (Intal) is usually inhaled as a powder or a mist and is used in the prevention of both hayfever and asthma. Often it has to be applied for several weeks before any benefit is achieved. Some people with gastro-intestinal allergies are claiming benefit from taking sodium cromoglycate by mouth, also as a preventive medicine.

The other agents which have a place in the management of severe allergic reactions are the steroids (see p. 219). These have the ability to suppress or minimise most inflammations, and this is certainly true of the allergies.

Other forms of allergy There are two other forms of allergy which deserve a brief mention. The first is the situation in which the body develops an allergy to its own tissues. This is thought to be the situation in the *auto-immune* disorders. These include rheumatoid arthritis, ankylosing spondylitis, lupus erythematosus and polyarteritis nodosa. These conditions do not benefit from the antihistamines, but the steroids play an important part in their management.

Many other agents are either in use or under investigation as a means of reducing or eliminating the destructive inflammatory processes. Some treatments go so far as to remove the lymphocytes or the plasma cells from the body.

The other form of allergy relates to the problem of *tissue rejection* in organ transplants. Transplanted organs are matched to the recipient as far as possible, but will almost inevitably be regarded by the body as a foreign substance and so induce antigen/antibody-type reactions. The success or otherwise of such procedures is very dependent on the ability to control such responses. Unfortunately, in interfering with these reactions, we also interfere with the body's normal response to bacteria so that any infections which occur have to be dealt with promptly and effectively, and of course heroic efforts are made to prevent infection getting established in the first place.

4.4 Medicines for the mind and nervous system

'It is my own practice to avoid drugs as much as possible; and I more frequently find it difficult to persuade people from using them, than to induce them to take them. But I hope that you will not believe me to be distrustful of the power of drugs to do real service to the sick under proper circumstances. I am far otherwise. And in reference to this point, I wish to tell you that your success in the use of medicines may depend somewhat on the temper with which you give them. You must be hopeful and feel an interest in them. Do not, like a cold stepfather, leave them to make their own way in the world; but watch them in their course'
— James Jackson, MD, *Letters to a Young Physician*, 1855

Over the years the human race has sought chemical means to try to alleviate emotional suffering. Almost every race has discovered some agent which alters the way in which people feel about themselves or about external events. Thus the South American chews the coca leaf, the Asiatic uses betel nut, or smokes opium, the Arab uses hashish, while the Western world favours alcohol and tobacco, the latter originally obtained from the North American Indian. Modern ingenuity has added to the list, or modified old agents.

The most common need seems to be to reduce anxiety. Most of the powerful painkillers (analgesics) have this property, and laudanum, which is an opium derivative, was widely used for this purpose 100 years ago and more. The bromides and chloral were also used extensively for anxiety until the introduction of the *barbiturates*. The latter were a major breakthrough and their use was widespread until the introduction of safer substances. As with the powerful analgesics (see Chapter 4.7, Medicines for the relief of pain, pp. 252–3), medicines which relieve anxiety have a tendency to produce dependence and this has been particularly evident with the barbiturates. Most of the agents which reduce anxiety are capable of inducing sleep if the dosage is sufficient. A medicine which will promote sleep is known medically as a *hypnotic*. In a similar way, most of the agents which are used as hypnotics will have an anxiety-reducing property if given in a lesser dosage.

Tolerance A particular problem with all these medicine is the development of *tolerance*. This means that the patient's body adapts to the medicine so that more and more has to be given in order to achieve the same effect. When a patient develops a dependence on a medicine, he or she is likely to experience adverse effects when the medicine is withdrawn. If the dependence is a physical one, these adverse effects will commonly take the form of physical symptoms. Thus the patient who is dependent on barbiturates may experience withdrawal symptoms that include extreme restlessness, and even convulsions. Uncontrolled and unsupervised withdrawal in such circumstances, sometimes referred to as 'cold turkey', can be a very dangerous procedure.

Psychological dependence is the psychological counterpart, and the patient may experience overwhelming anxiety associated with the realisation that this emotional prop is being withdrawn. In general, psychological dependence seems to occur earlier than physical dependence and is usually rather easier to contend with.

Emotional basis Medical practitioners soon come to learn that many of the ailments patients bring to the surgery have an emotional basis. In Chapter 2.4, The emotions and disease (p. 77) are listed some of the conditions where emotional stress is believed to play a significant part. Most of these conditions will be alleviated to a greater or lesser extent by the use of agents which reduce anxiety. In many cases the results are quite spectacular and sometimes people who have been unable to cope with work and have become semi-invalids are able to resume meaningful and useful lives. The most frequent and least severe symptom of anxiety is tiredness, and often such patients will come to the doctor requesting a 'tonic' or vitamins to give them more vigour.

Masking symptoms

Much debate within the medical profession has centred on whether it is legitimate to use anxiety-relieving medicines when it is clear that all that is being provided is symptomatic relief and the root cause of the problem is possibly being ignored. It can be likened to painting over rust. All may appear to be well, but deep down and now out of sight, the trouble continues. Some would even claim that in the long term the patient is actually worse off.

Medical students today are taught that they should not prescribe these agents except on a short-term basis to tide people over particular crises and that every effort should be made to establish the reasons for the anxiety and to find alternative means of coping with it. In an effort to identify the root causes, doctors often have to ask their patients some very personal questions. Do not be surprised at this, but try and answer honestly and fully. If you do withhold information, that is your privilege, but you should explain to the doctor that you would rather keep some things to yourself.

Some people appear to be constitutionally prone to anxiety and all means of control, other than medicines, seem in vain, however hard the doctor and patient strive. The doctor must then remember that he or she has a responsibility to alleviate pain (even emotional pain) where that is possible, tempering this with the old Latin nostrum *primum non nocere*, which means 'first do no harm'.

It becomes a matter of discussion and the weighing up of the pros and cons and then trying to make a joint decision which is in the best interest of the patient and not designed simply

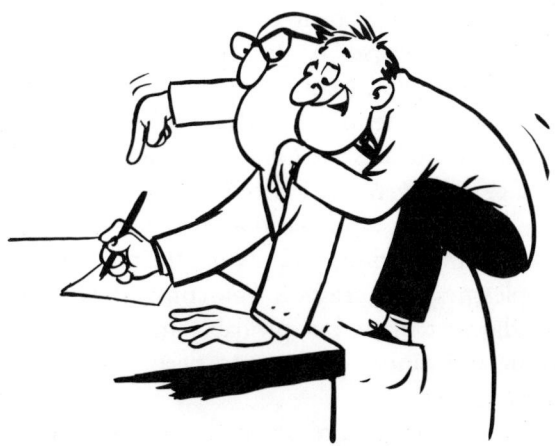

to get the patient 'off the doctor's back'. Such a decision also needs to take into account the development of tolerance already alluded to, the potential for dependence and the fact that often the relief of symptoms is of short duration. There are also the intrinsic side-effects of the medicine chosen. The same considerations have to be observed before commencing a patient on medication designed to produce sleep. The elderly are at particular risk as often such agents can produce confusion.

The principal medicines used in the treatment of anxiety are the benzodiazepines, and the most widely used would be diazepam (Valium). The first one to achieve popularity was chlordiazepoxide (Librium). Latterly there have been many variations on the theme, including lorazepam (Ativan) and oxazepam (Serepax). They have few side-effects, but rapidly produce dependency. Many medicines given for sleeplessness are also benzodiazepines. These include chlormezanone (Trancopal), flunitrazepam (Rohypnol), flurazepam (Dalmane), nitrazepam (Mogadon), temazepam (Euhypnos) and triazolam (Halcion). Also used sometimes as a means of relieving anxiety are the phenothiazines previously mentioned as a treatment for schizophrenia. The dosage of course is much smaller. Most phenothiazines have antihistamine properties and so are useful in allergies, but they are also valuable in the treatment of nausea, vomiting and giddiness. The phenothiazines seem rather less likely to cause dependence but have more side-effects. Probably the most alarming side-effect is a disorder similar to Parkinson's disease which is usually reversible, but very occasionally not.

The most frequently used phenothiazines would include chlorpromazine hydrochloride (Largactil), fluphenazine (Anatensol), pericyazine (Neulactil), perphenazine (Trilafon), prochlorperazine mesylate (Stemetil), promazine (Sparine), thioridazine hydrochloride (Melleril), and trifluoperazine dihydrochloride (Stelazine).

Sleeplessness (insomnia)

Most patients who have sleep problems do not require medication and the doctor should always try to establish the background to the problem.

Some people have problems with sleep because they expect to sleep too long. Need for sleep seems to diminish with age. The problem of sleeplessness is compounded by worry about it. If sufferers can achieve relaxation (see p. 192) they can often be almost as rested after a night of insomnia as if they had slept. Many people will sleep better if they are physically tired, so a brisk walk or a game of tennis each day may be of considerable assistance. It is wise to avoid anything which stimulates the mind prior to retiring and that includes exciting television, domestic disputes and even tea, coffee and other drinks which contain caffeine. It is claimed that tryptophane — an amino-acid — has sleep-inducing properties. Milk is a rich source of this and a warm milk drink certainly has the reputation of being an aid to sleep.

A frequent cause of sleeplessness is depression. Sometimes the depression leads to difficulties in getting off to sleep in the first place, but probably more often the patient wakes in the early hours of the morning and cannot get back to sleep. The condition usually disappears when the depression is controlled.

In fact some depression is apparently a result of chronic anxiety and if that is successfully dealt with, the depression lifts. Because of this, some of the anxiety-relieving medicines gained an early undeserved reputation as antidepressants. On the other hand, many of the medicines which are used to alleviate anxiety, rather than improving depression, actually make it worse. Clearly the response depends on the nature of the depression — another example of why medicines which are very effective for one person may not suit another.

Antidepressants

Possibly one of the greatest medical breakthroughs in the last few decades has been the development of antidepressant medicines. Formerly doctors had very little treatment that was effective for significant depression. Electro-convulsive therapy (ECT or 'shock treatment') was one of the few treatments which seemed to help, but was disliked by many patients. Psychiatrists believe ECT still has a small place for those patients who do not respond to other measures, but these days it is used very sparingly.

Tricyclics The group of medicines which have been used most widely in depression are known as the *tricyclics* and the first to be extensively used was imipramine (Tofranil). The exact means by which they work is still uncertain, but it would appear that for the cells of the brain to function normally, it is necessary that certain amine-type substances be present in sufficient quantity. It would seem that depressed patients have a deficiency of these amines and that the tricyclics make available to the cells an increased quantity of these naturally occurring substances. Other tricyclics are amitriptyline (Laroxyl, Tryptanol, Elavil), nortriptyline (Allegron, Aventyl), clomipramine (Anafranil), protriptyline (Concordin, Vivactil), dothiepin (Prothiaden), doxepin (Sinequan) and trimipramine (Surmontil). It would thus seem that the tricyclics have a facilitating role, in a way, remedying a deficiency. In this sense these medicines can be likened to insulin and its role in the body's utilisation of sugar. In the absence of adequate amounts of insulin, patients develop diabetes.

Unfortunately the benefits of antidepressants are not usually immediate and because the medicines have certain side-effects which develop before any improvement is seen, some people stop the treatment before reaping the rewards. Doctors, knowing this, usually introduce the treatment gradually so that the side-effects do not hit the patient too hard, and some tolerance to them can develop. The worst side-effect of the tricyclics for most people tends to be drowsiness and doctors have learnt that because of this and the fact that they have a prolonged action, it is best to give most, if not all, of the tablets at night. In fact this can be helpful for, as mentioned earlier, many depressed people experience difficulties with sleep, and something which tends to promote sleep is often welcomed so long as the drowsiness does not 'hang over' and persist throughout the next day.

Side-effects The other side-effects of tricyclics are similar to the effects of the medicine called atropine. These include an often troublesome dryness of the mouth and sometimes difficulty with focussing the eyes. Constipation can also be a problem but this is often a feature of depression anyway. Older men who have prostate problems may find that these are aggravated. Rapid beating of the heart can occur. People usually have to persevere with the tricyclics for three or four weeks before they are rewarded with the lifting of the spirits which commonly is the response to this treatment. Sometimes this change of mood is so gradual that patients think it has occurred spontaneously and so discontinue the treatment. Usually such patients then slowly drift back into their former depressed state. Of course, ultimately most depressions do resolve without treatment, but the patient may suffer much before this occurs.

Recently a modified form of the tricyclics has been introduced with a view to improving their effectiveness and reducing the side-effects, e.g. maprotiline (Ludiomil) and mianserin (Tolvon). These are the *tetracyclics* — not to be confused with the antibiotics known as tetracyclines.

It is unusual for people to become dependent on antidepressants.

Depression is a strange disorder and probably has more than one cause. Certainly many depressions seem to be based on external events, for example a bereavement. Others seem to have no known origin — the depression just seems to well up from within the person. The latter have never really been explained. Some psychiatrists suggest they are a response to suppressed anger. Others consider that the depression is a learnt but abnormal way of coping with life; yet others believe, as already mentioned, that this depression is due primarily to a biochemical abnormality in the cells. The response to medication would seem to support at least in part the latter suggestion.

It used to be thought that the depressions which were clearly a response to external events did not respond to medication, but recent studies suggest that the tricyclic medicines can help even these.

Mono-amine oxidase inhibitors

There is another family of medicines which are used for depression. These are known as the *mono-amine oxidase inhibitors* (MAO inhibitors). Again, these seem to affect the availability to the cells of certain amines by interfering with the natural breakdown (by a process known as *oxidation*) of these substances. These medicines tend to work a little more rapidly than the tricyclics, but they have even more severe side-effects for some people. Sometimes they work well in patients who have shown no response to the tricyclics. The side-effects are mostly brought on as a result of the patient taking certain foods when they are on the medicine.

Here is some standard advice which is given to patients about to commence these medicines:

'While taking this medicine and for 14 days after your treatment finishes, you must observe the following instructions.

1. Do not eat **cheese, pickled herring** or **broad-bean pods**.
2. Do not eat or drink **Bovril, Oxo, Marmite, Vegemite** or any similar **meat or yeast extract**.
3. Eat only **fresh foods** and avoid food that you suspect could be stale or 'going off'. This is especially important with **meat, fish, poultry** or **offal**. Avoid **game**.
4. Do not take any other **medicines** (including tablets, capsules, nose drops, inhalations or suppositories), whether purchased by you or previously prescribed by your doctor, without first consulting your doctor or your pharmacist. *Note*: Treatment for coughs and colds, pain relievers, tonics and laxatives are medicines.
5. **Avoid alcoholic drinks**.

'Keep a careful note of any food or drink that disagrees with you, avoid it and tell your doctor. Report any unusual or severe symptoms to your doctor and follow any advice that your doctor gives you.'

It also seems desirable that the tricyclic-type medicines should not be combined with the mono-amine oxidase inhibitors except very occasionally under strict medical control. Certain other medicines do not combine well with the mono-amine oxidase inhibitors, and these include: the antidiabetic tablets, morphine and allied painkillers, guanethidine sulphate, ephedrine, amphetamine, tryptophan, fenfluramine, levodopa, reserpine and most decongestants.

Bedwetting

Curiously, the tricyclic medicines have been found to be helpful in what appears to be quite a different context. This is *nocturnal enuresis*, the very distressing situation of children losing bladder control at night and so wetting the bed. For some children such treatment seems to be the only method that will work. However, many authorities do not favour the use of such powerful medicines for such a purpose, despite the low dosage usually required. It is often suggested that, if used at all, then tricyclics should only be used for a few weeks, perhaps to tide the patient over a special occasion such as a camping trip, and then discontinued. Most such children ultimately gain control of the bladder but usually not without a lot of embarrassment and much extra laundering of bedclothes. Bedwetting is not considered abnormal until after the age of five and even after that, many will become dry spontaneously.

Lithium

There is one other substance which to most researchers' surprise has been shown to be helpful in certain depressions. This is lithium. Most of us recognise that we go through phases when we feel exceptionally good ('on a high') and then we go through times when we feel rather low ('a down'). In some people these natural highs and lows seem to be exaggerated. These people are spoken of as *manic-depressive*. I recall one patient who was thus afflicted and who, when she was in the manic phase, would be up at 5 am every day, working happily in her garden and getting a tremendous amount done. A few weeks later, when the cycle had reversed, she would be lethargic and tearful and her husband frequently could not persuade her to get out of bed all day.

People such as this often show a dramatic improvement on lithium salts. Lithium is a simple element not unlike sodium, which is the principal component of common table salt. Lithium carbonate or lithium citrate are the usual forms used and they must be administered with care and discretion because there are many hazards if the dose is excessive. Long-term use can sometimes lead to thyroid problems, and the use of diuretics or the presence of vomiting may produce difficulties as a result of increased concentration in the bloodstream. Anybody who is taking lithium regularly should have frequent blood tests to monitor the level of lithium in the body.

Medicines which act on the nervous system

There are certain medicines which act by stimulating the nervous system. The best known of these is *caffeine*, which is present in tea and coffee. This is regarded as one of the safest substances known, but people vary widely in their sensitivity and some people will avoid tea and coffee because of the unwanted effects that they experience. Others will drink either beverage in great quantity just for the extra nervous energy and the alertness that caffeine provides. The side-effects include excessive and prolonged wakefulness, increased urine output, tremulousness, increased stomach acidity and sometimes irregular or rapid beating of the heart. Some people, accustomed to a high intake of caffeine in tea or coffee, will experience bad headaches when these substances are discontinued.

Amphetamine A much more potent stimulant is *amphetamine*. In the past this has been used by students to keep awake and so prolong their studies; by long-distance drivers to prevent themselves falling asleep at the wheel; and by overweight people to help them lose weight. Unfortunately this substance has a rapid ability to give people a sense of wellbeing which is habit forming. Furthermore, after the artificial 'high' that is experienced there is a 'let-down' period when users feel jaded and enervated. Latterly amphetamine has been eagerly sought for illicit purposes and has been nicknamed 'speed'.

As a general rule it is very unwise of doctors to prescribe amphetamines except for one or two very rare conditions, and then only with suitable precautions. In the writer's view the risk of dependence ('addiction') is so great, and the consequences so serious, that the use of the amphetamines cannot be justified in the treatment of obesity. It is said that certain other medicines, e.g. diethylpropion hydrochloride (Apisate, Tenuate), mazindol (Sanorex) and phentermine hydrochloride (Duromine, Ionamin, Umine) provide much less stimulation and that the risk of dependence is much less. However, they are not without risk altogether and in the author's view should be avoided. Fenfluramine hydrochloride (Ponderax) is not a stimulant and some consider it free from these hazards. However, as has already been discussed in Chapters 2.4 and 2.5 on dieting, the way to weight loss is not found in a bottle.

Epilepsy (fits)

Another group of medicines which act on the nervous system are those which are used to control *epilepsy*.

Epileptic attacks arise as a result of sudden spontaneous abnormal electrical discharges within the brain. Anti-epileptic medicines are used to suppress these unwanted discharges, which can cause the sufferer great embarrassment and can, of course, be very dangerous if the patient is in a hazardous environment. The attacks are often alarming to onlookers, and for this reason much unnecessary stigma is attached to epilepsy. In the more severe forms of epilepsy patients usually become unconscious for some time. Contrary to popular opinion, epilepsy is not related to insanity and many famous people have been epileptic, among the better known being Dostoevsky and Julius Caesar.

The medicines which are used for epilepsy are frequently very similar to those which are used as tranquillisers and they too often have the capacity to cause drowsiness. At one time medicines known as bromides were widely used and these caused acne, among other side-effects. The barbiturates which are best known for their use in producing sleep are still used extensively in the management of epilepsy, although seldom now for insomnia. If the dosage is too great, speech becomes slowed and the gait uncoordinated. It is possible to adjust the dosage to the best possible level in the bloodstream by appropriate blood tests. Phenobarbitone, phenytoin sodium (Dilantin, Epanutin) and primidone (Mysoline) are the three most widely used barbiturate-type medications. Sometimes phenytoin can produce overdevelopment of the gums and dental attention may be required.

In an acute attack of epilepsy one of the most useful agents is diazepam (Valium) which of course is one of the best known tranquillisers. In these circumstances the diazepam is usually injected directly into the veins.

Another medicine which is often used is carbamazepine (Tegretol). This is less inclined to cause drowsiness than the barbiturates. It is an interesting substance in that it helps many patients who experience the very distressing and disabling stabs of pain that occasionally occur as part of a facial neuralgia known medically as neuralgia of the trigeminal nerve (the fifth cranial nerve). This pain seems to be due to a sudden discharge of impulses along the pathways of this nerve which carries pain sensations from most of the skin of the face. The pain is often precipitated by touching a trigger-point, usually in the middle of the face or in the mouth. It is sometimes so severe and persistent that patients become suicidal.

Petit mal 'absences' There are other forms of epilepsy, different from the major attacks causing prolonged unconsciousness (known as *grand mal*) mentioned above. One of these is known as *petit mal* (French for 'little sickness') and usually consists merely of brief 'absences'. This means that the person — usually a child — experiences a brief spell when for an instant he or she is unaware of his or her surroundings. A moment or two later concentration returns and the person resumes where he or she left off. Medicines which are often used to prevent absences are ethosuximide (Zarontin) and Sodium valproate (Epilim). Sodium valproate has the advantage that it can be used for both petit and grand mal. (The two conditions sometimes co-exist.)

It is very important that patients on medication for epilepsy should not suddenly discontinue treatment. Any changes which are made to their dosage should be made gradually as otherwise attacks may be precipitated. If in doubt about changes in treatment, always ask your doctor first.

Parkinson's disease

A disorder of the nervous system which is potentially disabling is Parkinson's disease. In its more severe forms the diagnosis of this is quite easy. The patient will commonly have a continuous movement of the hands (described medically as 'pill rolling') and sometimes a persistent nodding of the head. If the patient uses the hands or turns the head, the shaking stops until movement ceases. Associated with all this is an apparent limitation of the movements of the face which seem to reduce the range of expression. Sometimes the picture presented to the doctor is less obvious and the shaking (tremor) is not a prominent feature. A lack of expression in the face and a certain difficulty with some movements, such as turning over in bed at night, may be the only indications that something is amiss.

Research has shown that this relatively common disorder is due to an abnormality in a localised area of the brain known as the *substantia nigra*. Again the problem is a chemical one. It seems that a substance known as dopamine, which appears to be produced as a means of passing messages from one part of the brain to another, is in short supply. This leads to an imbalance in the impulses passing through certain of the nerves of movement and hence the spontaneous and unwanted movement. Treatment is designed to correct the imbalance. Unfortunately it does not interfere with the insidious progression of the condition.

Causes The damage to the brain cells which causes these problems is usually thought to be due to a poor blood supply, although some cases follow 20 or more years after a virus inflammation of the brain known as encephalitis. One particular epidemic of virus which was specially active shortly after World War I was responsible for many cases.

Many cases of Parkinson's disease benefit greatly from the administration of a substance called levodopa (Larodopa). This agent is converted in the body to dopamine and this then makes up the deficiency that exists. It is usually given in association with another medicine known as carbidopa (the combination being known as Sinemet) or benserazide (the combination being known as Madopar), which prevent the breakdown of levodopa, thus enabling an adequate amount of it to reach the brain. As a result, a smaller amount of levodopa is likely to be effective and there is a reduced chance of side-effects. For effective use, skilful balancing of the two medicines may be necessary. As with the treatment of epilepsy, it is very unwise to stop treatment abruptly.

An incompatibility Mono-amine oxidase medications (used for depression) should not be given at the same time as levodopa. People with Parkinson's disease who respond well to levodopa are likely to notice an improvement lasting a couple of years, but after that the inexorable decline continues.

Another medicine which apparently stimulates the nerve cells in the same way as levodopa but which has a different structure is bromocriptine (Parlodel). It is used mostly for those people who for one reason or another are not able to take levodopa. Other medicines with a small effect in Parkinson's disease are amantadine hydrochloride (Symmetrel), orphenadrine hydrochloride (Disipal), benzhexol hydrochloride (Artane, Pipanol), and benztropine mesylate (Cogentin).

4.5 The antibacterial medicines ('antibiotics')

'One of the first duties of the physician is to educate the masses not to take medicine'
— Attributed to Sir William Osler (1849-1919)

The term *antibacterial medicines* relates to those substances which are used to destroy bacteria (germs). These represent one of the greatest medical advances of the twentieth century. Regrettably, we have very few agents which will help in eradicating that other major group of infecting organisms, the viruses.

Viral infections

Many infections frequently seen in medical practice have a viral cause. The common cold is one; influenza, measles, German measles, hepatitis, chickenpox and glandular fever (infectious mononucleosis) are others. The antibacterial medicines have no place in these conditions and may even cause harm unless there is a bacterial infection in addition. There are now some medicines which help to fight viral infections but they are of limited value and useful in only a few situations such as the treatment of the herpes viruses (e.g. cold sores and shingles).

The result of all this is that there is seldom any reason for giving antibacterial medication (i.e. antibiotics or chemotherapeutic agents) to a patient with a common cold, 'the flu', or other viral infection.

Fortunately the body usually has the capacity to cope with viral infections, but occasionally a patient is overwhelmed and death occurs. A situation where the virus usually seems to beat the body's defences is AIDS — a virus infection which interferes with the body's ability to produce its own immunity. (See pp. 276-8.) 'AIDS' is an acronym for 'acquired immunodeficiency syndrome'.

Terminology The first of the antibacterial medicines to be produced was a *sulphonamide*. This is a chemical substance and so is sometimes referred to as a *chemotherapeutic agent*. The purists would confine the term *antibiotic* to those antibacterial medicines which have an origin in biological substances. The difference is a minor one and many people tend to group them all together under the general term 'antibiotic'.

Penicillin, identified by Alexander Fleming and developed by H. W. Florey, was the first of the antibiotics, coming as it did from the mould *Penicillium notatum*. Since then, many other antibacterials have been discovered, and older ones modified and improved.

The problem for the doctor is to determine, first, which infections are likely to be amenable to antibacterial medication, and then, which antibacterial will be the most suitable in the particular circumstances. Each antibacterial medicine has its own range of activity; no single one is capable of destroying, or eliminating, the whole range of bacteria. Sometimes bacteria which are initially sensitive to a particular antibacterial, lose that sensitivity and develop a resistance. This is thought to be due in many cases to the giving of an inadequate dose.

An animal analogy The situation may be likened to that in which one might set out to kill rats. One could conceive of a colony of rats which had some ability to cope with the usual form of rat poison. If rather less poison was laid than was desirable, all the rats would probably have what was available, but it is reasonable to suppose that the weak ones would be killed while the strong ones would survive and multiply. In this way one could anticipate that a stronger race would develop, with even greater powers to cope with fresh supplies of poison. Whereas initially the colony varied in its strength, now it would be uniformly strong and the rats would become more of a problem than hitherto. A similar situation may well exist with bacteria and this is why doctors plead with their patients to take the full course of treatment at the recommended dosage. Unless the antibacterial disagrees with you in some way, always take the whole quantity prescribed.

The spectrum The range of effectiveness of an antibacterial is often referred to as its *spectrum*. A 'wide spectrum' antibiotic is one which is effective against a large range of bacteria. The reason why amoxycillin has proved so popular is the breadth of its spectrum of activity.

Like all other medicines, antibiotics can have troublesome or even dangerous side-effects. One otherwise excellent antibiotic, chloramphenicol, has been almost abandoned in most countries because of the effect it can have on the production of white cells from the bone marrow. It is still often used locally in the eye for infections such as conjunctivitis and as eardrops. Apparently, in these situations, little or none is absorbed and so the marrow is not at risk.

Some antibacterials act by killing the bacteria outright (*bactericidal*), while others act by merely preventing the reproduction of the bacteria (*bacteriostatic*). If two antibacterials are given at once, it is usually better not to combine a bacteriostatic and a bactericidal one.

It becomes clear that the decision about who should get which antibiotic can be a very complex one and certainly people should not be treating themselves with antibiotics without adequate knowledge. Often when I suggest a particular antibacterial to a patient, he or she will say to me 'I had that before and it didn't work'. It would seem that patients suppose that the antibiotic acts on them rather than on the bacteria.

Whether an antibacterial works in any particular situation depends very much on the nature of the bacteria and not on the person who has the infection. The same person may on one occasion have a bacterial infection which is cured by a particular antibacterial and on another occasion a similar infection caused by different bacteria which are completely resistant to that same antibacterial, and as a result they remain unwell. Having said that, it should in fairness be stated that some people do seem to have a susceptibility to certain bacteria, e.g. as a cause of infection in the urine, and as a result one might expect the infection to respond to the same antibacterial each time. However, even the same bacteria may develop the ability to resist an antibacterial that was previously effective.

Penicillin

Penicillin in its various forms is for most people a very safe antibiotic, but some patients do get allergic reactions and very occasionally these can be so severe as to be fatal. More often the allergy is a mild one and takes the form of a rash. Unfortunately, once a person has developed an allergy to penicillin, it is considered wise never to use it again on that patient except under very closely supervised conditions, and then only in an extreme emergency. It seems reasonable to suppose that the more often a person takes penicillin the more likely it is that an allergy to it will occur. This is why penicillin and other antibacterials should be used sparingly and you should not try to pressure your doctor into giving you one when he or she thinks it is unwarranted.

Of course, some people are required to take prolonged courses of antibacterials; the use of penicillin in people who are susceptible to rheumatic fever is a good example. Rheumatic fever is a condition which can be very destructive to the valves of the heart. It seems to be due to an abnormal response by the body to a fairly common infection with bacteria known as β haemolytic streptococci. This susceptibility is at its greatest between the ages of five and 15 years. Within this age group, anybody who has a sore throat caused by the streptococcus for more than about seven days should have preventive treatment by penicillin. This treatment should be continued for ten days if the streptococcus is to be completely eliminated from the throat. If this regime is carried out, the chance of developing rheumatic fever is very remote. However, once a person has had one rheumatic fever attack, any subsequent infection with the offending streptococcus may well stimulate a further attack. It is for this reason that such people are placed on long-term continuing treatment with penicillin and it is very fortunate for us that the streptococcus does not seem to have developed any resistance to penicillin.

Semi-synthetic penicillins Biochemists have been successful in altering the chemical structure of the naturally occurring penicillin, thus making more effective antibiotics. These are the *semi-synthetic penicillins*. Some staphylococci produce a substance called *penicillinase* which is capable of rendering penicillin ineffective. Flucloxacillin sodium (Floxapen) has been developed in order to overcome the effects of penicillinase. Flucloxacillin is not destroyed by stomach acid and so can be taken by mouth.

Ampicillin (Penbritin) is not effective against staphylococci which produce penicillinase, but has a wider spectrum of activity than ordinary penicillin. Amoxycillin (Amoxil) is a further derivative of ampicillin which has much the same range of activity, but is better absorbed when taken by mouth. It can even be taken when there is food in the stomach.

A more recent development is the addition of a substance called *clavulanic acid* to the amoxycillin. Clavulanic acid also inactivates penicillinase and so this combination has a very wide range of activity. The combined preparation is known as Augmentin.

If a person develops an allergy to any one form of penicillin, it is likely that he or she will find this same reaction is stimulated by all other forms of penicillin.

The cephalosporins

A fungus known as *cephalosporium* has been responsible for providing another group of antibiotics called the cephalosporins. The cephalosporins have many features in common with the penicillins and there is even some cross-sensitivity so that about 10 per cent of people who are allergic to penicillin are also allergic to cephalosporins and vice versa. Nevertheless, they make a good alternative to penicillin and in some situations are more effective than the penicillins.

The most commonly prescribed cephalosporins for use by mouth are cefaclor (Ceclor), cephalexin monohydrate (Keflex) and cephradine (Velosef).

Throat infections Happily, most people with throat infections — even with the β haemolytic streptococcus — have natural defences which lead to the infection clearing up in fewer than seven days, so that usually neither throat swabs nor antibacterials are necessary.

For those people who require prolonged protection from the β haemolytic streptococci, it is important that they take penicillin by mouth every day without fail, or if their memories are not good, that they have regular, long-acting injections of penicillin. Unfortunately, after many years of such preventive treatment some people become very casual and careless about their penicillin-taking and often stop altogether. The results can be very serious.

Diagnosis

As far as possible, antibacterials should not be given until after a definitive diagnosis is made, i.e. the doctor is sure about the nature of the disease being treated. Occasionally a patient may have a severe infection and be so very ill that the doctor may decide to give an antibacterial without making a proper diagnosis. This should be a rare occurrence, for often after the antibacterial has been given, it becomes even more difficult to make a diagnosis because it has altered the manifestations of the disease — yet another reason why people should not treat themselves. If the treatment is only partially successful, this may make it very hard to know what further action to take.

Modern sulphonamide treatments

These days the most widely used sulphonamide is co-trimoxazole, often known as either Bactrim or Septrin. These tablets contain both a sulphonamide and another substance known as *trimethoprim* which has an action on the folic acid utilisation of the bacteria and so enhances the activity of the sulphonamide against those bacteria which use folic acid — a vitamin. In fact, trimethoprim can be used on its own, particularly for infections of the urinary system. Co-trimoxazole as a consequence has a wide spectrum of activity and is used extensively in medical practice. As with all medicines, co-trimoxazole is not without side-effects, but these are fairly rare, although allergic rashes are by no means uncommon.

Bowel infections

Most bowel infections do not require antibacterials as the bowel seems to be very effective in coping with them. Such infections usually manifest themselves in the form of diarrhoea. In fact, antibacterials can sometimes worsen the situation by disturbing the natural balance which exists between bacteria and certain yeasts which colonise the normal bowel. These organisms live in harmony together (symbiosis) and cause no trouble unless an imbalance occurs. Antibacterials will kill bacteria whether they are normal inhabitants or not, and an overgrowth of yeasts may itself lead to diarrhoea and/or skin infections around the bowel opening and genitals. Because of this, some people recommend that patients who are given antibacterials by mouth should be advised to take yoghurt at the same time, for this, if it has not been sterilised, contains most of the organisms necessary to re-colonise the bowel. These days this advice is seldom given because it does not seem to take long for new colonies to establish themselves naturally.

Typhoid   One type of infection of the bowel, which is fortunately very rare, is that caused by salmonella, and the most severe of these is that responsible for typhoid. Such infections usually warrant antibacterial treatment and co-trimoxazole and amoxycillin are both effective.

Other uses for the sulphonamides include the treatment of chest and urinary tract infections. The sulphonamides also have a role in preventing skin infections after burns, but in these circumstances they are usually applied directly to the damaged area.

Tetracyclines

Another group of medicines which has had a wide popularity for its broad spectrum of activity is the *tetracycline* series. Until the advent of amoxycillin, the tetracyclines were probably the most widely prescribed antibiotic. They still have an important place but are avoided in children because of the staining, and even a failure of normal development of the teeth, which they sometimes cause. The damage in children is particularly severe antenatally if large doses are given to the mother in the course of pregnancy. The tetracyclines should also be avoided in cases of kidney failure as this may be worsened by their use. This effect on the kidneys does not seem to occur with doxycycline and minocycline.

Over the years many bacteria have developed a resistance to the tetracyclines but they are still effective in the treatment of chlamydia, rickettsia (which causes Q-fever), mycoplasma and brucella organisms. They are also capable of destroying the haemophilus influenzae organism which is responsible for much respiratory infection — particularly bronchitis.

Another common use for the tetracyclines is in the management of acne — the troublesome pimples that affect so many adolescents. Resistant cases of acne nearly always improve with prolonged use of tetracyclines. The action seems to go beyond killing the bacteria which play a part in causing acne and seems to extend to an effect on the associated inflammatory reaction of the skin itself. (See p. 183.)

Erythromycin

Another useful antibiotic is *erythromycin*. This has a range of activity rather similar to penicillin and is often used in its stead for patients who have developed an allergy to it. Erythromycin is also capable of killing many of the staphylococcal organisms which have developed a resistance to penicillin. It is apparently effective in Legionnaire's disease if instituted early enough. Chlamydia organisms and mycoplasmas are also sensitive.

Aminoglycosides

There is a further group of antibiotics known as the *aminoglycosides*. This group includes gentamicin, kanamycin, neomycin, streptomycin and tobramycin sulphate, among others. These too have a wide range of activity and will attack many bacteria which are not affected by penicillin. Streptomycin and kanamycin are usually effective against the organism responsible for tuberculosis. Unfortunately they are not well absorbed from the bowel and as a result cannot be given by mouth. Therefore except in bowel infections, they must be administered by injection.

All of this group tend to be harmful to the ears, the organs of balance, and the kidneys, and where possible they should be given for a short time only. Certainly they should not be given concurrently with either of the diuretic medicines, frusemide (Lasix) or ethacrynic acid (Edecrin), which themselves are capable of producing similar damage.

Gentamicin is the first choice of many doctors for the treatment of serious infections with those organisms which are described as 'gram negative' when they are stained for microscopic examination using gram's stain — a system used for differentiating certain broad categories of bacteria.

Neomycin is widely used by local application in the treatment of skin infections. Framycetin is similar to neomycin and also applied locally, as is gentamicin. If a skin allergy develops towards one of these agents, it usually occurs with the others as well.

Metronidazole (Flagyl)

There are a number of other antibacterials which have specialised uses but it would be confusing and unhelpful to review them all.

However, there is one medicine which is perhaps worthy of mention because of the extraordinary range of its activity. This is metronidazole (usually marketed as Flagyl). This is effective against those bacteria which are unable to tolerate oxygen — the so-called anaerobic bacteria — as well as some protozoa. Anaerobic bacteria are a cause of some bowel infections and so-called non-specific vaginal discharge.

Protozoa are not bacteria at all; they fall into the category of *parasitic microbes*. The best known protozoa are: giardia lamblia which is capable of causing severe diarrhoea; trichomonas, which causes a specific vaginal discharge and irritation (see also section 3.24, pp.174–7); entamoeba histolytica, which can also lead to diarrhoea; and trypanosoma, which in tropical areas is a cause of sleeping sickness. Metronidazole is widely used in the treatment of the first two of these disorders.

Nitrofurantoin and nalidixic acid

There are certain substances which have an antiseptic action on bacteria in the urine but which have little or no action on bacteria in any other part of the body. Nitrofurantoin (Furadantin) is such a substance. It is best taken during or after meals, or with milk, as it is less likely to cause stomach upsets under these circumstances. It is not given to people whose kidney function is deteriorating and is more effective if the urine is slightly acid.

Nalidixic acid (Negram, Mictral) is another urinary antiseptic which is used particularly when the urine is infected with Bacterium coli organisms (sometimes known as Escherichia coli). Some people who have repeated urinary infections find that they can keep such infections at bay by taking a small dose of nitrofurantoin or nalidixic acid every day. Others achieve the same result by keeping the urine acid by taking say, ascorbic acid (vitamin C) regularly. Another agent, Citravescent, is used when it is important to keep the urine alkaline.

Antiviral agents

Unfortunately medical science has had very limited success in its search for anti-viral agents. It may be that the problem of AIDS will heighten interest and stimulate even greater research efforts. Actually a small amount of progress *has* been made and there is a substance, acyclovir (Zovirax), which is effective in the treatment of herpes simplex (cold sores) and to some degree in the treatment of herpes zoster (shingles) and chickenpox. Curiously, the last two conditions seem to be different manifestations of the same virus. Shingles sometimes makes its appearance early in life, particularly in persons whose immunity is reduced as a result of some other concurrent disorder such as leukaemia or cancer, or even when immunity is being artificially suppressed with a view to discouraging rejection of an organ transplant.

Acyclovir is only effective if given very early in the course of the infection. It may be given by mouth or through the bloodstream by injection into the veins in serious cases. It can also be administered by local application to the developing sore on the skin.

Idoxuridine (Herplex, Stoxil) is another antiviral agent which has a place in the treatment of cold sores and shingles. Unfortunately it cannot be taken by mouth. It too must be given very early in the disease and is used most frequently when the herpes involves the eye.

Amantadine Amantadine (Symmetrel) is yet another antiviral (this time taken by mouth only) which is used mostly in the prevention of a form of influenza known as 'influenza A'. It has also been used in the treatment of shingles.

Antifungal agents

Antifungal medicines represent another area of importance. Over the years many agents have been found to be effective in the management of fungal and yeast infections. The spores of these organisms, which are somewhat similar to seeds, are present in the atmosphere and infection is probably most commonly acquired from the floors of showers and swimming pool surrounds. The spores develop and thrive in any environment which is regularly moist, warm and protected from direct sunlight. Many of the body's crevices and folds fulfil these conditions admirably. Poorly ventilated shoes and moist sweaty feet make a perfect environment and fungal infections between the toes are commonplace. Other frequent sites are the groin, the armpits, beneath the breasts of overweight women, the vagina, and the penis, particularly in the uncircumcised.

Some fungal infections are acquired from animals and it is said that hedgehogs are almost invariably carriers. Dogs and cats often have these infections and can give their guardians the fungal infection known as ringworm. There is some doubt as to whether ringworm passes from one human host to another.

The best known yeast which acts as an infecting agent is candida albicans, sometimes known as monilia. This commonly invades the vagina and is also often found under the nails. It is also the cause of thrush in babies. Most fungal and yeast infections can be dealt with by local applications accompanied by a reversal of the environmental conditions described above as favourable to their growth.

Gentian violet One of the most effective local agents is gentian violet. This actually also has antibacterial properties which may be valuable when there is a mixed infection, as often occurs. The problem with gentian violet is that it is a most pervasive dye. This is fine when it comes to getting into skin crevices and the like, but it is disastrous if it spills on to carpets or stains bedclothes. For this reason it is not used as widely as it once was. Nystatin (Mycostatin) is a substance produced by certain bacteria which has similar effects on fungus infection but is not antibacterial. It is used for infections of the mouth and bowel with candida albicans. Sometimes it is given in conjunction with antibiotics in an effort to prevent the imbalance in the growth of organisms that may occur with the use of antibiotics, already discussed on p. 239. Pessaries are available for vaginal application.

There are a number of new antifungals which are used either locally or by mouth; clotrimazole (Canestan), ketoconazole (Nizoral) and miconazole (Daktarin) are among the best known of these. They also may be administered by pessary and in this form are very effective in dealing with vaginal infections. In such infections it is wise to treat the sexual partner as well, as otherwise prompt reinfection is common. Simultaneous treatment by mouth is only necessary in very resistant cases. Clotrimazole is not used by mouth but the other two are available in tablet form for this purpose.

Acid/alkali balance The benefits of local treatment of the vagina by antifungals are enhanced if the normal acid/alkali balance is maintained. In order to do this, a mild acidifying agent is desirable. There are a number of commercially available preparations, but many people find they can achieve the same object by the use of dilute vinegar or even yoghurt.

A small tampon can be placed briefly in a warm solution of dilute vinegar. The tampon is then placed in the vagina before it has had a chance to swell appreciably. Such a procedure should ensure that the total surface of the vagina is adequately covered.

People who have poor immunity to infection, as in AIDS and some other conditions, may have widespread fungal infections which are very hard to eradicate. Such infections sometimes respond to an antifungal agent known as amphotericin B. This can also be given directly into the bloodstream through the veins (i.e. intravenously).

Resistant skin infections — particularly of the ringworm type and those which involve the fingernails — often settle very satisfactorily with a prolonged course of griseofulvin (Grisovin). Griseofulvin is not helpful when the infection is due to candida albicans. In the case of fingernails, the treatment usually has to be continued for at least six months — sufficient time for the nails to grow out from the nailbeds to their normal length without infection.

4.6 Medicines for treating high blood pressure and circulatory disorders

'From inability to let well alone: from too much zeal for the new and contempt for what is old; from putting knowledge before wisdom, science before art, and cleverness before common sense, from treating patients as cases, and from making the cure of the disease more grievous than the endurance of the same, Good Lord deliver us'.

— Sir Robert Hutchison, *British Medical Journal*, 1953

As is discussed elsewhere, high blood pressure can have a damaging effect on the blood vessels. There is now evidence that the chance of a stroke can be considerably reduced if blood pressure over 110 diastolic (see p. 244) and possibly lower levels, is controlled. It is possible that the chances of a heart attack due to blockage of the arteries to the heart may also be reduced, but this is less certain.

There are two components to the blood pressure. One is the pressure in the blood vessels when the heart is contracted (systole) and the other is the pressure when the heart is relaxed after a beat (diastole). Accordingly, the first pressure is known as the *systolic* pressure and the second the *diastolic* pressure. The evidence suggests that both these levels are important but that a high diastolic pressure is probably more damaging than a high systolic pressure. Certainly the systolic pressure seems to be subject to much more fluctuation and will often rise when the patient is experiencing anxiety, as before an examination, or after strenuous exercise. Usually when a person is relaxed and rested the systolic pressure will fall back to normal levels.

Faintness

Warmth seems to cause blood vessels to relax and as a consequence a fall in blood pressure occurs. Many people, when they suddenly stand up after being in a reclining posture for some time, will experience a sensation of light-headedness or faintness. This is due to a delay in the body's adaptation to the new posture, such that for a few moments there is an inadequate amount of blood getting to the brain. This is likely to be more pronounced in hot weather. Some people will actually collapse in a faint on such occasions. Most faints are caused by a reduced circulation of blood to the brain due to a slowing of the heart, a relaxation of the blood vessels leading to a fall in blood pressure and sometimes a measure of pooling of blood in the lower extremities.

The best treatment is to place the patient on the ground and elevate the legs. This will encourage the return of blood to the upper extremities, particularly the brain. *Do not sit up a fainting patient.*

Faintness is a common side-effect of the treatment of blood pressure and if it occurs, the same management is appropriate. In fact, provided it does not interfere with the patient's activities, a slight light-headedness when on treatment for blood pressure should be seen as an indication that the patient is getting a significant response to treatment. In fact, it is usually a sign that no further drop in the blood pressure is likely to be tolerated by the patient.

There is much debate in medical circles about what constitutes normal blood pressure. It is known that the blood pressure tends to rise with increasing age and this may be partly because the vessels become firm and less elastic and so find it difficult to accommodate the extra fluid forced into them when the heart contracts. The systolic pressure (associated with contraction of the heart) is the component which changes most with age. Some doctors, as a rule-of-thumb, suggest that the upper limit to be regarded as normal for the systolic pressure should approximate to 100 plus the patient's age, in mm of mercury.

Thus for a 50-year-old person, 150 might be thought of as the upper limit of normal. Nevertheless, this is a rather arbitrary figure and most people are wise to leave to their own doctor the decision as to what deserves to be treated in their particular case. The same applies to the pressure when the heart is relaxed (i.e. diastolic). Here there is usually much less variation. Most young people will have a pressure around 70 or 80 mm of mercury and many doctors would feel that if the pressure is over 90 in a person under 40, this is an indication that treatment should be started. On the other hand, if the patient were over 60, something like 100 mm of mercury in the diastolic pressure is probably going to be considered the lowest suitable for treatment. When the doctor records the blood pressure it is written 120/80 or 200/100, with the systolic pressure as the first figure and the diastolic following after.

Taking blood pressure

The instrument used for taking the blood pressure is a *sphygmomanometer*. The doctor will place a cuff around the patient's arm and blow it up until it reaches a level at which there is a complete obstruction to the blood passing into the arm. The doctor then listens with a stethoscope over the blood vessels of the elbow and nothing will be heard until the pressure in the tourniquet-like cuff is reduced a little and the systolic pressure is just sufficient to let enough blood through to generate a pulsing sound. This level of pressure is then noted as the systolic pressure. The pressure in the cuff is then slowly released until the stream of blood is such that again no noises are heard. The point when the pulsing sounds are no longer heard in the stethoscope corresponds to the diastolic pressure.

No one knows for sure the reason for the behaviour of these sounds but the method seems to be reasonably accurate, although sometimes there is discussion about the exact point at which the sounds cease to be of significance.

Most high blood pressure (i.e. *hypertension*), is of unknown cause and is referred to as 'essential hypertension'. Occasionally it is due to kidney disease or some abnormality of the adrenal glands. This is spoken of as 'secondary hypertension'.

As high blood pressure is caused mostly by a narrowing of the arteries, treatment is usually directed towards dilating the blood vessels or reducing the volume of fluid within them.

Diuretics

Probably the most widely used treatment for high blood pressure today would be medications which increase the output of urine. These are known as *diuretics*. (See also pp. 256–7.) Initially these do have an effect on the volume of the blood and this reduces the blood pressure. However, after a few weeks the body seems to adjust to this and the blood volume returns to its former level. However, the blood pressure often remains down, and this is thought to be due to dilatation of the arteries. In some people diuretics are used alone, but more often these are given in combination with some other medication. In these circumstances, the diuretic seems to reinforce the action of the other agent, often enabling the dose to be kept low, and so avoiding side-effects.

Diuretics do not seem to lower the blood pressure in people who have not got an abnormally elevated blood pressure. The contraction (i.e. tightening) of the muscles in the walls of the arteries seems to be under the control of the nervous system. The part of the nervous system involved is often referred to as the *autonomic nervous system*. This name is given to it as it is that part of the nervous system which acts autonomously, i.e. independently of the wishes and will of the person.

This is in contradistinction to the voluntary nervous system over which we have considerable control and which is responsible for all movement which we deliberately initiate.

Autonomic nervous system control The contraction of the type of muscle (smooth muscle) that controls the diameter of blood vessels is under autonomic nervous system control and this means that it is influenced by the minute electrical impulses passing through these nerves. At the end of these nerves *adrenalin (epinephrine)* and a similar substance called *nor-adrenalin (nor-epinephrine)* is produced and these substances can have a direct effect on the muscle. Curiously, the action of nor-adrenalin seems always to cause contraction and constriction but the action of adrenalin varies in different sites. This is believed to be due to differing ways by which this substance is received in the various tissues. Certain medicines have the ability to interfere with this action of adrenalin and adrenalin-like agents on the muscle activity. When this is primarily on the contraction of muscles of blood vessels, the medicines that prevent the action are known as *alpha-adrenergic blocking agents* or *alpha-blockers*. When this is primarily on the heart (which is also smooth muscle and really is formed as a complex development of the blood vessels) they are known as *beta adrenergic blocking agents* or *beta blockers*.

In some circumstances, if the action of the nor-adrenalin is blocked, the adrenalin, then acting alone, actually has the effect of dilating the blood vessels (vasodilator). Other medicines do not act directly on the muscle, but prevent the release of adrenalin or adrenalin-like substances from the autonomic nerve endings. Guanethidine sulphate (Ismelin) is such a substance, but is seldom used nowadays.

Yet others prevent the transmission of nervous impulses across the junctions between nerves in the autonomic nervous system. These are sometimes referred to as the 'ganglion blockers'. Hexamethonium and mecamylamine (Inversine) are examples of this sort of medicine but they also are seldom used today.

Dual-acting medications Some medications appear to act in more than one way. Methyldopa (Aldomet) is such a one. Not only does it prevent the release of adrenalin-like substances by the autonomic nerves but it also has an action on the brain and spinal cord ('central effect') which is beneficial in patients with high blood pressure. Rauwolfia and medicines derived from it also appear to reduce the level of adrenalin and adrenalin-like substances in the brain and spinal cord. Reserpine and Serpasil are examples and these were once widely used in the management of high blood pressure.

Of course, the situation is considerably more complex than stated here and in some instances the exact mode of action remains uncertain. It needs to be remembered, too, that adrenalin has a number of other actions in the body. One of these is the relaxation of the smooth muscle in the bronchial tubes which form the air passages to the lungs. In asthma one of the problems is the contraction and tightening of these muscles, which are not under voluntary control. Adrenalin and similar substances have an important use in relaxing these muscles. However, if the patient has had beta-blocking medications (q.v.), the adrenalin will not work on the muscle and the patient finds the treatment is ineffective. For this reason, people who are suffering from high blood pressure and who are also asthmatic should not be given beta blockers.

In a similar way, adrenalin has the ability to assist in the release of glucose (blood sugar) from the stores of glycogen in the liver. If a diabetic is given insulin in excess by mistake, this ability of the liver to produce extra glucose via the body's adrenalin is very important in stabilising the level of glucose in the bloodstream. Again, if the patient is on a beta-blocking agent, this action will not be possible. (See also p. 270.) The autonomic nervous system not only controls the smooth muscle in blood vessels, heart and bronchial tubes; it also has actions in other sites and as a result, agents which are designed to block these actions may at the same time block other functions elsewhere. Thus certain of the treatments used for high blood pressure also reduce the activity of the smooth muscle in the walls of the bowel, leading to constipation. Others have an effect on the glands which secrete saliva, leading to a very dry mouth. Yet others can affect sexual function, sometimes causing impotence in men.

Side-effects

It is very important that anybody who is treated for high blood pressure should inform their doctor of any side-effects so that the treatment can be changed or the dosage modified. It is questionable whether it is worth having life prolonged by treatment if the quality of that life is seriously impaired.

Some of the treatments for high blood pressure dilate the blood vessels more directly. Hydralazine hydrochloride (Apresoline) is one such. It is usually used with a beta-blocking medicine as the latter has a slowing effect on the heart, whereas hydralazine has a tendency to cause an increase in the heart rate. Hydralazine is believed to increase the effectiveness of the vasodilatory actions of adrenalin alluded to earlier. It is often used where the kidneys are not functioning too well as it increases the blood flow to these organs.

Other medications for blood pressure include clonidine hydrochloride (Catapres) which is like methyldopa in that it appears to act directly on the brain. It is also used extensively in the prevention of migraine but in smaller dosage (e.g. Dixarit). It should never be stopped suddenly as this can lead to an abrupt and severe rise in blood pressure which can be dangerous.

Minoxidil (Loniten) is reserved for the treatment of severe blood pressure. It produces its effects by dilating the arteries and there is an associated increase in the rate of the heart beat which can be undesirable if the heart is already weakened. Like hydralazine, it is customary to give it together with a beta blocker and a diuretic. Applied locally to the scalp, a lotion of this substance (Regaine) has been found to stimulate hair growth.

Prazosin (Hypovase, Minipress) is not a beta blocker, but an alpha blocker. This causes dilatation of blood vessels but little or no increase in the heart rate. Apart from its use in blood pressure, it is sometimes prescribed for people prone to spasm of the blood vessels to the arms and hands, i.e. Raynaud's syndrome.

Verapamil, nifedipine and diltiazem are used most frequently for controlling an irregular heart beat. They all have some effect on blood pressure by causing dilatation of the arteries. These agents also have a place in the treatment of angina.

There is a substance known as angiotensin, which is produced in the liver, which can react with another substance from the kidney called renin. The combination acting on the blood vessels produces constriction of the arteries and consequent elevated blood pressure.

Certain medicines acting on angiotensin have been found to interfere with this reaction, and by dilating the arteries, lead to a fall in blood pressure. Captopril (Capoten) and enalapril maleate (Renitec) work in this way. Unlike most medicines which dilate arteries, there is no extra work required of the heart. They are often used when other medicines fail to bring the blood pressure under control.

Other uses for vasodilators

Dilatation of arteries has other uses in addition to lowering the blood pressure. Arteries to the brain and to the heart are of particular importance. When there is insufficient blood (and hence oxygen) getting to the brain, the patient may feel faint or, if there is a total blockage, may suffer brain damage. If the area affected in this way has an important function, the patient may lose that function. Thus if it affects nerve pathways controlling movement, the patient will be paralysed and is said to have had a *stroke* (otherwise known as a *cerebrovascular accident*). Sometimes the paralysis is short lived, and the episode is referred to as a TIA which stands for *transient ischaemic attack*. Ischaemia is a word for diminished blood supply.

When there is insufficient blood to the heart, the patient will usually, initially, experience a tight pain in the chest. This is heart pain brought about by the lack of oxygen in the heart muscle and it is known as *angina* or cardiac ischaemia. If this angina is very severe, the heart muscle may be permanently damaged and the nervous supply of the heart may be interrupted.

In these circumstances the patient is said to have had a heart attack or *coronary*. If the damage is severe, the heart may be weakened and even destroyed. If the nerve pathways supplying the heart muscle are involved, there may be interruption of the nervous impulses that control the heart with the result that the heart beats erratically or perhaps stops altogether.

The arteries which supply the heart, known as the *coronary arteries*, seem to be particularly prone to suffer from the changes to their lining known as *atheroma* (or *atherosclerosis*).

Glyceryl trinitrate Some medicines capable of dilating arteries are used in the treatment of both high blood pressure and angina, while others seem to be more effective for one or the other. One that is used particularly to dilate the coronary arteries is *glyceryl trinitrate* — which chemically is closely related to the explosive nitroglycerine. This substance comes in the form of a small pellet (known as Trinitrin, Nitrobid, Nitrostat or Anginine) which is placed in the mouth and chewed. The fragments are then supposed to be put under the tongue where the active ingredients are rapidly absorbed. Within about 30 seconds many patients will experience some relief from their angina. If the pain goes before all the tablet is used, it is a good idea to spit out the remainder. Often sufferers find that it is helpful to place one of these tablets under the tongue in anticipation of some extra activity which it is thought will probably produce the pain of angina. In this way they will often circumvent the distress that it can cause.

Because of the dilating effect that can occur in arteries other than those of the heart, this medicine is capable of lowering the blood pressure for a short period of time and occasionally a patient will faint after using glyceryl trinitrate. Other patients find that the tablet leaves them with a persistent headache.

Usually angina sufferers learn how much they need and find that the advantages that the tablets offer greatly outweigh the side-effects. Quite recently some new methods of administering glyceryl trinitrate have been developed, including aerosol sprays and skin applications. The latter have the advantage of prolonged action, but often the body seems to develop a tolerance to them.

Other long-acting agents There are some other long-acting medicines similar in structure and action to glyceryl trinitrate. These include isosorbide dinitrate and isosorbide mononitrate and pentaerythritol tetranitrate (Mycardol, Peritrate). Other medications which can be used for their long-acting vasodilatation, but which act in a different way, are nifedipine (Adalat), diltiazem (Cardizem) and perhexiline maleate (Pexid).

The beta-blocking medicines referred to above in connection with the treatment of high blood pressure have a special place in the prevention of angina. The exact way they work in this situation is uncertain but it is known that they have a slowing effect on the heart rate and they reduce the workload of the heart. It may be that in this way they compensate for the diminished blood supply to the heart.

Medicines for circulation problems

Certain medicines which dilate blood vessels are used extensively in people who have a deficient blood supply to their arms or legs. These substances are referred to as *peripheral vasodilators*. Sometimes the poor circulation to the arms or legs is due to spasm of the blood vessels. The smooth muscle in the walls of the vessels contracts in response to a cold environment. This contraction may persist even after the affected area of the body is returned to a normal temperature. Some spasm of this sort is normal in anyone in response to cold, but in some people it is excessive, often causing the affected limb to go completely white and then, when the circulation has improved a little, very blue. The blueness is caused by the presence of blood which has lost most of its redness because it no longer has sufficient oxygen, and the patient is said to be *cyanosed*.

Reactions to cold It is interesting that a contraction or spasm of the arteries to the heart, i.e. *coronary vasospasm* can be induced in susceptible people by a cold environment, and some recent studies suggest that cold on the face is the most important trigger. Such people usually experience heart pain, i.e. angina.

Raynaud's disease is the condition which follows when cyanosis occurs as a consequence of abnormal spasm of blood vessels to the limbs, also usually due to cold. Sometimes a similar situation is brought on by the use of ergotamine, which is given as treatment for migraine. A poor circulation in the limbs is much more often due to *atheroma* — the same changes in the arteries that are the major problem in coronary artery disease. This, as discussed on p.46, appears to occur most frequently in people who have a high blood cholesterol for whatever reason. Unfortunately diabetics are specially prone to such blockages in their arteries, particularly, it would seem, if they are careless and do not control their blood sugars well, but sometimes in spite of their very best efforts. (See also Chapter 6, Diabetes mellitus.)

Exceptionally poor circulation When the blood supply is exceptionally poor, death of tissues will occur and this is the most common cause of *gangrene* in the limbs. If the loss of blood supply to the limbs is insufficient to cause gangrene, it may still cause pain on movement of muscles. Thus some people find that they can only walk a relatively few steps before they get pain in their calves. They soon learn that if they stop walking for a short time, the pain will go and they can then walk a similar distance again before experiencing the pain once more. This is known as *intermittent claudication*. The impressive word 'claudication' merely means 'limping', which I suppose is the result if the patient tries to continue walking with the pain present. The amount of help which people with intermittent claudication and/or incipient gangrene can get from vasodilation is strictly limited. Some preparations such as Ronicol and Hexopal are derived from nicotinic acid. Another agent, cyclandelate (Cyclospasmol), is more frequently used when the circulation to the brain is impaired. Isoxsuprine is used similarly in the form of Defencin or Duvadilan. Although some claim excellent results, many physicians doubt the value of these agents also. Curiously, one of the best dilators of the peripheral circulation is alcohol and this is sometimes prescribed for patients with such problems.

However, it must be realised that except where spasm is a major factor, the possibilities of increasing the blood flow are not good. As the arteries get older, they seem to become more rigid and the inner lining becomes thickened and obstructed with atheroma. It is rather optimistic to expect much improvement in the circulation as a result of relaxing the muscles in the walls of these vessels. There is some evidence that very small doses of aspirin, taken regularly, may help to prevent the formation of clots which usually represent the last stages of blood-vessel obstruction.

Migraine

As already mentioned, there are some medicines which produce a constriction of the arteries and there is one condition where this seems to be a helpful action — *migraine*. (See also Chapter 3.3 on headaches.)

Migraine is a curious disorder of the blood vessels to the brain. It appears to start as a narrowing of the blood vessels —and at this stage the patient may experience a variety of symptoms, but most commonly a sensation of flashing lights or palisades — followed by a compensatory dilatation of the arteries. It is in the latter phase that the severe throbbing headache is experienced. Thus one of the most effective treatments in migraine is the use of ergotamine to contract the diameter of the blood vessels and so relieve the throbbing headache. Ergotamine is obtained from ergot, which occurs naturally, growing on certain grains. Unfortunately ergotamine is not very well absorbed and various means have been adopted to hasten this process. Thus, as well as in the ordinary tablets to be swallowed and absorbed from the stomach, ergotamine is available as an aerosol so that it can be inhaled; there are tablets to place under the tongue for absorption through the tissue of the mouth, and there are preparations known as suppositories for insertion into and subsequent absorption from the rectum, i.e. back passage. When ergotamine is taken to excess, there is the possibility that it will cause gangrene of the fingers and toes. Some people find that it nauseates them or even causes vomiting. Prolonged use can actually cause headache directly or may induce headache when it is withdrawn suddenly. The sooner treatment is started in an attack, the more effective it is likely to be.

Absorption Many migraines respond well to simple treatment with ordinary painkillers such as aspirin or paracetamol, provided they are absorbed rapidly. Unfortunately the activity of the bowel and stomach is usually reduced during a migraine attack. This problem can often be overcome by giving a substance that speeds the emptying time of the stomach, e.g. metoclopramide (Maxolon), at the same time as the painkiller. Metoclopramide has another advantage in that it often prevents the nausea, i.e. sick feeling, which is a common characteristic of a migraine attack.

When a patient suffers from both high blood pressure and migraine, the symptoms often seem to improve when the blood pressure is brought under control. In addition to this some of the agents used in the treatment of high blood pressure also seem to have a specific action in migraine, usually as a preventive measure, i.e. prophylaxis. Beta-blockers are one such, but it must be remembered that many migraine sufferers also experience asthma and as explained on p. 246, these medicines can block the treatment of an acute asthma attack and so are unsafe in such people. Only some beta-blockers are effective.

Clonidine (Dixarit) is considered by some to be helpful, but sometimes causes, or even makes worse, depression, and can lead to wakefulness.

The taking of medicines on a regular basis to prevent migraine is not recommended unless the patient averages more than one attack monthly. Continuous ergotamine is particularly undesirable. As tension plays a part in migraine, some patients find that manoeuvres designed to relieve tension are helpful (see p. 192) while others resort successfully to tranquillisers. The latter are usually habit-forming and should, of course, be used only with the greatest of discretion.

4.7 Medicines for the relief of pain

'My heart aches and a drowsy numbness pains my sense as though of hemlock
I had drunk or emptied some dull opiate to the drains'
— John Keats, *Ode to a Nightingale*

The most commonly used medicines for the relief of physical pain are aspirin and related agents which have already been discussed in Chapter 4.3, Anti-inflammatory agents. These are safe in most circumstances and not habit-forming. Paracetamol is another pain-relieving medication that is not habit-forming.

Most other medicines used for pain relief are derivatives of opium which comes from the poppy. These are probably all habit-forming to a greater or lesser extent. Unfortunately it would seem that the greater the capacity to relieve pain, the greater the tendency to produce physical or psychological dependence (addiction). The most powerful, and therefore the most prone to induce the drug habit, is heroin, and the least likely is probably codeine. Chemical manipulation of codeine can be used to produce a substance equally as addictive as heroin and so restrictions have been placed on the availability of codeine in some countries. The product of this illegal chemical manufacturing is often referred to as 'homebake'.

Morphine and pethidine (Demerol, Meperidine) are two of the most frequently administered painkillers. They are both very effective for this purpose and are vitally important in the treatment of shock.

Narcotics

By definition a *narcotic* is a medicine which produces sleep or stupor. Physicians usually reserve the term for opium and those agents derived from it and use the term *sedative* for other medicines which reduce the level of consciousness. The term *hypnotic* is used for medicines which are given primarily to induce sleep. Legal usage tends to include marijuana in the category of a narcotic, but it is not in any way related to opium. It apparently has some potential to make its users drowsy and gives them a sense of wellbeing.

A drug such as morphine appears to act in several ways. Its most important use is to alter the appreciation of pain. This appears to occur regardless of whether the patient is conscious or unconscious. Secondly, there is a sedative effect, i.e. the patient is made to feel drowsy and less anxious, and if the dose is large enough the patient may actually go to sleep. Even while the patient is still experiencing pain, there is also a sense of being apart from it and not being worried by it. The patient has the feeling of being a bystander in the situation. Unfortunately in addition to its pain-relieving properties, morphine has some important side-effects.

Obviously the tendency to cause dependence is the greatest worry. The commonest immediate problems are a feeling of nausea and even vomiting. Sometimes there is depressed breathing, which can be dangerous in people whose breathing is already impaired, as in asthma. Depression of respiration is the usual cause of death in overdosage. The cough reflex is also suppressed so that secretions may accumulate in the lungs and lead to infection, e.g. pneumonia or bronchitis. A constriction of the ducts from the gallbladder to the bowel, induced by morphine, can cause or aggravate gallbladder pain. The activity of the bowel is reduced and this can lead to severe constipation.

Frequent use of morphine leads to tolerance, so that larger and larger doses have to be taken in order to produce the same effect. Addicts often misjudge the dose necessary to give the feelings which they enjoy and die as a consequence.

Many modifications of morphine have been produced chemically but all have some tendency to cause dependency. Some, however, are less likely to cause nausea and vomiting and some are less inclined to cause constriction of the ducts of the gallbladder.

The following are painkillers which are related to opium and hence morphine: hydromorphine (Dilaudid), methadone (Dolophine), pethidine (Demerol, Meperidine), dextropropoxyphene hydrochloride (Darvon, Doloxene), pentazocine hydrochloride (Talwin, Fortral) and buprenorphine (Temgesic). They are all best avoided by people who either have a dependency problem or are at risk of developing one. For those people unfortunate enough to develop dependence there are in most countries many agencies set up to help them overcome the habit. The problems are basically the same as those associated with alcoholism and the general practitioner should be able to help any sufferer to get into the system. (See also pp. 106–19.)

4.8 Medicines for the heart

'For a perfect sight of the old medicine, let me conduct you to the bedside of Charles II: With a cry he fell. Dr King who fortunately happened to be present, bled him with a pocket knife. Fourteen physicians were quickly in attendance. They bled him more thoroughly; they scarified and cupped him; they shaved and blistered his head; they gave him an emetic, a clyster and two pills. During the next eight days they "threw in" fifty-seven separate drugs; and towards the end, a cordial containing forty more. This availing nothing, they tried Goa Stone, which was a calculus obtained from a species of Indian goat; and as a final remedy, the distillate of human skull.'

— Sir Andrew Macphail, 'The Source of Modern Medicine', *British Medical Journal*, 1933

Digoxin and the treatment of heart failure

Among the best and oldest known of medicines for the heart is digitalis. This has already been mentioned as derived from the foxglove, but usually it is administered in refined form as either digoxin or digitoxin. This substance is a good example of the way in which medications have to be carefully monitored and the dose modified according to circumstances. Getting the dosage just right for any one person is very critical if success is to be achieved.

Digoxin has two principal actions on the heart:
1. A mechanical strengthening of the action of the heart (*inotropic action*).
2. A slowing of the heart by influencing a structure in the heart known as the *pacemaker*.

The first seems to occur as a result of changes in the sodium and calcium balance within the cells of the heart muscles. The slowing that occurs to the heart rate is less marked in normal persons — who are not usually given digoxin anyhow — than in those whose hearts are under strain and not coping well. Doctors tend to use the alarming term *heart failure* when what they mean is that the heart is under strain and that symptoms of breathlessness or fluid retention are occurring as a result.

If it is the *left side* of the heart which is under strain, as occurs in advanced high blood pressure and often after a *coronary thrombosis* (i.e. heart attack or *myocardial infarction*), the main symptom is of breathlessness and the doctor hears moist crackling sounds (*crepitations*) at the lung bases on listening with a stethoscope. X-rays of the chest will reveal typical changes also.

When the *right side* of the heart is under strain, the most obvious sign is that the ankles are swollen. The doctor will also look for engorgement of the veins in the neck and enlargement of the liver. It must be remembered that there are many other causes for such symptoms and signs.

When a person has both right- and left-sided 'failure' that person is said to have *congestive heart failure*. The essential problem is that because the heart is not coping very well, there is a back pressure which extends to the smallest blood vessels (capillaries). This back pressure may be thought of as forcing fluid out of the circulation into the tissues and the fluid which accumulates in those situations is known as *oedema*.

The kidney also experiences some of this back pressure and does not function so effectively. Less fluid is excreted from the body and this leads to even more back pressure and a vicious cycle is established. The way this vicious cycle is broken is to either —
1. encourage the kidneys to remove more fluid from the body,
2. strengthen the action of the heart,
3. reduce the work the heart has to do, e.g. by slowing the rate of the heart or reducing the resistance against which the heart has to work,
— or 1, 2 and 3 together.

Digoxin is probably the best known of the agents which strengthen the action of the heart and as already mentioned, has the advantage that it also slows the heart's rate.

The kidneys are encouraged to remove more fluid by agents known as diuretics (see also pp. 256-7) and the resistance against which the heart has to work is likely to be influenced by blood-pressure-lowering agents when high blood pressure (hypertension) is a problem, and also by blood-vessel dilators (vasodilators).

A number of factors have an influence on the efficacy of digoxin. The first is absorption into the body. People vary in the amount which passes from the gut into the bloodstream. Thus the presence of certain antacids given for indigestion may reduce the amount absorbed. Digoxin is passed through the liver and the kidney in the course of its time in the body. Changes in either of these sites can influence the concentration of it in the body, the effect of kidney damage being particularly noteworthy. Elderly people usually require much smaller dosages than young adults.

When the potassium level in the bloodstream falls — as it sometimes does with certain diuretics (see below) — the effect of digoxin is enhanced. The same applies to a low concentration of magnesium or a high concentration of calcium. When the dosage of digoxin is too great for an individual, the first sign is often nausea. Later there may be palpitations (i.e. an abnormal awareness of the beating of the heart), muscle weakness, tiredness, headache and restlessness. Very occasionally people suffer from *xanthopsia*, which means that everything they see has a yellowish appearance. Of course, most of these symptoms can be caused by other things as well.

It is clear that the doctor has many matters to take into consideration and it requires a nice judgement to ensure that patients get the advantages of this remarkable medicine without the side-effects.

The doctor will be checking the pulse and the heart sounds and looking for abnormal rhythms of the heart which may develop when the dosage is excessive.

Digoxin is probably at its best in the treatment of a condition called *atrial fibrillation*. In this situation the upper chambers of the heart, known as the *atria*, develop a rapid and usually inefficient beat which is much faster than, and out of sequence with, the lower, more muscular part of the heart, known as the *ventricles*. Digoxin is often able to slow down this rapid beating and restore the action of the heart to normal, or near normal. The amount of digoxin that is required may be influenced by the simultaneous use of other medicines which also have a slowing effect on the heart, e.g. the beta-blockers (q.v.). It is sometimes helpful for a test to be done which will measure the level of digoxin in the bloodstream and it is usual to keep the level at 1–2 microgrammes per litre.

Diuretics

These agents reduce the fluid in the body and this action is helpful in heart 'failure' and in high blood pressure. They have an influence on the sodium and potassium levels in the bloodstream and in the body cells. The exact reasons why the kidney does not excrete adequate amounts of sodium (salt) and water in heart failure, remains uncertain. It is obvious, however, that the accumulation of fluid that results is harmful and the relief which these agents afford is usually dramatic.

Many people dislike having to make frequent trips to the toilet, which is the usual response to these medicines. As a result they often discontinue them prematurely. The reward is often acute and frightening episodes of breathlessness (dyspnoea).

If the amount of fluid retained is not great, usually a mild diuretic such as bendrofluazide, (Neo-Naclex), cyclopenthiazide (Navidrex), chlorothiazide (Saluric, Diuril, Chlotride) or chlorthalidone (Hygroton) is adequate. If there is much fluid, a stronger agent such as frusemide (Lasix) is usually best. The action of the latter is usually complete in about two hours. The longer-acting diuretics are the ones favoured for use in high blood pressure. Hygroton may be given on alternate days.

Unfortunately there is a tendency for potassium to be lost to the body at the same time as the water. The doctor needs to keep an eye on the potassium levels in the bloodstream, particularly with the stronger agents, and sometimes potassium supplements by mouth are desirable. Combined preparations are available and agents such as Navidrex K are popular. This is bendrofluazide together with potassium. (The chemical symbol for potassium is K.) Another widely used preparation is Slow K, which is a potassium salt presented in such a way that it is slowly released to the body and less irritating to the gut. Not every patient needs additional supplements of potassium. Certain foods are also good sources of potassium, e.g. bananas, oranges and raisins (see p. 101).

It has already been mentioned that a low potassium level tends to increase the action of digoxin, possibly to a toxic level. As diuretics are commonly given with digoxin, careful surveillance by a doctor is essential.

There are a few diuretics which do not cause potassium loss at all; amiloride (Midamor) and triamterene (Dytac, Dyrenium) come into this category, as does spironolactone (Aldactone). These, however, are relatively weak diuretics and although sometimes they are adequate on their own, they are usually used in combination with a stronger agent.

There is one other problem with diuretics, and that is the tendency of most of them to produce abnormalities in glucose (sugar) metabolism in persons with a tendency to diabetes (q.v.). This is reversed when the diuretic is discontinued.

Medicines to treat irregularities of the heartbeat

The beating of the heart is controlled by minute electrical impulses which pass through the nerves which supply the heart. These impulses can be recorded on an instrument called an *electrocardiograph* (ECG or EKG for short). These impulses, in turn, usually originate in a structure known as the *pacemaker*. If there is any interruption to the passage of the electrical impulses through the heart, as may occur when the blood supply is cut off (e.g coronary thrombosis or myocardial infarct), the rhythm of the heart may change, or even stop altogether. A variety of agents have been found to be capable of influencing the ability of the nerves to conduct electrical messages. Each has its own advantages and disadvantages and much skill must be exercised in determining which one will be the most effective in any particular circumstance.

Digoxin is one such drug which usually leads to the slowing of a too rapidly beating heart. Given in excess, it can itself lead to irregularities. It seldom works well when the rapid pulse is brought on by an over-active thyroid gland (thyrotoxicosis).

Another agent is lignocaine (Xylocard). Lignocaine is usually injected into the veins in certain severe abnormalities of heart rhythm. Other agents which are used in appropriate circumstances are: flecainide (Tambocor); mexiletine (Mexitil); tocainide (Tonocard); procainamide (Pronestyl); disopyramide (Rhythmodan); amiodarone (Cordarone X); phenytoin (Dilantin), which is also used to quell the abnormal electrical impulses in the brain in epilepsy; verapamil (Civicor, Isoptin, Veradil); and the beta-blockers (see p. 245).

Some of these are more effective in treating abnormal rhythms in the upper part of the heart (the atria) and others in the lower part of the heart (the ventricles). If the heart rate is excessively slow following a heart attack, often atropine is indicated.

Many people have minor irregularities of the heart and often these are of no real consequence. It is usually only when an irregularity causes the heart to work harder that treatment is necessary.

Certain serious irregularities which fail to respond to agents such as the above can be corrected by what is known as *cardioversion*. In this situation a considerable direct-current electric shock is applied to the heart.

People whose heartbeat remains uncontrollably slow can sometimes be helped by an artificial pacemaker. This battery-operated implant sends electrical impulses through the heart, thus replacing or working in conjunction with the natural pacemaker. Metal detectors interfere with the action of pacemakers and persons fitted with them have to get special permission to avoid the hazards presented by such security devices at airports. Leaking microwave ovens and arc welders should also be avoided.

4.9 Medicines used for the gastro-intestinal system

'I have finally kum to the konklusion, that a good reliable sett ov bowels iz wurth more tu a man than enny quantity ov brains'
— *Josh Billings: His Sayings*, Henry Wheeler Shaw, 1818–85

A wide variety of agents are used in an effort to ameliorate symptoms having their origin in the gut. Many of these have been touched upon before. Thus in the chapter on nausea, attention has been drawn to the various medicines of the phenothiazine group which are used to reduce the distress caused by this symptom. Certain allied medicines actually have the effect of increasing the appetite. Cyproheptadine hydrochloride (Periactin) is one such. It has been noted that many people on tricyclics (see p. 228) and other anti-depressants also put on weight. In some cases this may be partly due to the fact that they are feeling better and eating well once again. However, there seems to be a definite appetite-inducing action which is independent of this. It does not follow that people on these medicines will inevitably gain weight but rather that they have to be very careful about what they eat if they do not wish to put on weight.

Probably the most widely used medicines for the gastro-intestinal system are the various agents designed to combat *excess acidity*. Stomach damage and ulceration seems usually to be related to an excessive production of the normal hydrochloric acid and other substances such as pepsin which help in digestion. At one time there was little available except the antacids to combat the activity of these agents. These were principally compounds containing aluminium (e.g. aluminium hydroxide), calcium (e.g. calcium carbonate) and magnesium (e.g. magnesium carbonate). Sometimes bismuth was used. In an emergency, short-term use of sodium bicarbonate (baking soda) is possible.

There are literally dozens of antacids available and many of them can be bought over the counter without a doctor's prescription. There is evidence that antacids can be helpful in healing duodenal ulcers, but there is some doubt about their effectiveness in the case of gastric ulcers. With a duodenal ulcer the pain relief obtained is usually clear cut and prompt but of only limited duration. Almost all patients with duodenal ulcer will wake at night with pain below the sternum (breastbone). Antacids are also helpful for people who are experiencing symptoms as a result of the regurgitation of the acid stomach contents on to the oesophagus (gullet).

Recently several very potent agents have been developed which actually prevent the stomach producing excess acid. The best known of these are cimetidine (Tagamet, Contracid) and ranitidine (Zantac). Often only one dose of two tablets each night for a month is enough to permit an ulcer to heal. Pirenzepine dihydrochloride (Gastrozepine) is another agent which reduces the secretion by the stomach of acid and other substances which participate in the digestive process.

Tri-potassium di-citrato bismuthate or DCB (De-nol) is a substance which works in several ways and is very effective in encouraging ulcer healing. It is believed that it adheres to the ulcer and protects it from acid. It actually also reduces the quantity of some of the substances which play a part in digestion and possibly kills certain bacteria which are now thought to contribute to ulcer formation. Since it also adheres to food, it is particularly important that this substance, which comes in both tablet and liquid form, should be taken well before meals. People taking this also need to know that it will darken their bowel motion. Sucralfate (Antepsin, Carafate) works in a similar way, protecting the ulcer from further damage and so enhancing healing. It is also known to absorb bile.

Carbenoxolone is derived from liquorice. It is believed to increase the availability and thickness of normal stomach mucus. In this way it helps in the healing of both gastric and duodenal ulcers. Unfortunately it also causes the body to retain salt and water and this can embarass the heart, particularly in those people whose heart is already under strain. Too much liquorice can have the same effect.

Most of the other agents used in gastro-intestinal disorders are discussed in the sections dealing with common symptoms, particularly those on abdominal pain, nausea and diarrhoea, and also in the chapter on the emotions and disease, p. 77.

Constipation

Perhaps a word relating to constipation should be included here. Constipation is a very common complaint which causes much anxiety. As mentioned elsewhere, any sudden change in bowel habits which persists more than a few days requires evaluation. Often it is simply related to a change in diet or to reduced exercise. However, occasionally it is due to significant disease which must be diagnosed and treated.

The factors which help to maintain bowel regularity are:
1. bulk in the diet,
2. fluid,
3. exercise.

It is also important to develop a pattern of opening the bowels regularly and usually the best idea is to make a point of going to the toilet at the same time each day, preferably shortly after a meal. It is, of course, possible at times to ignore the call to open the bowels and after a while the urge passes. The faeces then remain in the bowel and their fluid contents are absorbed. The longer they remain in the bowel, the harder and drier they become. This is not harmful in itself but may result in severe constipation and much difficulty and discomfort in ultimately passing the motion. Straining is not good for the body and can also lead to tears in the tissues around the anus or aggravate haemorrhoids (piles). Clearly it is wise not to allow the bowel motion to get to this state.

By watching the diet, drinking adequate fluid and getting sufficient exercise most people can keep themselves regular and very few should have to resort to *laxatives*, which is the name given to medicines designed to make the bowels move.

Sometimes patients are required to take medicines which are themselves constipating and many analgesics (i.e. painkillers) come into this category.

Laxatives can work by:
1. irritation,
2. providing bulk,
3. osmotic action,
4. softening.

Of the irritants, castor oil would probably be the best known. Others include cascara, senna (senna tea, Senokot), fig and aloes. Phenolphthalein, bisacodyl (Dulcolax) and danthron (Dorbanex) also come into this category. Long-term use of these can be damaging to the bowel, so they should be used very sparingly.

Bulk providers include bran which unfortunately also gives many people flatulence, and such things as Isogel, Metamucil and methylcellulose, whose use is described in Chapter 2.4 in the section on the irritable bowel.

Magnesium sulphate (Epsom salts), magnesium hydroxide and magnesium carbonate all have the effect of drawing fluid to themselves by osmotic pressure. This fluid acts as bulk in the bowel and stimulates bowel activity. Lactulose (Duphalac, Cephulac), which is a sugary substance, also acts osmotically.

Finally there are the softeners which become emulsified with the bowel motion and so render it easier to pass. Liquid paraffin acts in this way and is a constituent of Petrolagar, and so does dioctyl sodium sulfosuccinate (Docusate, Dioctyl, Coloxyl, Colace).

Where constipation is chronic and long-term use of laxatives is inevitable, the one which is currently thought to be least damaging to the bowel is lactulose, which is marketed as Duphalac.

For an account of the agents used in diarrhoea see Chapter 3.25, Nausea, vomiting and diarrhoea, pp. 177–9.

5. Contraceptives

'We want far better reasons for having children than not knowing how to prevent them'

— Dora Russell, *Hypatia*, 1933

The contraceptive pill

The contraceptive pill is now widely accepted as a safe and effective means of controlling fertility. It is probably better avoided by women with the following problems:

1. A history of clots occurring in the legs or any other part of the body.
2. A history of heart disease.
3. A history of liver disease.
4. A history of breast cancer.
5. Cigarette smokers (especially over 35 years of age).

It does seem that in women predisposed to the formation of blood clots, that tendency is enhanced by taking pills containing oestrogen (see below). Smoking is also a risk factor, as it too increases the chances of clot formation, particularly in the coronary (heart) or cerebral (brain) blood vessels.

Some ideas which have been laid to rest include the belief that there should be occasional breaks from the pill. These are unnecessary. Furthermore, it appears to be perfectly safe to start the pill in early adolescence and if it is required, continue until the menopause. As with other medications, the general principle is to use the smallest dose which is effective.

Main constituents of the pill

Most pills contain two main constituents which are either the same as or mimic the hormones which are produced naturally in the body. One of these is an *oestrogen* and the other is a *progestagen*. The commonly used oestrogens are ethinyl oestradiol and mestranol and the former is almost twice as powerful as the latter.

There are two major groups of progestagens (see later).

Most progestagens have a weak male hormone-like (i.e. *testosterone*) action and all progestagens in use have a slight *anti-oestrogen* effect as well as their own particular characteristics. This *anti-oestrogen* effect reduces the activity of any oestrogen which is present in the pill, but curiously, in the process of breaking down in the body, some progestagens actually also produce mild oestrogen-like effects.

Here is a list of things which can occur if the balance of hormones in the pill is not correct for a particular person.

Too much oestrogen
1. Bleeding in mid cycle, i.e. between menstrual periods.
2. Heavy periods.
3. Nausea and vomiting.
4. Weight gain before periods.
5. Increase in breast size.
6. Excessive mucus discharge from the uterus (womb).
7. Migraine headaches and/or other headaches.
8. Irritability.
9. Development of pigment spots (chloasma)
10. Recurrent thrush.
11. Mild blood pressure elevation.

Too much progestagen
1. Very slight periods.
2. Absent periods.
3. Increased appetite.
4. Persistent weight gain.
5. Breast tenderness and increased size.
6. Dry vagina.
7. Depression.
8. Decreased desire for sex.

Too much androgen (testosterone-type effect) — usually minimal or absent
1. Acne.
2. Oily skin and hair.
3. Increased body hair.
4. Increased desire for sex.

It must not be assumed that anyone who is suffering from these symptoms and who is also on the pill is necessarily getting these signs and/or symptoms as a result of the pill, but such a possibility must be considered when seeking a cause. Nor should it be assumed that because you are on a pill which contains say, testosterone equivalents, you will experience the features associated with testosterone excess. The doses of all the hormones are so small that the number of women suffering the effects of excess from any of the hormones is very small indeed and relates to differing individual responses.

The following shows approximate ethinyl oestradiol (i.e. oestrogen) equivalents of the progestagens:

Progestagen	ACTION Oestrogen-like	Anti-oestrogen
Norethisterone	1.0	10
Norethisterone acetate	1.5	100
Ethynodiol diacetate	5.0	4
dl-Norgestrel	0	74
Levonorgestrel	0	148

Thus norethisterone acetate has one and a half times the oestrogen-like effect of norethisterone but 10 times the anti-oestrogen effect.

Values for desogestrel, which is derived from lynoestrenol, are hard to obtain. It is said that levonorgestrel and desogestrel are of approximately equal strengths; desogestrel has no male hormone or oestrogen-like properties. Lynoestrenol has a very weak male hormone-type action.

The following shows approximate methyl testosterone (male hormone) equivalents of the progestagens.

Protestagen	Testosterone equivalents
Norethisterone	1.6
Norethynodiol	0
Norethisterone acetate	2.5
Ethynodiol diacetate	1.0
dl-Norgestrel	7.6
Levonorgestrel	15.2

Thus norethisterone acetate has two and a half times the testosterone-like action of ethynodiol diacetate.

Oestrogen content of some commonly used contraceptive pills

The following table gives the most commonly used pills. The brands are listed in order of their decreasing content of oestrogen.

	Oestrogen content	Progestagen content
Ovulen 1.0	100 μgm mestranol	1000 μgm ethynodiol diacetate
Ovulen 0.5	100 μgm mestranol	500 μgm ethynodiol diacetate
Anovlar	50 μgm ethinyl oestradiol	4000 μgm norethisterone acetate
Gynovlar	50 μgm ethinyl oestradiol	3000 μgm norethisterone acetate
Lyndiol	50 μgm ethinyl oestradiol	2500 μgm lynoestrenol
Ovostat	50 μgm ethinyl oestradiol	1000 μgm lynoestrenol
Ovulen 1/50	50 μgm ethinyl oestradiol	1000 μgm ethynodiol diacetate
Norinyl-1	50 μgm mestranol	1000 μgm norethisterone
Restovar	37.5 μgm ethinyl oestradiol	750 μgm lynoestrenol
Brevinor-1 / Synphasic	35 μgm ethinyl oestradiol	1000 μgm norethisterone
Brevinor	35 μgm ethinyl oestradiol	500 μgm norethisterone
Femulen		500 μgm ethynodiol diacetate
Noriday		350 μgm norethisterone

Because there is a difference in the way the body uses the various progestagens and because there is difficulty in comparing exactly the actions of the two major types of progestagen, a second table is given for the levonorgestrel group.

	Oestrogen content	Progestagen content
Nordiol	50 μgm ethinyl oestradiol	250 μgm levonorgestrel
Neogynon / Eugynon / Ovral	50 μgm ethinyl oestradiol	50 μgm norgestrel
Microgynon 50	50 μgm ethinyl oestradiol	125 μgm levonorgestrel
Biphasil	50 μgm ethinyl oestradiol 50 μgm ethinyl oestradiol	50 μgm levonorgestrel (11 tabs) 125 μgm levonorgestrel (10 tabs)
Marvelon	30 μgm ethinyl oestradiol	150 μgm desogestrel
Nordette / Microgynon 30	30 μgm ethinyl oestradiol	150 μgm levonorgestrel
Femodene	30 μgm ethinyl oestradiol	75 μgm gestodene
Triphasil	30 μgm ethinyl oestradiol 40 μgm ethinyl oestradiol 30 μgm ethinyl oestradiol	50 μgm levonorgestrel (6 tabs) 75 μgm levonorgestrel (5 tabs) 125 μgm levonorgestrel (10 tabs)
Microval		30 μgm levonorgestrel
Microlut		30 μgm levonorgestrel

Desogestrel is less anti-oestrogenic than levonorgestrel and therefore the oestrogen strength of Marvelon is greater than those which are lower on the table. Gestodene is very much the same as desogestrel.

Although it is usual to start with the smallest effective dose of both oestrogen and progestagen, there may be particular circumstances which lead the doctor to recommend a stronger pill. Thus a person who has a problem with acne may benefit from a higher-than-average dose of oestrogen, or a person suffering from heavy periods may do better on a pill containing more progestagen.

Contraceptive injections Some women prefer the convenience of an injection and so accept a three-monthly dose of Depo-Provera which is a pure progestagen (medroxy progesterone acetate). Such women usually have no periods while they are on Depo-Provera, and of course, if they have side-effects from the first injection, have to put up with these for three months until the dose is all absorbed.

Because of the wide range of products available, it can be seen that if anyone experiences a side-effect as a result of imbalance of the various constituents of the contraceptive pill, it is possible to look at the table of signs and symptoms and determine which component should be altered to minimise or eliminate the problem. For example, if the problem is heavy bleeding, an attempt may be made to control this either by reducing the oestrogen content or increasing the progestagen proportion of the pill.

Starting the contraceptive pill

Pills tend to be made up in 21-day or 28-day format. In fact in most packs there are only 21 active pills and the other seven are inactive. The 28-day packs have the advantage that the user does not have to stop and start the pill. She simply gets into the habit of taking a tablet every day.

As a general rule, the active agents should be started on day one of the cycle. If women starting the combined pill for the first time begin on the first day of their period, they will have immediate and effective contraception. Should they wait until about the fifth or seventh day after the period starts, as was formerly advised, they will require additional protection (see barrier methods) until at least seven days of pill-taking have passed.

The progestagen-only pill is a little different. It is used particularly when oestrogens are not desirable, especially if there is a history or risk of clots occurring. Thus older women who are smokers will probably experience fewer side-effects from the progestagen-only pills. These pills are slightly less reliable for contraception and the timing of the dosage is more critical — they must be taken within two hours of a selected time each day. Like the combined preparations, they are started on the first day of menstruation and then continued every day without a break. The user should not consider herself adequately protected until she has been taking the progestagen-only pill for at least 14 days.

If someone is changing from the combined pill to the progestagen-only pill, there should be no break between taking the last combined pill and commencing the first progestagen-only pill, regardless of whether the period has appeared. The progestagen-only pill has the advantage that it can be started within a few weeks of childbirth even when a woman is breastfeeding. Although breastfeeding provides some protection from further pregnancy, the protection is incomplete. The combined pills adversely affect the production of milk, so the progestagen-only pills, which don't have this action, have a place in this situation.

With all types it is very important that the user should not forget to take the pill. With the combined pills, the time is not quite so critical, so if a pill is missed in the evening, the user is usually still protected, provided the missed pill is taken the next morning, i.e. within 12 hours. Apparently the risks of pill omission are greatest at the beginning or end of the cycle rather than in the middle, and seven days without active pills at the beginning or end is the maximum consistent with safe contraception. Ovulation may occur if the gap is greater than this. If there is any doubt, it is probably best to institute some other form of contraception for the rest of the month. Clearly it is wise to get into the habit of taking the pill at a fixed time each day, e.g. just before brushing one's teeth.

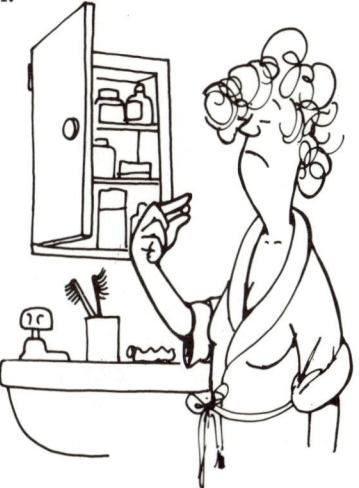

Certain situations may render the pill less effective. Thus a woman with a stomach upset may vomit the pill before it can be properly absorbed, or a severe diarrhoea may prevent it being absorbed into the body. Occasionally certain medicines also seem to interfere with the absorption or the utilisation of the pill and the following have all been blamed from time to time: antibiotics — particularly amoxycillin; certain tranquillisers, e.g. chlorpromazine; certain anti-epileptic agents, e.g. phenytoin; anti-inflammatory agents, e.g. phenylbutazone; antifungals, e.g. griseofulvin; some diuretics, e.g. spironolactone; large doses of vitamin C. Such interference is rare, but is sufficient reason for women to mention to their doctor that they are on the pill if the doctor is about to prescribe.

When first starting a patient on the pill the doctor will usually take out a full history relating to the regularity and amount of menstruation, any inter-menstrual loss, vaginal discharge and so on. The doctor will also want to know about such things as migraine headaches, clots in blood vessels, liver disease or jaundice, problems with the pituitary gland, diabetes, depression, epilepsy, kidney disorders, hearing problems (otosclerosis), whether the patient uses contact lenses and whether the patient smokes — all things which need to be taken into consideration before starting anyone on the pill.

Many doctors will recommend a full pelvic examination. This affords an opportunity to inspect the neck of the womb (cervix), as it is not uncommon for some changes, e.g. an 'erosion', to occur here when patients are on the pill. Additionally, certain non-malignant growths may be found in the uterus. They are sometimes sufficient reason not to use the pill. The doctor will also take the blood pressure so that there is a base-line reading available, should a woman be found to have an elevated blood pressure subsequently.

Many doctors like a follow-up visit, one or two months after starting the pill. Thereafter usually a check once every six months is adequate. At follow-up visits the doctor will again take the blood pressure, and an enquiry will be made about the side-effects due to oestrogen, progestagen and testosterone-like actions. The doctor will also check for weight gain. Approximately every three years, but more frequently if thought desirable, a cervical smear and pelvic examination is usually done. This is also a good time for a check of the breasts for lumps. Unfortunately this association of examinations for cancer with follow-up for the pill often leaves women with the impression that there is some association between these cancers and the pill. Such is not the case; it is merely a convenient opportunity to do these examinations and may save a woman the bother of having to make a special visit for this purpose.

OTHER CONTRACEPTIVES

Barrier methods

The contraceptive pill is only one of many ways of preventing pregnancy. Devices which present a barrier to the passage of the sperm into the womb have been used for contraception for many years. The best known of these would be the *sheath* or *condom*. These days this is usually made of rubber, and designed to enclose (or sheath) the erect penis (male organ). At the end of the sheath there is a space where the ejaculated semen is collected. The major anxiety with this method is that the condom may be punctured and the fluid escape, or that the condom may come off the penis as it is withdrawn from the vagina at the end of intercourse. The risk of pregnancy is further reduced if the female uses a *spermicide* as an additional precaution. A spermicide is a substance designed to destroy the spermatozoa in the ejaculate. The use of the sheath has recently increased in popularity as it seems to provide some protection from STDs (sexually transmitted diseases) and it is hoped may help prevent the spread of AIDS. The efficacy of condoms can be increased by the use of a spermicide in the structure of the condom as well as in the vagina. Many men dislike the use of condoms as they consider that they reduce sensation and so detract from the pleasure of intercourse.

Another barrier method is the *diaphragm*. This, too, is usually made of rubber and is designed to fit in the vagina in such a way that it is held firmly over the neck of the womb. Initially it needs to be properly fitted by a doctor or nurse so that it does not slip out of place during intercourse. It also needs to be in place before intercourse occurs as it is a fiddly thing to insert and unlikely to be satisfactory if this is attempted in the heat of passion. The diaphragm is usually used in conjunction with a spermicide. It is considerably less reliable than the condom.

A device similar to the diaphragm is the so-called 'Dutch Cap' which is designed simply to fit snugly over the cervix and prevent the entry of seminal fluid. It is seldom used today.

Intra-uterine devices

Another contraceptive technique involves the use of *intra-uterine devices* (IUDs). These are usually made primarily of plastic and they are inserted by a trained person right into the cavity of the uterus. The principal action is to prevent the fertilised ovum (egg) from implanting itself in the inner lining of the uterus. The most commonly used IUDs contain a small amount of copper which seems to enhance the effectiveness of the device, but it remains unknown exactly how an IUD works. Although not quite as effective as the contraceptive pill for preventing pregnancy, it is nevertheless very reliable and provides a cheap and usually worry-free method of contraception.

Very occasionally there are complications. In a few patients, usually during the insertion process, the IUD goes right through the wall of the uterus and sometimes an operation is required to retrieve it. There is also the rare complication of infection in the uterus, apparently related to the presence of the IUD. Most women will experience a moderate increase in their monthly menstrual loss after an IUD has been inserted, and for a few days after the insertion there is likely to be an ache in the pelvis. The great advantage of an IUD is that women can largely forget about contraception, merely checking after menstruation to ensure that the device is still in place by feeling the telltale 'threads' which remain at the cervix when it is properly located. The doctor or nurse who inserts the IUD should give instructions on how to make this check. If it is decided to dispense with the IUD it is quite easy to remove it by pulling on the 'threads', but this should not be attempted by the wearer.

Other methods

Despite the best efforts of all, there will be some people who forget or fail to take precautions and so run the risk of unwanted pregnancy. For these there are two other options. If the mistake is recognised within 72 hours, it is possible to take the *'morning after' pill* and so prevent successful implantation of the fertilised ovum. These days this usually takes the form of extra doses of the contraceptive pill and most general practitioners are prepared to give details of how this should be done in order to be effective. The extra doses frequently cause nausea and often treatment to counteract this is given concurrently.

If pregnancy does ensue, another option for some people is *abortion*, but in order to be safe this must be achieved within 12 weeks of the onset of the pregnancy. Each country has its own rules governing the legality of abortion. In some it is available on request, whilst in others it is only acceptable if the pregnancy presents clear and significant risk to the physical or mental health of the mother or, alternatively, there is evidence that the unborn child is likely to be physically or mentally abnormal.

Abortion is not without hazard to the mother and should not be seen as an alternative to the use of contraception. Many women suffer all the symptoms of loss (see p. 173) after an abortion and others are overwhelmed with guilt. Few doctors are comfortable with abortion but many see it as causing less human misery for all involved than continuing the pregnancy and then bringing up or relinquishing an unwanted child.

'Safe period' identification

Some people are reluctant to use any of the foregoing contraceptive methods and the Roman Catholic Church officially forbids them. Such people often seek ways by which they can identify times within the menstrual cycle when intercourse is unlikely to lead to pregnancy. Techniques for identifying a 'safe period' have improved with advances in our knowledge about fertilisation but their use must always be recognised as more likely to lead to pregnancy than the less natural methods described above.

Pregnancy cannot occur if the woman does not produce an ovum, i.e. egg. This is known as *ovulation* and usually occurs about half way between two menstrual periods. Furthermore, the ovum has a limited life, the exact duration of which remains uncertain, but probably it lives for two to three days only. One could thus anticipate that for a few days after menstruation, before ovulation occurs, a person who was not taking other precautions would be fairly safe from pregnancy. Similarly if the menstrual cycle was a typical and regular one, the chances of pregnancy would be small for a few days prior to menstruation. Unfortunately the time of ovulation is quite variable but there are ways by which it can be identified with reasonable accuracy. A few women regularly get lower abdominal pain at the time of ovulation and some even get a slight 'spotting' of blood from the uterus at this time. The pain is known as 'mittelschmerz', which is German for 'little pain' and if it is recognised and occurs regularly, this can be a useful indication of the time of ovulation.

Other women learn to identify the time of ovulation by taking their vaginal or rectal temperature each morning immediately upon waking and before getting out of bed. This temperature, which should be read with great care and accuracy, is known as the *basal temperature*. If this is accurately recorded on graph paper it usually becomes apparent that at the time of ovulation there is a small, but definite rise in the basal temperature which is sustained over the next several days. Unfortunately infections such as the common cold can also cause fluctuations in temperature and lead to confusion.

The Billings method Perhaps the best way to determine the time of ovulation is the method devised by Dr Evelyn Billings. Dr Billings drew attention to the changes that occur in the mucus that is produced in and around the cervix, i.e. the neck of the womb, throughout the menstrual cycle. It was noted that immediately after menstruation women observed a sensation of dryness, but after a few days the sensation changed to one of wetness and the mucus took on the consistency of egg white. It was determined that this time of wetness preceded and included the time of ovulation and hence of fertility. Once the sensation reverted to one of dryness with thick mucus only, it was considered that there ceased to be a risk of pregnancy. When it is remembered that adequate mucus is necessary for the effective transport of sperm to the uterus, this seems a very logical and simple guide to fertility which apparently also has a reasonable degree of reliability. It is suggested that a couple should maintain abstinence from sexual intercourse through the period of 'wetness' and for three days after its cessation.

Unfortunately the character of the mucus can sometimes be altered by medicines and the vaginal secretions that occur with sexual excitement. However, with experience and after regular charting of mucus characteristics it is said that most women can come to identify successfully when they are at greatest risk of pregnancy. Of course, this information can also be used by women who are seeking to become pregnant. If they can accurately identify the time of ovulation, they should attempt intercourse particularly in the two to three days immediately after it occurs. This will be the time when the chances of pregnancy are at their greatest.

Sterilisation

Other than total abstinence, the most effective method of contraception is sterilisation. This can be achieved in the female by cutting and occluding the fallopian tubes, or in the male by doing much the same thing with the vas deferens. The fallopian tubes are the tubes which convey the ovum from the ovary where it is formed to the body of the uterus. The vas deferens are the tubes which convey the sperm from the testes to the urethra and penis.

Because the fallopian tubes are in the abdomen, the sterilisation procedure tends to be a more complicated one in women than in men. Furthermore, for some reason which remains unexplained, many women seem to experience period problems after their tubes are tied. Sometimes this leads to them subsequently requiring removal of the uterus (i.e. hysterectomy). Tying the vas is a simple procedure and can be done on an outpatient basis under local anaesthetic. There are few complications.

These procedures should be regarded as permanent and should not be considered unless the couple concerned are quite sure that they want no more children. In fact, operations designed to reconstitute both the vas and the fallopian tubes are frequently performed, but success cannot be guaranteed.

Neither procedure has any physical effect on a person's sexual interests or capabilities, other than preventing pregnancy.

6. Diabetes mellitus

'An ill manner of living and chiefly an assiduous and immoderate drinking of cider, beer or sharp wines; sometimes sadness, long grief, also convulsive affections and other inordinations and depressions of the animal spirits . . .'
— Thomas Willis on the causes of diabetes, 1679

The common feature of all forms of *diabetes mellitus* is the presence of an abnormal amount of glucose in the bloodstream. Everybody has some glucose in their blood, and the amount present is kept within fairly strict limits by a substance called *insulin* which the body produces naturally. Diabetes occurs when certain cells of the organ known as the *pancreas* (sometimes referred to as the 'sweetbreads') fail to produce enough insulin for the needs of the body.

Sometimes this is because the production of the hormone insulin is less than it should be, resulting in a need for this substance to be administered by injection; at other times it is due to an increase in the body's requirements for insulin, usually associated with overweight. Where there is an increase in the body's requirements, the problem can often be remedied by bringing the weight down to what is regarded as ideal for the height and build of the sufferer. Alternatively, the pancreatic cells may be stimulated to produce more insulin, or the insulin which is already present may be made more available to the cells of the body which need it.

In 1922 when Frederick Banting and Charles Best discovered that a deficiency of insulin was the cause of diabetes, and effective replacement became available to the public, the lives of millions of diabetics were revolutionised. Insulin is now available in many forms and the aim is to provide the body with an amount of this substance sufficient to keep the level of sugar (glucose) in the blood as constant as possible.

The level of glucose tends to rise somewhat after meals and falls a little on exertion and even more with starvation. The liver contains a moderate store of a substance called *glycogen*, which can be broken down to glucose should the need arise. Adrenalin (epinephrine) plays a part in this, usually under the influence of another hormone, also produced in the pancreas, called *glucagon*. In effect, insulin and glucagon act in opposite directions, thus ensuring that there is a balance between utilisation and storage of glucose (via insulin) and the breakdown of glycogen (via glucagon) from the liver. This type of self-regulatory mechanism is referred to as *homeostasis* and a study of the physiology of the body reveals the presence of many such systems.

Unfortunately, in conditions where insulin is not present to facilitate the proper use and storage of glucose, the reaction tends to go the other way and the glycogen stores in the liver are quickly used up. Thereafter the body has to secure its energy from other sources than glucose via glycogen and so fatty tissues are drawn upon. When this occurs, certain unwanted byproducts known as *ketones* are produced which are very toxic to the body and in pregnancy can sometimes be lethal to the baby.

Diabetic coma

The presence of ketones in the bloodstream and urine of the diabetic is considered a serious sign and is usually associated with nausea, vomiting and laboured breathing. Later, as a result of the combination of a high blood sugar and the ketones, the patient becomes increasingly tired and may lapse into coma. Usually before this there is a marked thirst and excessive urination. This leads to severe dehydration. The patient is very ill and nearly always requires hospitalisation. The coma that occurs is known as *diabetic coma* and these patients urgently need insulin and correction of the dehydration. There is usually a marked loss of salt and potassium and this needs replacement also.

Another form of coma can occur as a result of an excess of insulin. This may occur when a diabetic has a dose of insulin, and then omits a meal, or when the insulin dosage is excessive, or occasionally when the body has used up an unexpectedly large amount of glucose as a result of strenuous exercise. Most patients get a warning that such a coma is in the offing, but a few become unconscious suddenly.

The usual early indications of impending coma due to low glucose are the development of a headache, sweatiness, rapid pulse, hunger and light-headedness. The patient may give the impression of being intoxicated. If identified promptly, these symptoms can usually be averted by the sucking of a glucose tablet, or the administration of a drink containing sugar in some form. Care should always be taken to make certain that the patient is capable of swallowing, lest some fluid go into the lungs.

If a person becomes unconscious treatment should be by injection — either of glucagon, or else some glucose directly into the veins.

It is useful to compare the features of the two types of coma, as the treatment of each is clearly very different.

Diabetic coma *(High glucose=hyperglycaemia)*	**Insulin coma** *(Low glucose=hypoglycaemia)*
Very dry skin, dry tongue	Sweaty, moist tongue
Dehydrated	Not dehydrated
Deep breathing	Normal breathing
Slow onset	Abrupt onset
Requires insulin	Too much insulin
Often low blood pressure	Usually raised blood pressure
Urine contains glucose/ketones	Urine usually free of glucose/ketones

Very unusually, even non-diabetics, after severe, prolonged exertion, may experience some of the symptoms of low blood sugar (hypoglycaemia).

The tendency to diabetes seems to be inherited. A few cases follow upon an attack of mumps or some other viral illness which sometimes affects the pancreas. Most people who have an absolute deficiency of insulin, and thus require injections of replacement insulin, develop the problem in early life and so this type of diabetes is often referred to as *juvenile diabetes* or *insulin dependent diabetes mellitus* (IDDM), or *Type I diabetes*.

The diabetes which develops most frequently in association with excess weight is due to a relative lack of insulin and by contrast is often referred to as *maturity onset* or *non-insulin dependent diabetes mellitus* (NIDDM), or *Type II diabetes*, since it usually occurs later in life. In theory, many sufferers of the latter could have their diabetes controlled by getting their weight down to normal and persevering with a restricted diet. If patients are able to cooperate with this weight reduction and dietary restriction, they can sometimes be regarded as cured of the diabetes, although still requiring surveillance. However, many people do not seem to have the willpower to get their weight to normal levels and maintain a strict dietary regime. Such people are now usually satisfactorily controlled by tablets, as are those who remain diabetic even when their weight is normal.

Modern developments in treatment

The first progress towards treatment by mouth instead of by injection occurred when some French physicians observed that some of their patients who were taking certain of the sulphonamide antibacterials exhibited a fall in their blood sugars. Further research on the sulphonamides led to the development of tolbutamide (Rastinon, Diatol, Orinase,) and like insulin, this has dramatically improved the lives of many diabetics. It has now been shown that this substance and others like it, e.g. chlorpropamide (Diabinese), glibenclamide (Daonil, Euglycon), glipizide (Minidiab), tolazamide (Tolinase) and gliclazide (Diamicron) stimulate the pancreas to produce more insulin as well as allowing the insulin produced to work better, i.e. overcome some of the resistance many diabetics develop to the action of insulin.

Later came another development with the introduction of the biguanides, e.g. phenformin and metformin. These work in a slightly different way and usually also help to curb the appetite. Sometimes they cause diarrhoea.

The overall aim of treatment is to keep the blood sugar within what are believed to be normal limits, viz, 4–7 millimoles per litre. Most authorities believe that by doing so, the risk of developing the complications of diabetes can be minimised.

Whether treatment be by tablets or insulin injections, the dose has to be adjusted to suit the individual. The size of the dosage will vary according to the food intake and the amount of exercise. The dosage of insulin is much more critical than that of the tablets. Meals must never be omitted except on the instruction of a doctor, e.g. before an operation. The same can be said of the treatment, insulin in particular should never be omitted. A common mistake is to discontinue insulin because of vomiting. In fact the insulin should be given as usual and steps taken to ensure that the patient gets an adequate amount of nourishment subsequently. This may require the sucking of sweets or other readily available sugar, normally denied the diabetic.

Testing methods

Progress at all times is followed by regular examinations of the urine or the blood. Many diabetics achieve good control of their condition by testing their urine three or four times daily. Nowadays, self-monitoring of blood tests is usually preferable to urine tests as this indicates more accurately the level of sugar at the time of the test. Furthermore, in some people the amount of sugar in the urine does not reliably relate to the amount of sugar in the blood. Nevertheless, in appropriate subjects, and correctly done, urine sugars can give an excellent indication of blood sugar control. The urine is usually tested just before a meal. Preferably the bladder should be emptied half to three-quarters of an hour before the sample to be tested is passed. Ideally, the patient on tablets should show no evidence of sugar in the urine at any time. Because of new techniques in the estimation of sugar in the blood, this method has recently been recommended for many diabetics and is not difficult.

Whatever procedure is used, the results, and the time, of the tests should be recorded in a notebook so that the doctor can check progress and make modifications to dosage or diet as required.

It is seldom helpful to test for sugar only once a day, particularly if this is always done at the same time. Some diabetics are so well controlled that their tests never show evidence of a raised blood sugar level. Nevertheless, it is wise to vary the time of testing frequently to make sure that the good control is maintained throughout the 24 hours, particularly before taking food and two hours after meals.

Some people, usually in the older age groups, are fortunate enough to be able to find a long-acting insulin preparation so suitable that a single injection affords good control throughout the 24 hours. More often a mixture of a long-acting and a medium- or short-acting insulin is used. Many people require two or more injections daily to provide satisfactory control. A recent development is the slow, continuous injection of minute quantities of insulin by automatic in-dwelling injection devices. In this manner the input of insulin by the normal pancreas is mimicked.

The complications of diabetes

By careful control it is hoped to avoid the complications of diabetes. These can be grouped under two principal headings:

1. Those that relate to the increased susceptibility to infection afforded by an increase in sugar in the bloodstream and urine, e.g. boils, urinary infections, fungal infections of the genitalia, etc.
2. Those that relate to the effect of diabetes on the blood vessels. This can involve the smallest blood vessels (i.e. capillaries) of various organs, e.g.

      eyes → haemorrhages, cataract;
      kidneys → a condition called nephrosis;
      nerves → loss of sensation, numbness, etc., especially in the legs

or the larger blood vessels, e.g.

      coronary arteries → heart attacks;
      cerebral arteries → stroke;
      limbs → gangrene.

Patients who develop diabetes require careful instruction as to proper diet, help in adjusting the dosage of insulin or tablets and encouragement to test themselves regularly for evidence of elevated blood sugar. Meticulous care of the feet, often with the help of a podiatrist, is also important.

The doctor will also be very interested to know if the patient has been having symptoms consistent with a low blood sugar. Diabetics require frequent examination for evidence of any complications, particularly those which involve the eyes, kidneys, the nervous system or the circulation. The general practitioner with the usual equipment available in the office can detect major changes in the eyes, but usually it is best for them to be checked every one or two years by an eye specialist.

The kidneys can be checked by blood and urine tests, and blood pressure is of special importance for when there is hypertension as well as diabetes, damage to the blood vessels is likely to be aggravated. Examination of the nervous system requires a check of the reflexes and a search for any evidence that sensation has been lost in any site. Finally, an examination of the pulses is desirable to assess the state of the circulation in the feet.

A blood test which estimates what is known as *fructosamine* gives an indication of how good diabetic control has been over the last two weeks.

Here is an indication of some of the insulin preparations and their duration of action:

Type and name	Onset (hours)	Peak action (hours)	Duration (hours)
Fast-acting, 'regular' (soluble)	0.5–1	3–6	6–10
Medium-acting, NPH (Isophane)	1.5–3	6–12	18–24
Lente	1–3	6–12	24–48
Long-acting, ultralente	4–6	18–24	≥ 36

and the tablets:

Name	Duration (hours)	Dose frequency
Tolbutamide (Orinase, Rastinon)	6–12	2–3 × daily
Acetohexamide (Dimelor, Pramidex)	12–18	1–2 × daily
Tolazamide (Tolinase)	12–14	1–2 × daily
Glipizide (Minidiab, Glucotrol, Euglucon)	up to 24	1–2 × daily
Glibenclamide (Daonil, Diabeta)	up to 24	1–2 × daily
Gliclazide (Diamicron)	up to 24	1–2 × daily
Metformin hydrochloride (Glucophage)	up to 24	2–3 × daily

Dietary recommendations usually suggest that there should be a maximum of 25 kilocalories per kilogram of ideal body weight. Thus for a 70 kg ideal body weight (see p. 86) the kilocalorie intake would be 70×25 — 1750 kilocalories daily: 50–55% of this should be in the form of carbohydrate; 15% protein; and 30% fat.

Intake of cholesterol should be 200–300 mgm daily (see p. 100) or less. In general, the following foods should be avoided or kept to a minimum: sugar, glucose, jam, honey, marmalade, syrup, treacle, chocolates, sweets, cakes, pastries, biscuits; tinned fruit in syrup, crystallised fruits; sweetened fruit squash, fruit juices and cordials; lemonade, Pepsi or Coca-Cola, Ribena, bitter lemon, ginger ale, tonic water, sherry and wines, port, liqueurs.

These are foods containing very readily available sugars. Many drinks today have artificial sweeteners and these are usually acceptable.

Diabetics on insulin and some on tablets should always carry with them some form of readily available sugar, e.g. glucose tablets, to combat hypoglycaemia (low blood sugar). They should also carry in a purse or wallet information about their condition and what to do if they are found unconscious or unable to speak.

7. AIDS (acquired immune deficiency syndrome*)

'Prevention is everybody's business because we have in our midst one of the greatest threats to human health — perhaps second only to the threats of nuclear war. AIDS is a new disease. Old preventive approaches won't work; new ones are called for'
— Dr Paul Goldwater, *AIDS: the Risk*, 1986

Over the centuries the world has witnessed many devastating epidemics, among the worst being plague, typhus, influenza and poliomyelitis. Some diseases seem to wax and wane in their severity and some communities seem to have more natural resistance than others. Scarlet fever was once a greatly feared illness, whereas today it is usually very mild. The Maori people died by the hundred when they were first exposed to measles.

AIDS, however, is a new viral disease which threatens to outdo them all. It is caused by a virus which invades the cells and interferes with the body's ability to produce antibodies. As a result, the resistance to other infections and to certain malignant growths is greatly reduced and the sufferers often die from chest or bowel infections which would readily be overcome by most other people who did not have the disease, or from cancers which are seldom seen in other circumstances. Occasionally people have disorders of their immunity system from other causes, for example as a result of treatment designed to prevent the rejection process in organ transplants. In these circumstances the diminution in immunity is deliberately induced and usually carefully monitored and furthermore it is reversible. Unfortunately, so far there seems to be no cure for AIDS and once the immune deficiency is established, it progresses relentlessly.

There is some evidence that the progression may be slowed by certain medicines and several are currently under trial. These include phosphonoformate (PFA), azidothymidine (AZT), zidovudine (Retrovir), dideocytidine which is similar to zidovudine and a protein, peptide T. These all seem to be beneficial and we can only hope that they will eventually lead to something which is completely effective in eliminating the virus and restoring the body's immunity.

The virus which causes AIDS has been designated HIV which stands for *human immunodeficiency virus*. How, then, is this virus spread?

---

*A syndrome is a recognised and characteristic grouping of symptoms indicative of a particular disease.

Blood is the body fluid which seems most likely to spread AIDS. Semen and secretions from the cervix may also carry the virus. Saliva and tears could theoretically be responsible, but seem to offer very little risk. AIDS sufferers should not be organ donors. Most people seem to acquire the virus as a result of sexual intercourse with someone suffering from the disease, and anal (i.e. via the back passage) intercourse seems to present a greater risk than vaginal intercourse.

Another major cause of AIDS spread is the sharing of needles by people who are dependent on drugs. Drug addicts can reduce their risk substantially by always ensuring that they use new and sterile needles when they take their drugs by injection.

In the past it has been possible to become infected with AIDS as a result of a blood transfusion. Fortunately it is now possible to test blood to ensure that the donor was not suffering from AIDS. There is a catch to this, however, because after becoming infected with the virus, it usually takes some months before the blood of the sufferer shows the changes which indicate the presence of the virus. It is thus just possible that blood could contain the virus and not show evidence of the infection. Nobody who thinks they could possibly have been infected by AIDS should consider giving blood until at least six months after the event. It is worth noting that it is not possible to *contract* AIDS by donating blood.

We still do not know whether everybody who is infected with the virus will develop a full-blown AIDS but it seems likely that many will do so.

How can one avoid catching AIDS?

1. Allow sexual intercourse to occur only between non-infected partners who are faithful to each other. It is safest to stay with one known partner and avoid all casual sex.
2. Avoid sharing needles for injections of any kind or for tattooing or ear piercing.

For anyone who is unable to comply with these recommendations, the risk is reduced but not eliminated by wearing a condom for intercourse; not practising anal intercourse; the avoidance of oral sex; the avoidance of intimate sexual kissing (wet kissing).

An infected woman can pass AIDS to her unborn baby during pregnancy and possibly by breastfeeding.

It is probably wise not to share razors or toothbrushes as these are often contaminated with blood.

It is said that AIDS cannot be caught by normal everyday contact with an infected person. Many people will have seen pictures of the Pope hugging a child with AIDS. The virus is not passed from one person to another by shaking hands, hugging or dry kissing, nor is it passed by touching articles used by an infected person, e.g. clothes, toilet seats, door knobs, towels. There is no evidence of it being transmitted by insects such as mosquitoes or lice.

Children are not at risk of catching AIDS from other children who carry the virus, through normal day-to-day contact such as occurs at school.

It usually takes several years after the infection is acquired before the symptoms of AIDS appear, but some people have a brief feverish illness somewhat like glandular fever, a few weeks after infection. This settles down and it is usually many months before anything else happens.

When the fully developed disease does appear, it can take many forms. It should be remembered that there are numerous other conditions which can cause similar symptoms and signs. If you are in any doubt about the nature of a medical problem that you have developed, you should check it out with your general practitioner who, if it is thought necessary, will arrange for the appropriate tests to be done. Alternatively you could go to the nearest clinic for sexually transmitted diseases (STD or VD clinic).

Some of the more common symptoms and signs of AIDS

Swelling of the lymph nodes in groins, armpits or neck which remain for two months or longer;
Prolonged tiredness which cannot be explained by stress, depression or some other disease;
Repeated infections, particularly herpes (cold sores), shingles, boils or influenza;
Persistent fevers and sweats;
Unexpected, unexplained weight loss;
Prolonged diarrhoea;
Breathlessness and cough which persists;
Skin problems, particularly discoloured raised blotches or bumps (which may also occur in the mouth).

Sufferers from AIDS require a great deal of counselling and support. Apart from general practitioners, there are today many agencies which can help. The psychological reactions that the AIDS patient experiences are predominantly the response to loss coupled with guilt (see p. 173). Special advice and instructions are available for people undertaking the nursing care of AIDS patients.

8. Dementia (including Alzheimer's disease)

The cardinal sign of dementia is a loss of memory for things which have occurred in the recent past. Despite this, many elderly people suffering from dementia have a very clear memory of events which happened in their youth. Usually in the early stages of dementia there are personality changes and patients may give evidence of being suspicious of others and irritable. Often they withdraw into themselves, demonstrating a lack of insight and a loss of their sense of humour.

There are several causes of dementia, which is sometimes spoken of unkindly as 'brain rot' but the most frequently diagnosed is that due to Alzheimer's disease. This condition seldom occurs before 45 years of age and its cause remains unknown, although it seems that some people probably inherit a predisposition to it. Some authorities believe that a rare virus infection is the precipitating agent.

True dementias have to be distinguished from conditions resulting from depression (q.v.), deafness, and delirium (e.g. from infection) or even a gross deficiency of the hormones produced by the thyroid gland (i.e. hypothyroidism or myxoedema). It is also most important to make sure that the symptoms do not arise as the result of the administration of medicines such as tranquillisers, sleeping tablets and antihistamines.

Apart from Alzheimer's disease, other causes of true irreversible dementia include brain damage from prolonged alcohol excess, chronic syphilis, diminished blood supply to significant parts of the brain (cerebral atherosclerosis), brain tumour and a number of rare disorders of the nervous system (e.g. Huntingdon's chorea). Although depression may mimic dementia, a true dementia is usually accompanied by depressive features.

Most dementias are slowly progressive (although those due to a deficient blood supply to the brain may occur abruptly), and it is common for Alzheimer's patients to have early signs of the condition for up to 18 months before medical aid is sought. The total duration of this disorder from diagnosis to death is usually around five years.

Features of dementia which are particularly distressing to relatives include confusion, a tendency to wander, restlessness and problems with sleeping, and aggressiveness. The latter usually manifests itself as an unwillingness to cooperate with those who seek to help.

As yet there is no cure for dementia. The best that can be offered is tender loving care, attention to hygiene and diet, protection from injury and sometimes medication in an effort to reduce wandering or other prominent symptoms. In the late stages incontinence is a particular problem and usually institutional care becomes necessary. Often it is then safest for these patients to sleep on a mattress on the floor.

There are excellent organisations, such as the Alzheimer's Disease and Related Disorders Society (ADARDS), which have been set up to help those people who have the responsibility of caring for patients with dementia.

APPENDICES

APPENDIX 1

A brief review of common laboratory tests

'He is a great physician who above other men, understands diagnosis'
— Jacob Bigelow (1786–1879), *Nature of Diseases*

Blood tests
These may be divided into *those which evaluate the cells and other particles in the blood* and *those which estimate a variety of substances dissolved in the blood fluid (i.e. serum)*. The blood *plasma* is the serum plus the clotting agent, *fibrinogen*.

Tests on the particulate elements within the blood are usually done in the investigation of anaemia or clotting disorders and are the province of the *haematologist*, while tests on the chemical substances in the serum related to various body disorders are the province of the *biochemist*. Both of these specialties come broadly within the term *pathology*, a name given to the scientific study of the alterations to the body produced by disease.

Haemoglobin This is the pigment in the red blood corpuscles (known as *RBCs* or *erythrocytes*) which carries oxygen to the body. If there is a shortage of red blood cells, the haemoglobin will be found to be low. Iron is necessary for the production of haemoglobin and so a low haemoglobin may be the result of an inadequate intake of iron. This is known as *iron deficiency anaemia*. Anaemia is said to be present whenever there is a fall in the red blood corpuscles and/or haemoglobin content of the blood. Foods which are rich in iron are listed on p. 101.

The haemoglobin may also be low if there has been bleeding, e.g. heavy periods, bleeding stomach ulcer, childbirth, nose bleed, cancer of the bowel, injury, etc. The diagnosis of anaemia is only a first-level diagnosis and it is always necessary to do other investigations to determine the reasons for the anaemia. Occasionally it is due to a failure of the bone marrow to form red blood cells.

In a few people there is an excess of red cells and hence an abnormally high haemoglobin level. One such condition is *polycythaemia vera*, in which the increase in the number of red cells is spontaneous. More often the increase in red cells is a response to a need for more oxygen, as occurs in people who live in a rarefied atmosphere such as the Andes. It also occurs in people with lung disorders, e.g. chronic bronchitis and emphysema, where there is a problem in getting adequate oxygen from the air through the walls of the lungs and into the bloodstream. The presence of more red cells enables such exchange of oxygen and carbon dioxide as is possible, to be more efficient.

The normal level of haemoglobin in the bloodstream varies with age and sex. Here are the usual values:

     Adult male 135–180 g per litre
     Adult female 115–165 g per litre

The size of the red cells can also be important in making a diagnosis. They tend to be smaller than normal (i.e. *microcytic*) in iron-deficiency anaemia and larger than normal (i.e. *macrocytic*) in pernicious anaemia and anaemia due to a deficiency of a vitamin known as folic acid. To assist in this diagnosis, it is possible to measure the *mean corpuscular volume* (MCV). This is the average volume of a red-blood corpuscle. It is low in iron-deficiency anaemia and high in pernicious anaemia.

White cell counts It is often useful to have a count of the white cells in the blood. There are several types of white cell, the commonest usually being the *neutrophils*. They tend to be increased in numbers in certain bacterial infections and often they are low in viral infections. This is not an invariable rule, however, and some virus infections such as herpes zoster (i.e. shingles) may cause a high neutrophil count. Apart from infections, many other conditions can influence the number of neutrophils present. The normal range is 2,500–6500 per cubic mm (i.e. 40–60 per cent of the total number of white blood corpuscles).

Another common white cell is the *lymphocyte*. Lymphocytes tend to be increased in chronic infections. Atypical lymphocytes are frequently found in infectious mononucleosis (glandular fever). Certain lymphocytes have a special role to play in the development of immune reactions, i.e. antigen-antibody. In glandular fever, for example, the lymphocytes are actively producing antibodies against the glandular fever virus. The normal range is 1500–3500 per cubic mm (i.e. 20–40 per cent) of the total number of white blood corpuscles.

The *monocyte* is another specialised white cell. Monocytes tend to be low in those with chronic infections. The normal range is 200–800 per cubic mm (i.e. 4–8 per cent of the total white blood count).

The white blood cell population also includes *eosinophils* (normal range 50–400 per cubic mm, i.e. 1–3 per cent of the total white count), and *basophils* (normal range 10–100 per cubic mm, i.e. 0–1 per cent of total white count). Eosinophils are particularly notable in allergic disorders and parasitic infections such as worms.

Platelets Platelets are tiny cells which are essential for blood clotting. They tend to be high in certain blood disorders including polycythaemia, already mentioned. A reduction in platelet numbers increases the tendency to bruise easily or even to bleed spontaneously. Increased platelet numbers can sometimes predispose to clot formation (thrombosis). The normal number of platelets range from 150,000–350,000 per cubic mm.

Blood clotting is a very complex process involving many blood constituents, and the investigation of a bleeding tendency involves many tests. Some of the substances involved in clotting are formed in the liver and this is one reason why in advanced liver disease there may be bleeding problems. Investigation of a bleeding disorder involves tests to measure both platelets and blood proteins (e.g. prothrombin, see p. 286.).

Erythrocyte sedimentation rate (ESR) When a tube filled with blood is allowed to stand, the red blood corpuscles will sink to the bottom. The rate at which this sedimentation occurs has always been of great interest to doctors. The exact reasons why the rate varies in certain conditions has never been fully determined, but active disease often gives rise to a high ESR. The higher the rate, the greater the activity. A raised ESR is often a chance finding which may alert the doctor to search more aggressively for an underlying disorder. On the other hand, a low sedimentation rate cannot be taken as absolute evidence that all is well, although considered in association with other tests it may be quite reassuring.

The sedimentation rate tends to be particularly high in the so-called 'auto-immune' diseases, of which rheumatoid arthritis is the best known. A continued fall in the ESR in an established case of such a disorder is often a good indication that the condition is improving.

The ESR is also elevated in pregnancy and has a tendency to rise with advancing years. The normal values are:

Children	0–20 mm per hour
Adult male	0–10 mm per hour
Adult female	0–20 mm per hour
Elderly	0–30 mm per hour

Biochemistry

There are literally dozens of tests which can be done on the serum for specific purposes. Only a selection of the most frequently used are included here. They are listed alphabetically.

Alkaline phosphatase (ALP) (Normal 10–75 international units per litre or 4–14 King-Armstrong units per 100 ml.)
This tends to be increased in certain bone diseases, of which the most common in adults is a condition called Paget's disease — occasionally a cause of deafness in the elderly. It is high in children when their bones are growing. Where there is a blockage of the ducts from the gallbladder to the intestines, there is usually an increase in the level of alkaline phosphatase.

Amylase (Normal 70–300 international units per litre or 80–200 Somogyi international units per 100 ml.)
This is a substance produced in the pancreas. An increase in the serum usually indicates some sort of damage to the pancreas. This is particularly notable in acute pancreatitis, which is often a result of gallstones in the bile ducts, or alternatively overindulgence in alcohol. Mumps is another possible cause of pancreatitis.

Bilirubin (Normal 1–20 micromoles per litre or 0.1–1.1 mgm per 100 ml.)
Elevations of this substance, which is really the manifestation of bile in the blood, are seen particularly when there is obstruction to the free discharge of bile from the liver. This may

occur when there is liver disease or obstruction to the bile ducts. Sometimes it is due to an excessive destruction of red blood corpuscles by the body, resulting in overloading of the liver.

Cholesterol (Normal 1.2–7.0 millimoles per litre or 115–280 mgm per 100 ml.)
This substance probably plays a part in causing coronary artery disease, as is discussed in Chapters 2.5 and 2.6 on diet. Some people exhibit a tendency to a high cholesterol and they are usually more prone than average to heart disease. Such people are said to suffer from *hypercholesterolaemia*. Cholesterol elevation bears some relationship to the intake of fats. It is also increased in persons suffering from a deficiency of thyroid gland secretions, in many people with diabetes, certain liver disorders and in nephrosis, which is a kidney disease resulting in the excessive secretion of proteins by the kidney.

Creatinine phosphokinase (CPK) (Normal 50–100 international units per litre.)
This is a substance which is produced when the muscles are damaged. Even an injection into a muscle may cause a rise. It is particularly useful to identify the presence and amount of heart damage following a coronary thrombosis (i.e. myocardial infarction, otherwise known as a heart attack).

Creatinine (Normal 0.06–0.11 millimoles per litre or 0.6–1.5 mgm per 100 ml.)
This is a sensitive indication of kidney function. When it is elevated there is usually something wrong with the kidney's ability to excrete waste products.

Glucose (Normal 3.5–6.0 millimoles per litre or 60–100 mgm per 100 ml in the fasting patient.)
When the fasting level of glucose is elevated, it suggests the possibility of diabetes. Sometimes it is high when the thyroid gland or the adrenal gland are overactive. Certain medicines, particularly diuretics, can cause a rise in glucose in the blood.

If more detailed information is required, it is sometimes useful to repeat the test at approximately half-hour intervals for two hours after the patient has been given 75 g of glucose by mouth. This is known as a *glucose tolerance test* or GTT. After two hours the serum glucose should have returned to the fasting level.

Iron (Normal male 15–30 micromoles per litre or 75–180 microgram per 100 ml; female 14–28 micromoles per litre or 65–170 microgram per 100 ml.)
The serum iron is likely to be low in iron deficiency anaemias. It is high in certain other anaemias and in a condition known as *haemochromatosis*.

Lipids (Normal 400–600 mgm per 100 ml after a 12-hour fast.)
These tend to be elevated in certain inherited conditions known as *hyperlipidaemias*. The use in diagnosis of high-density lipoproteins and low-density lipoproteins is discussed in Chapter 2.6. It is believed that excessive low-density lipoproteins increase the risk of coronary artery disease.

Potassium (Normal 3.5–5.2 millimoles per litre or 3.5–5.2 milli equivalents per litre.)
This mineral tends to accumulate in the blood when the kidneys are malfunctioning. It is likely to be lower than normal in conditions in which large quantities of body fluids are lost. Vomiting and diarrhoea may cause low potassium and so may the use of diuretics (medicines given to reduce the fluid in the body by causing the kidney to excrete more urine). An increase

in steroids in the body also leads to a decrease in potassium. Potassium and sodium appear to have an inverse relationship; when the sodium is high the potassium is low, and vice versa.

Prothombin time (Normal 12–16 secs)
This test is done in the evaluation of clotting disorders and as a means of determining the effectiveness of treatment with certain medicines which are used to prevent blood clotting (i.e. anticoagulants). The value is also increased in liver disease. Often the value is expressed as a ratio relative to a normal person. The normal range is therefore approximately 1.0 (range 0.8–1.2). The target prothombin ratio (PR) for treatment with the anticoagulant warfarin (Marevan) is 2.0.

$$\text{Prothrombin ratio} = \frac{\text{Prothrombin time of patient on treatment}}{\text{Prothrombin time of a normal person}} = \frac{24}{12} = 2$$

Sodium (Normal 137–150 millimoles per litre or 137–150 milli equivalents per litre.)
The level of the sodium (i.e. salt) has an influence on the amount of water in the body. When the body is dehydrated, this can be due to lack of water or lack of sodium. The sodium level in the body may be increased when patients have an increase in the level of steroids in their body.

Thyroid function tests (Normal free thyroxine 0.8–3.0 micrograms per 100 ml or 10–40 nanomoles per litre.)
This test is done as one of several to evaluate if the thyroid gland is producing enough of its secretion, thyroxine, for the needs of the body. Deficiency of thyroxine leads to loss of energy, apathy, increased weight and a marked sensitivity to cold. Too much (i.e. *thyrotoxicosis*), causes weight loss, intolerance of heat, tremulousness and racing of the heart. In some cases there is a tendency to increased prominence of the eyes and the so-called 'thyrotoxic stare'.

Urea (Normal 3.2–6.6 millimoles per litre or 20–40 mgm per 100 ml.)
This has similar significance to the measurement of creatinine and is used primarily in the diagnosis of kidney disorders. The amount of protein in the diet has an influence on urea levels in the blood. It may appear to be high when the body is short of fluid, as in dehydration.

Uric acid (Normal male 0.25–0.42 millimoles per litre or 3.2–8.1 mgm per 100 ml; females 0.17–0.36 millimoles per litre or 2.2–7.1 mgm per 100 ml.)
Done principally in the evaluation of gout. Uric acid also tends to be increased when the kidney is not excreting waste products normally.

Urine tests

The urine was probably the first body fluid to be subject to testing. The early physicians would taste the urine and noted that some people, whose output was particularly copious, passed urine which was sweet to the taste, while others were relatively tasteless. Those which were sweet to the taste were said to have diabetes mellitus and those which were tasteless were said to have another condition, diabetes insipidus. Subsequently it was found that the sweet taste was glucose.

We now sometimes test the urine chemically for glucose as a simple way of detecting diabetes mellitus. Generally glucose should not appear in the urine at all, but occasionally it appears as a result of anxiety or tension. Diabetics often control their dose of insulin by regularly testing the amount of sugar in their urine, but this not as reliable as a blood test.

The urine may also be examined for the presence of white blood corpuscles. When present in considerable numbers these indicate the presence of infection. Such urine is then cultured with a view to identifying the organism responsible for the infection, preferably before treatment is started. Sometimes an infection may cause the presence of red blood corpuscles in the urine (i.e. *haematuria*) as well as white blood corpuscles. There can be many other causes of haematuria and if not explained by infection, it always requires a full investigation.

Also regularly looked for in urine is the presence of the protein, *albumin*. This is present in small quantities in infections, but when seen in abundance suggests the possibility of an important kidney disorder known as *nephrosis*.

APPENDIX 2
The infectious diseases — a summary

Disease	Time from contact to start of disease	Period of infectivity to others	Features
Measles (Rubeola, morbilli)	7–14 days	2–4 days before rash to 2–5 days after onset	Brown-red spots becoming confluent, red eyes, runny nose.
Rubella (German measles)	14–21 days	Just before rash appears until rash disappears	Pink spots less inclined to confluence than measles. Mild illness.
Chickenpox (Varicella)	14–21 days	A day or two before symptoms, until last spot has crusted over	Colourless blisters on red surround. Occurs in crops.
Infectious mononucleosis (Glandular fever)	10–30 days	Uncertain	Occasionally a rash similar to measles or scarlet fever.
Scarlet fever	3–5 days	1 day before symptoms until 2–3 weeks after	Pink colour of skin, strawberry-like tongue
Mumps	14–24 days	Just before symptoms until glandular swelling disappears	Usually swelling of the parotid glands just in front of the ears.
Whooping cough	7–21 days	Just before symptoms for at least 4 weeks	Typical whoop associated with cough; vomiting.

APPENDIX 3

Cardiopulmonary resuscitation — some questions and answers

(Based on the recommendations of the American Heart Foundation)

Q. Assume that you have just encountered a patient who has collapsed from unknown causes. What will be your first action?
A. Check if patient is conscious.
Q. If the patient is unresponsive and lying awkwardly, what will be your next action?
A. Make sure the patient is on his or her back (i.e. supine) on a firm surface. The floor is better than a bed.
Q. What is the next step?
A. Check that the patient is breathing. If necessary, open the airway by tilting the head in such a way that the tongue is away from the roof of the mouth.
Q. If the patient is not breathing, how do you proceed?
A. Commence mouth-to-mouth respiration, i.e. rescue breathing.
Q. How should rescue breathing be done?
A. Pinch the nostrils and make a seal with your mouth around the patient's mouth so air will not escape as you blow in. Check that the chest rises with every breath.
Q. What is likely to be your greatest concern at this stage with respect to respiration?
A. One is always concerned that the patient may vomit and obstruct the passage of air.
Q. How many breaths should be given in the first instance?
A. Give four breaths initially.
Q. What is the next step?
A. Check the pulse. This is usually best felt in the neck over the carotid artery as it passes between the Adam's apple and neck muscles.
Q. If the pulse is absent or questionable, what should you do next?
A. Commence external cardiac massage?

Q. What is the mechanism of external cardiac massage?
A. The heart is squeezed between the sternum (i.e. breastbone) and the spine. In this way, an artificial circulation is produced.
Q. Where is the pressure applied?
A. The lower end of the sternum. Fit your middle fingers into the notch where the lower ribs meet the sternum. Place the heel of the hand next to those fingers, put the other hand on top so that the heels of both hands are parallel and the fingers directed away from you. Now, keeping your elbows straight, apply pressure straight down — using the weight of your body.
Q. How far should the sternum be depressed?
A. In an adult, approximately 4 to 5 centimetres (1½–2 inches).
Q. How many chest compressions per minutes should you aim for?
A. 80. This allows for intervals when mouth-to-mouth respiration can be given.
Q. How many chest compressions should be given between mouth-to-mouth respiration?
A. 15, if you are working alone.*
Q. How many breaths should you give between each cycle of 15 chest compressions?
A. 2.
Q. After a minute of this cycle of chest compressions and mouth-to-mouth respiration, what should you do?
A. Check to see if a pulse is obtainable.
It should be re-checked every few minutes thereafter.

---

*Note: If 2 people are working together, 1 breath is given for every 5 chest compressions. There is no interval in the chest compressions (60 per minute).

Acknowledgements

Many people have given support, advice and helpful criticism in the development of this book. The following have assisted in reviewing appropriate sections:

Dr Phillip Barham
Dr Michael Cooper
Dr Rick Cutfield
Mrs Margaret Gibson-Smith
Mrs Lynn Gillanders
Dr Wilma Grant
Mrs Trish Gribben
Dr Nick Holford
Dr Judith Johnson
Mrs Deirdre Kent

Dr Bob Large
Ms Kerry Maher
Professor Colin Mantell
Dr Roy Morris
Dr Paul Ockelford
Ms Merren Parker
Mrs Yvonne Partridge
Dr Alex Thomson
Dr Bill Tucker
Professor Rae West

All of these have given me the benefit of their knowledge and expertise and I am very grateful to them. If there remain any errors of fact, these are my responsibility and not that of my advisors.

I would particularly like to pay tribute to the encouragement to pursue this project given me by Mrs Margaret Gibson-Smith, Chief Librarian of the Philson Library at the Auckland School of Medicine, who perceived a real need for such a book.

My thanks also to Mrs Lynda Burgess and Ms Ruth Bliss who have laboured for so long and with such diligence on the preparation of the typescript and to Mrs Joy Browne and the staff of David Bateman Ltd, publishers, for their friendly and helpful cooperation at all times. Finally, my thanks to Lincoln Wakefield, now residing in Australia, who responded to a special request to provide the line drawings which so admirably complement the text.

Reading list

Childhood Asthma. Neil Buchanan, Hodder & Stoughton, 1986
How to Give up Smoking Forever. Deirdre Kent, Consumers Institute of New Zealand, 1986
Putting the Ill at Ease. Evelyn Wilde Mayerson, Harper & Row, 1976
Medicines. A Guide for Everybody. Peter Parish, Penguin, 1984
Family Medical Guide. A. M. Cooke (ed.), Longman, 1980
Sleep. Ian Oswald, Penguin, 1970
Alcoholism. Kessel & Walton, Pelican, 1972
The Doctors. Paul Ferris, Pelican, 1967
I'm OK — You're OK. Thomas Harris, Pan, 1979
Dying. John Hinton, Pelican, 1972
Bereavement. Colin Murray Parkes, Pelican, 1978
Questions & Answers on Death & Dying. Elizabeth Kübler-Ross, Macmillan, 1974
Modern Therapies. Binder, Binder & Rimland, Prentice Hall, 1976
Exercise, The Facts. E. J. Bassey & P. H. Fentem, Oxford University Press, 1981
Games People Play. Eric Berne, Penguin, 1964
The Pritikin Promise. Nathan Pritikin, Pan Books, 1983
Farley Goes to the Doctor. E. P. Kingsley, a Sesame Street/Golden Press Book, 1980
Nicky Goes to the Doctor. Richard Scarry, Golden Press, 1978
Nits & Other Nasties. Trish Gribben & David Geddes, Heinemann, 1982
Pyjamas Don't Matter. Trish Gribben, Heinemann, 1979
Book of Child Care. Hugh Jolly, George Allen & Unwin Ltd, 1975
AIDS: The Risk. Paul Goldwater, Penguin, 1986
The Billings Method. Controlling fertility without drugs. Penguin, 1980
Why me? Merren Parker, Australia & NZ Book Coy, 1981
To the Good Long Life. Morton Puner, Macmillan, 1978
A Time to Enjoy. The pleasures of ageing. William Dangott & Richard Kalish, Prentice Hall, 1979
A Time to Grieve. Merren Parker, Reed, 1987
How to Bring up Your Parents. Stanley Gold & Peter Eisen, Sun Books, 1969
The Family Doctor's Answer Book: A total guide to your child's health. A Matthew Cohen, Appleton-Century Crofts, 1980
The Psychology of Interpersonal Behaviour. Michael Angyle, Pelican, 1976

Counselling — A Skills Approach. E. A. Munro, R. J. Manthei, J. J. Small, Methuen Publications (NZ), 1979
Primary Health Care & The Community. John Richards, Longman Paul, 1981
Diabetes Explained. Arnold Bloom, MTP Press, 1982
High Blood Pressure. Peter Lewis, Churchill Livingstone, 1981
Coronary Heart Disease — The Facts. J. P. Shillingford, Oxford University Press, 1981
It's Your Body. Know What the Doctor Ordered — A Guide to Medical Testing. M. L. Fox & T. G. Schnabel, Charles Press Publishers, 1979
The Medical Risks of Life. Stephen Lock & Tony Smith, Penguin, 1976
The Good Health Guide. Open University, Pan Books, 1982
How to Live with Diabetes. H. Dolger, B. Seeman, Penguin, 1984
The Medical Maze. Ronald Bridger, Brick Row Publishing Coy, 1985

Index

Abbreviations, in prescriptions 206, 212, 214
ABC theory 199
Abdominal pain 130; in anxiety 81; importance of history 130; types of pain 24
ABO abnormality, screening 52
Abortion 268; recurrent 71; screening 53; in German measles 163
Abreaction 198
Abscess, in middle ear 150
Abstinence, in alcoholism 112
Academy of Family Practice (USA) 33
Accidents 43, 54f, 60, 61
Acetohexamide (Dimelor) 274
Acid/alkali balance 79, 242
Acid 258; regurgitation 132, 258; excess 131; on oesophagus 132; as cause of abdominal pain 131
Acid risings 132
Acne 182; effect of the pill 262; causes, treatment 182-3, 232, 239
Acquired haemolytic anaemia 221
Acquired immune deficiency syndrome (see AIDS)
Acupuncture, in smoking 117; for back 127
Acyclovir, method of use 160, 241
Adalat (nifedipine) 247, 248
ADARDS 280
Addiction 107; amphetamines 231 (see Dependence)
Addison's disease 219
Adenoids, in otitis media 149
Adolescence, and schizophrenia 196; and asthma 155; atopic eczema 164; and the contraceptive pill 261
Adoption 66
Adrenal gland, in hypertension 245
Adrenalin (epinephrine) 45, 245, 247; in maintaining glucose levels 270; in urticaria 144; in asthma 153
Aerosol, in asthma 154
Agitation, in depression 195
AIDS 241, 242, 267, 276
Air hunger 80
Al-Anon, objectives 113
Albumin 287
Alcohol 44; in coronary artery disease 44; in tension headache 137; motor vehicle accidents 45; as vasodilator 249; cause of ulcer 131, 133; effect on pancreas 109
Alcoholics 16; screening 60, 61; effects of withdrawal 108; physical damage 108
Alcoholism, definitions 108; at-risk persons 109; self-test 109; problems 279; CAGE test 110; acceptance 110; role of spouse 111; scapegoating 111
Alcoholics Anonymous 112; credo 113; 12 steps to recovery 114
Aldactone 256
Aldomet (methyldopa) 246
Alkaline phosphatase 284
Allegron (nortriptyline) 228
Allergens 143, 157, 222
Allergies 23; with aspirin 205; use of corticosteroids 221; rashes 143; nasal discharge 157
Allergy 222; to food 94; to medicines 206; gastro-intestinal 81; skin tests 94, 222; rashes 143
Allopurinol (Zyloprim), use in gout 172
Alpha-blockers (see Blocking agents) 245
Alpha-keri 164
Alrheumat (ketoprofen) 219
Aluminium hydroxide 258
Alupent (orciprenaline) 154
Alzheimer's disease 279
Amantadine (Symmetrel) 234; use in influenza A 241
Amiloride 256
Aminoglycosides 240
Aminophylline, in asthma 153
Amiodarone 257
Amitriptyline (Elavil) 228; use in migraine 139
Amoxil 122, 213, 236; effect on the contraceptive pill 266
Amoxycillin (see Amoxil) 213
Amphetamine 231; in overweight 86
Amphotericin 242
Ampicillin (Penbritin) 237
Amylase 284
Anaemia 282; screening for 57, 62; in cancer of the bowel 282; investigation of 282; cause of fatigue 140
Anafranil (clomipramine) 228
Analgesic 225; constipation 253
Anal hygiene 167, 177
Anal tag 167
Anatensol (fluphenazine) 227
Anger, response of baby 68; in depression 173; suppressed 195
Angina, causes 141-2, 247
Anginine (glyceryl trinitrate) 248
Angio-oedema 144
Angiotensin 247
Angor animi 141
Ankles, swelling, in heart failure 255
Anorexia nervosa 88, 180
Anovlar 263
Antabuse (disulfiram) 112
Antacids 258
Antenatal (prenatal) screening 51; classes 67
Antibacterials 235f
Antibiotics 19, 235; correct indication for use 136, 155; cause of thrush 176
Antibodies 222
Anti-clotting tablets, use with aspirin 250; prothrombin time 286
Antidepressants 228; effect on appetite 258
Antifungals 241; gentian violet 242
Antigen 222
Antigen-antibody reactions 222
Antihistamines 157; drowsiness 223, 279; in asthma 155; in vertigo 149; in nausea 177
Anti-inflammatory medicines 131; combination with diuretics 219
Antispasmodics 82
Antivert (meclizine) 149
Antiviral agents 241
Antra, in sinusitis 156
Anturan (sulphinpyrazone) 172
Anus, use of suppositories 210
Anxiety 190-5, 226; pregnancy related 66; symptoms 191; cause of acidity 131; cause of fatigue 140
Aphthous ulcers of the mouth 124; use of steroids 221
Apisate (diethylpropion) 231
Apresoline (hydrallazine) 246-7
Appendicitis 133f
Appetite, effect of medicines 86, 262; in depression 195
Appointment, with doctor 20; booking 21, 37; double 21; cancellation 21
Aprinox (bendrofluazide) 256
Aquacare 164
Arguments, as cause of stress 78
Artane (benzhexol) 234
Arteries, coronary 142, 247-8
Ascorbic acid (Vitamin C) 241
ASH 43
Aspirin 171, 205, 218, 252; in allergies 205; in asthma 155; in pregnancy 218; breast feeding 218; with anti-clotting tablets 250; in tension headache 137; in pain 218; in sore throat 124
Astemizole (Hismanal) 157, 223
Asthma 128, 152, 222; in children of parents who smoke 116; with aspirin 155; use of corticosteroids 221; dangers of respiratory depressants 155; cardiac 152; infection in 155; exercise 153; use of peak flow meter 153; diary 153; treatment 246; danger signs 155
Astringents 167
Atheroma, (see also Atherosclerosis) 46, 96, 99, 248, 249
Atherosclerosis, risk factors 46
Ativan (Lorazepam) 227

INDEX

Atopic eczema 83; use of steroids 164; in adolescence 164; in infancy 164
Atria 256, 257
Atrial fibrillation, with digoxin 256
'At-risk' patient, for alcoholism 109; breast cancer 75; cancer of the cervix 71
Atropine, side-effects 229; constipation 229; difficulty focussing 229; prostate problems 229; rapid heart beat 257
Augmentin 237
Auscultation 129
Auto-immune disorders 223; ESR in 284
Autonomic nervous system 245
Aventyl (nortriptyline) 228
Aversive conditioning 202
Azapropazone (Rheumox) 219
Azatadine maleate (Zadine) 157
AZT (azidothymidine) 276

Back, backache 127; injuries 125; problems in overweight 86; use of anti-inflammatories 127; slipped disc 124; gynaecological disorders 127
Bacteria, in bronchitis 135; resistance 236; gram negative 240; anaerobic 240
Bactericidal antibacterials 236
Bacteriostatic antibacterials 236
Bacteriuria, in pregnancy 53,69
Bactrim (cotrimoxazole) 238
Balance, semicircular canals 147
Baldness 247
Barbiturates 225, 232
Barium enema 179
Barium meal 131
Basal cell carcinoma (BCC), rodent ulcer, treatment 165-6
Basal temperature 268
Basophils 222, 283
BCG inoculation 75
Beclomethasone (Becotide) 157
Becotide (beclomethasone) 157
Bedwetting (see Nocturnal enuresis) 184, 203, 230
Behavioural therapy 201
Behaviour problems 58, 59, 60
Belief systems 199
Benadryl (diphenhydramine) 149
Bendrofluazide (Neonaclex) 256
Benemid (probenecid) 172
Benserazide (Madopar) 233
Benzhexol (Artane) 234
Benzoates, in allergies 144-5
Benzodiazepines 227
Benzoyl peroxide (Benoxyl) 182
Benztropine (Cogentin) 234
Bereavement, depression in 173
Berotec (fenoterol hydrobromide) 154
Beta-blockers (see Blocking agents) 245, 250, 257

Betnovate (betamethasone valerate) 220
Biguanides, in diabetes 272; diarrhoea 272
Bile 131
Biliary colic, cause 130-1
Bilirubin, normal values 284
Billings method 269
Biochemistry 282
Biphasil 264
Bipolar affective disorder 195
Bisacodyl (Dulcolax) 167, 260
Bismuth, as antacid 258
Blackhead 182
Bladder, control 230; cancer 116; infection 184; in smokers 116
Bleeding, screening for disorders of 53; of bowel 75-6; midcycle 268; causes 282
Blindness 163; with herpes 160
Blocking agents 245; place in migraine 250; contraindications 250
Blood count, in diagnosis of fatigue 140
Blood group, screening, Rh status 52; ABO abnormality 54
Blood, loss of 31; in faeces 76; clotting 286
Blood pressure, high 71; normal levels 244; indications for treatment 244; method of taking 244; in diabetic 271; low 148
Blood sugar, normal levels 272
Boils 159, 273
Bone cancer 125
Bone marrow, disorder with chloramphenicol 205
Bowels, bowel habits 75; screening for cancer 75; as cause of blood loss 76; looseness 134; looseness in anxiety 191; mucus 81; spasm 80; infection 239
Bran, cause of flatus 81; in constipation 260
Breast, cancer 72, 125; radiation 73; frequency of examination 73; ultrasound 73; mammography 73; hormones for cancer 72; pituitary suppression 72; ovary suppression 72; self-examination 73; risk factors 75; milk 88
Breast feeding, screening to encourage 53; use of aspirin 218; use of progestagen-only pill 265
Breath control 193
Breathing 256f; laboured with ketones 271
Brevinor 263
Bricanyl (terbutaline) 154
British National Formulary (BNF) 213-4
British Pharmacopoeia (BP) 214
British Pharmaceutical Codex (BPC) 213-4
Bromides 225

Bromocriptine (Parlodel) 233
Bronchial tubes, inflammation 129
Bronchiectasis, as cause of cough 129
Bronchioles 116
Bronchitis, chronic 116, 129, 135; depressants 253; as cause of polycythaemia 283; cough in 128
Bronchodilators, in cough 128
Bronchospasm 128
Brucella 239
Brufen (ibuprofen) 219
Bulimia 88
Bulk, inadequate 259
Buprenorphine (Temgesic) 253
'Burnout' 29
Burns 239
Butazolidine (phenylbutazone), effects on bone marrow 219

Caffeine, effect on sleep 228; side-effects 148, 231
CAGE test, for alcoholism 110
Calcium, food sources 100; in heart muscle 255; carbonate as antacid 258; in osteoporosis 187
Calculus, renal 130
Calls to doctor, out of hours, at house 20
Camcolit (see Lithium carbonate) 195
Canadian Task Force on Periodic Health Examination 51
Candida albicans (monilia), thrush 175; treatment 175-6, 242
Canestan (clotrimazole) 175, 242
Cancer, fear of 24; danger signs 48; of cervix 62, 64-5, 180; of breast 62-3; skin 62, 64-5; bone 125; bladder 62, 64-5, 116; mouth 64, 115; pre-cancerous changes 70; lung 75; throat 45; uterus 180, 186
Capillaries, in heart failure 255
Capoten (captopril) 247
Captopril (Capoten) 247
Carbamazepine (Tegretol) 232
Carafate (sucralfate) 259
Carbenoxolone, side-effects 259
Carbidopa (Sinemet) 233
Carbohydrate, in diet 84
Carbon dioxide, in hyperventilation 79
Carbon monoxide, in smokers 116
Carcinoma (see Cancer)
Cardiac asthma 155-6
Cardiac massage, method 289
Cardiomyopathy, in alcoholism 108
Cardioversion 257
Cardizem (diltiazem) 247-8
Care 34f, fragmentation of 38
Caries 210; screening for 59-61, 63; diet in 70
Carotid artery, compression in migraine 139
Cartilage, torn 170
Cascara 260
'Case finding' 51
Castor oil 260

Casual sex, risks 277
Catapres (clonidine) 186, 247
Cataracts 147; parathyroids 208; in diabetes 147, 273; with injury 147
Ceclor (cefaclor) 238
Cephalexin (Keflex) 238
Cephalosporin 123, 238
Cephradine (Velosef) 238
Cerebrovascular accident (CVA) 247
Cervical incompetence, after conization 71
Cervical smears 38, 70–1; frequency 71; method 70; after genital herpes 71, 161
Cervix, screening 61–2; at-risk patients 71; cancer 70–1; effect of pill 71; infection 174
Changing doctors 19
Check-ups 51f
Chemotherapeutic agents 235
Chest, disorders 128f, 152f; in overweight 86; pain 141
Chest infection, in children whose parents smoke 116
Chest pain, character, radiation, site 141
Chest X-ray, lung cancer 75; tuberculosis 75
Chicken pox (varicella) 159, 163
Child abuse 66; screening for 67; obtaining help 67
Child, newborn 53f
Childbirth, as cause of blood loss 282; effect on dysmenorrhoea 181
Children, going to the doctor 30f; unplanned 66; weight, length 54
Chlamydia, as cause of vaginal discharge, treatment 174, 239; in urethritis 185
Chloasma, with the pill 262
Chloral 225
Chloramphenicol, bone marrow disorder 205
Chlordiazepoxide (Librium) 227
Chlormezanone (Trancopal) 227
Chloroquin, cause of photosensitivity 171
Chlorothiazide 256
Chlorpromazine (Largactil) 227; action on the pill 266
Chlorpropamide (Diabinese) 272
Chlorthalidone 256
Cholesterol 285, 96f; in diabetes 274
Chronic obstructive respiratory disease (CORD), in smoking 116
Cigar smoking 115
Cimetidine (Tagamet, Contracid) 133, 160, 259
Cirrhosis 167; in alcoholism 108
Citravescent 241
Clavulanic acid 237
Clindamycin 183
Clinics 38
Clinoril (sulindac) 219
Clomipramine (Anafranil) 228
Clonidine (Catapres, Dixarit), in migraine 250; in hot flushes 186; in hypertension 247
Chloroquin, in rheumatoid arthritis 171
Chlotride 256
Clotrimoxazole (Canestan) 175, 242
Clots, with the pill 260; with oestrogen 186
Coal tar 165
Coca leaf 225
Codeine 129, 218, 252
Coffee 228, 231; as cause of acidity 131
Cogentin (benztropine) 234
Colace (dioctyl sodium sulphosuccinate) 260
Colchicine, use in gout 172
Cold (coryza) 135–7
Cold, as cause of spasm 249; as cause of cough 128
Cold sore (see Herpes simplex) 160, 174, 241; in AIDS 278
'Cold turkey' 107, 226
Colic, description 130
Colon, irritable 81
Coloxyl (dioctyl sodium sulphosuccinate) 260
Coma, with ketones 271; too much insulin 271; high blood sugar 271
Combined pill, changing to progestagen only 265; safety 261
Comedone 182
Common cold 135–7
Communication, non-verbal 28
Community-orientated care 33
Concentration, in depression 195
Concordin (Protriptyline) 228
Conditioning 202
Condom 266, 277
Confidence 18, 22
Confidentiality 15, 22
Confusion 17
Congenital dislocation of hip (CDH) 70; screening for 54–5
Congenital disorders of the heart; screening for 54–5; as cause of breathlessness 155
Congestive heart failure 255
Conization, for abnormal smears 70–1
Conjunctivitis 179
Constipation 166, 259; with analgesics 253; causes 229, 246; treatment 259
Contact dermatitis (see Contact eczema) 143, 222
Contact eczema, causes 143
Contact lens, and the pill 266
Continuity 15, 34
Contraceptives, oral 261; contraindications 261; starting 264; complications 180; effect of diarrhoea and vomiting 266; other medicines 266; constituents 263f; in dysmenorrhoea 181; barrier methods 266–7
Convulsions, with fever 31
Coordination 108
CORD (chronic obstructive respiratory disease), in smokers 116
Cordarone X 257
Coronary arteries 142, 247–8; thrombosis 254, 257; vasospasm 249
Coronary heart disease 46
Corticosteroids (see Cortisone) derivatives 220f; treatment card 221–2
Cortisone (see Corticosteroids) 219
Coryza (common cold), features 135–7
Cost benefit, of screening 50
Cost of care 16
Cotrimoxazole (Bactrim, Septrin) 238f; in acne 183, 238
Cough, causes, treatment 128–9
Cough centre, cough reflex 129, 253
Cough mixture, contents 129
Counselling, by social workers 37; psychologists 190; the Church 37
Cradle cap 164
Cream, as moisturiser 212
Creatine phosphokinase (CPK), screening for 61; in myocardial infarction 285; normal values 285
Creatinine, in kidney function 285; normal values 285
Crepitations, in lungs 254
Criteria, for screening 50
Crohn's disease 221
Cushing's syndrome 219
Cyanosis 249
Cyclandelate (Cyclospasmol) 249
Cyclizine (Marzine) 177
Cyclopenthiazide 256
Cyclospasmol (cyclandelate) 249
Cyproheptadine (Periactin) 258
Cystic fibrosis, screening for 54
Cystitis 184, 241; screening for 53; outlook in 69, 184

D-penicillamine, side-effects 171
D and C (dilatation and curettage) 180
Daktarin (miconazole) 242
Dalmane (flurazepam) 227
Dander, animal, as cause of allergy 157, 223
Dandruff 164
Danthron, as laxative 80, 260
Daonil (glibenclamide) 272, 274
DDT powder, in treatment of lice 162
Decongestants, nasal 157; in haemorrhoids 167
Defencin (isoxsuprine hydrochloride) 249
Dehydration, with ketones, with vomiting 178, 271
Delirium tremens, in alcoholism 108
Dementia 279
Demerol (pethidine) 252–3

De-nol (tri-potassium dicitrato bismuthate) 259
Dental decay (caries) 59f
Denver test, for development assessment 56, 58
Dependence 106; on drugs 225
Depo-provera 264
Depression, screening 53, 66, 173, 195; in alcoholism 109; relation to anxiety 191; in dementia 279; as cause of fatigue 141; diagnosis 195; in bereavement 173; treatment 228f; with the pill 262; resistance to disease 135; at menopause 185; in anorexia nervosa 88; with period 181; with clonidine 250
Deputising services 35
Dermatitis 143f, 158f; industrial 143; atopic (*see* Eczema) 164
Dermovate (clobetasol propionate) 220
Desensitisation 202
Deseril (methysergide) 139
Detachment, clinical 201
Development, delayed, screening for 55–7; questions for parents 67
Dextropropoxyphene (Doloxene) 253
Diabetes insipidus, urine testing 286
Diabetes mellitus 270; screening in pregnancy 51; diuretics in 85, 257; insulin 274; oral treatment 272; dehydration 271; mumps as cause 272; juvenile (IDDM) 272; maturity onset (NIDDM) 272; weight reduction 270; recording results 273; complications 159, 272; cholesterol in 285; fructosamine 274; coma 271; urine infections 184
Diagnosis 16
Diamicron 272
Diaper (napkin) rash 164
Diaphragm, for contraception 267
Diaphragmatic hernia 132
Diarrhoea 80, 177–8, 239; treatment 178; prolonged in AIDS 278
Diary, food 87, 95; asthma 153
Diastole 243–4
Diastop (diphenoxylate) 178
Diathermy 165
Diazepam (Valium) 106, 149, 227, 232
Diclofenac (Voltaren) 219
Dideocytidine, in AIDS 276
Diet 23, 46; screening for 52, 61f; in caries 70; reducing 84f; strict 89f; in constipation 260; in diabetes 274–5; in stomach ulcer 131; low residue 81; low salt in Meniere's disease 149
Diethylpropion (Apisate, Tenuate) 231
Dietitians, role of 38
Diflunisal (Dolobid) 219
Digestive system 25

Digitalis leaf 204
Digoxin 204, 254f; in thyrotoxicosis 257
Dilantin (phenytoin) 232, 257
Dilatation and currettage (D and C) 180
Dilaudid 253
Diltiazem (Cardizem) 247–8
Dimelor (*see* Acetohexamide) 274
Dioctyl sodium sulphosuccinate (Docusate, Dioctyl, Coloxyl) in constipation 260
Dioctyl (*see* Dioctyl sodium sulphosuccinate) 260
Diphenhydramine (Benadryl) 149
Diphenoxylate (Lomotil, Diastop) 178
Discharge, penis 185; vagina 174; with the pill 262
Disease, symptomless 49; tendency to cluster 51
Disipal (orphenadrine hydrochloride) 234
Disopyramide (Rhythmodan) 257
Dissatisfaction, with doctor 19
District nurse 38
Disulfiram (Antabuse), slow acting 112
Diuretics 85, 245, 256–7; in Meniere's disease 149; precipitates gout 171; in heart failure 255
Diuril 256
Diverticulitis, causes 134–5
Divorce, as factor in alcoholism 109
Dixarit (clonidine) 247, 250
Dizziness, in hypotension 148
Doctor 17; role 33
Doctor-patient relationship 17
Docusate (*see* Dioctyl sodium sulphosuccinate) 260
Dolobid (diflunisal) 219
Doloxene 253
Dopamine 233
Dorbanex (danthron) 260
Dosage 207
Dothiepin (prothiaden) 228
Double-blind trial 209
Down's syndrome, screening 52
Doxepin (sinequan) 228
Doxycycline 239
Drops, eye, ear, nose, methods of application 211
Drowsiness 155
Drugs 45; addiction to 252; dependence 226; screening for 53
Dulcolax (bisacodyl) 260; in haemorrhoids 167
Duodenal ulcer (*see* Ulcer) 131, 258
Duphalac (lactulose) 260
Duromine (phentermine) 231
Dusting powder 212
Duvalidan (isoxsuprine hydrochloride) 249
Dysmenorrhoea 181f
Dyspnoea 256
Dysuria 183

Dytac 256

Earache 31; causes 149–51
Eardrum, perforation 149
Ears, discharging 150; screening for defects of hearing 54
Ear drops 211f
ECG (electrocardiogram) 142, 257
Econazole (Ecostatin, Gynopevaryl) 175
Eczema, atopic 164; in otitis externa 151; infantile 164
Edecrin (ethacrynic acid) 240
Efudix (fluorouracil) 165
Ego 198
Elavil (amitriptyline) 228
Electrocardiogram (ECG or EKG) 257; in investigation of heart pain 142
Electro-convulsive therapy (ECT), *see* Shock treatment 196, 228
Emergency care 20, 35, 37
Emergency, what constitutes one 31
Emotion, emotional problems 77
Empathy 192
Emphysema, in smoking 116; as cause of polycythaemia 283; as cause of breathlessness 156
Encephalitis, in Parkinson's disease 233
Enalapril (Renitec) 247
Endocrine glands, in acne 182
Endocrine system 27
Endometriosis, treatment 181
Endometrium, in menstruation 179
Endorphins 194
Energy, requirements 85; food values 89f
Enteritis 177
Eosinophils 283
Epanutin (phenytoin sodium) 232
Ephedrine 154
Epigastrium 131
Epilepsy 232
Epilim (sodium valproate) 232
Epsom salts (magnesium sulphate) 260
Ergotamine, use in migraine 139, 250; dangers in angina 249
Erosion of cervix 266
Eructation 81
Erythrocyte, sedimentation rate (ESR or BSR) *see* ESR 284
Erythromycin 239; in penicillin allergy 123, 159; for chlamydia 176; in acne 183
ESR (erythrocyte sedimentation rate), normal values 284; in rheumatoid arthritis 171
Essential nutrients 93
Ethacrynic acid (Edecrin) 240
Ethics, medical 18
Ethosuximide, in petit mal 232
Ethinyl oestradiol 261f
Ethynodiol diacetate 263
Euglycon 272

Eugynon 264
Euhypnos (temazepam) 227
Eumovate (clobetasone butyrate) 220
Euphoria 77
Eustachian tubes, effects of blockage 135, 149, 157
Examination 16; clothing 21; internal 175
Exercise 102f; as aid to relaxation 194
Exocrine glands 182
External cardiac massage 289f
External pile (perianal haematoma) 167
Eye drops 211
Eyes 156f; screening for gonococcal infection 54; screening for squint 54–5, 59; check in diabetes 274; pain/irritation 179
Eyesight, focusing 60
Eyestrain, as cause of headache 138

Fabahistin (mebhydrolin) 157
Facial tenderness, in sinusitis 157
Facilitation 201
Faintness 247
Fallopian tubes 269
Family, care 15, 21, 34; definition 33; physician 32; therapy 203
Family practitioner, definitions 33
Faintness 148; as side effect of treatment for blood pressure 243, 247
Fatigue, causes 140–1
Fat, in diet 84
Fatty acids, essential, sources 93
Feldene (piroxicam) 219
Femodene 264
Femulen 263
Fenbrufen (Lederfen) 219
Fenfluramine (Ponderax) 231
Fenoprofen (Fenopron) 219
Fenopron (fenoprofen) 219
Fenoterol hydrobromide (Berotec) 154
Fertility 268
Fever with convulsions 31; in sinusitis 157; in otitis media (see Temperature); in AIDS 278
Fibrillation, atrial 256
Fibrinogen 282
Fibroids 71; effect on menstrual periods 180
Filter cigarettes 115
Fingernails, infection 161; pitting in psoriasis 165
Fits 232
Fixed drug rash 145
Flagyl (metronidazole) 176, 240
Flatus (wind) 81
Flecainide (Tambocur) 257
Floaters, in eye 147
Flooding 202
Floxapen (flucloxacillin) 159, 237
Flucloxacillin (Floxapen) 159, 237
Fluphenazine (Moditen) 227

Fluid, replacement in gastro-enteritis 178
Flunitrazepam (Rohypnol) 227
Fluorine, food sources 93
Fluorouracil (Efudix) 165
Flurazepam (Dalmane) 227
Flurbiprofen (Froben) 219
Folic acid 94, 283
Food, allergy 94; diary 87
Food poisoning 177
Foreign body, in eye 179
Formulation 212
Fortral (pentazocine) 253
Foxglove, tincture, extract 204
Framycetin (Soframycin) 240
Free association 198
Freud, Sigmund, and psychotherapy 198
Friar's balsam 157
Froben (flurbiprofen) 219
Fructosamine, as test of diabetic control 274
Fruit, use in reducing diets 92
Frusemide (Lasix) 240, 256
Fulcin (griseofulvin) 161
Fungal infection 161f, 273
Furadantin (nitrofurantoin) 240

Gallbladder, disease in overweight 86; pain 253; constriction of ducts with morphine 253; biliary colic 130
Ganglion blockers, hexamethonium, mecamyamine (Inversine) 246
Gangrene 249–50; in diabetes 273
Gardnerella vaginalis 175
Gastric ulcer (see Ulcer) 131, 258
Gastritis 177
Gastro-enteritis, causes, treatment 177
Gastrolyte 178
Gastroscope 132
Gastrozepine (pirenzepine) 259
General paralysis of the insane (GPI) 196
General practice 32f
General practitioner 14, 32; role in emotional disorders 191
Generic name vs trade names 11, 213
Genito-urinary system 25f
Gentamicin 240
Gentian violet 242; antibacterial, antifungal 175, 242
German measles (rubella) 288; screening 57, 163
Giardia lamblia 240
Giddiness, from ear drops 211; treatment 149
Glandular fever (infectious mononucleosis) 83, 122, 163, 288
Glaucoma 178–9
Glibenclamide (see Daonil) 272, 274
Gliclazide 272
Glipizide (Glibenese, Glucotiol) 272, 274
Globus hystericus 80

Glucagon, in low blood sugar 270
Glucophage (see Metformin) 272, 274
Glucose 270; in diabetes 270f; normal values 285
Glucose tolerance test (GTT) 285
Glue-ear 150
Glyceryl trinitrate 248; patch 211
Glycogen, stored in liver 270
Gold salts, side-effects 171
Gonorrhoea, screening 52, 54, 62, 185; infection of cervix 174
Gout 171–2; uric acid 286; in back problems 128
Grand mal 232
Granocol 82
Griseofulvin 161; action on the pill 266; in fungal infections 161, 242
Grisovin (griseofulvin) 161, 242
Group therapy 112
Growth chart 54–9
Growth disorders, screening for 54–5, 58–60
GTT (see Glucose tolerance test) 285
Guanethidine (Ismelin) 246
Guilt, in depression 195
Gullet (see Oesophagus)
Gynaecological, problems as cause of back pain 127; examination 175
Gynotrosyd (ticonazole) 176
Gynovlar 263

Haematology, tests done 282
Haemophilus influenzae 239
Haemoglobin 282; need for iron 282
Haemorrhoids (piles) 76; straining 259; and varicose veins 167; in pregnancy 167; treatment 166–7
Halcion (triazolam) 227
Haloperidol (Serenace) 197
Hallucinations, in alcoholism 108; in psychosis 196
Hand, foot and mouth disease 163
Hayfever 156, 222
HDL (see High density lipoprotein)
Headache 137–9, 185; with caffeine 231; with glyceryl trinitate 248
Health, WHO definition 42; change as a cause of stress 77
Hearing, screening 54, 59–61, 63–4
Heart 27; failure 129, 254; in rheumatic fever 122; as cause of cough 129
Heart attack (see Myocardial infarction) 141, 273
Heartburn 132
Heart disease, contraception in 261
Heat, effect on spasm 126
Height, as indicator of osteoporosis 65, 187
Hepatitis, cause of jaundice 131 cause of gastro-enteritis 177
Hepatitis B, screening for 54–5; inoculation 43, 57
Herbal remedies 204
Heroin, dependence 252
Herpes simplex (cold sore) 160, 241;

INDEX 299

effect of steroids 221; in eye 160; on cervix 174
Herpes zoster (shingles) 159, 241
Herpes, genital 160
Herplex (idoxuridine) 241
Hexamethonium 246
Hexopal (inositol nicotinate) 249
Hiatus hernia 132; in overweight 86
High blood pressure 61, 63-4, 71, 151
High density lipoprotein (HDL) 96
Hip fracture, in osteoporosis 187
Hismanal (astemizole) 157, 223
Histamine 222-3
History, medical 24-8; own words 28
HIV (see AIDS) 276
Hives (papular urticaria) 143-4
Hoarseness 48
Holistic care 34
Holmes and Rahe, life adjustment scale 77-8
Holocrine glands 182
'Homebake' 252
Home calls 15, 20
Homeostasis 270
Homosexuality, as factor in alcoholism 109
Hormones, in breast cancer 72; thyroid 286; in menstruation 180
Hospitalisation 17
Hot flushes, treatment, precipitants 186
Hunger, with low blood sugar 271
Hydrallazine (Apresoline) 246
Hydrochloric acid, in stomach 258
Hydrocortisone 168, 219; on face 220; varying strengths 220; in asthma 154; pellets for mouth ulcers 124
Hydromorphone 253
Hygiene, relation to cancer of cervix 71
Hygroton 256
Hyoscine (scopolamine) patch 178
Hypercholesterolaemia 46
Hyperglycaemia, in diabetes 271
Hyperkeratosis, usual sites, treatment 165
Hypersensitivity 222
Hypertension 151, 243f; screening 52; with the pill 262; (see also High blood pressure and Blood pressure, high)
Hyperventilation (overbreathing), symptoms 79-80
Hypnotherapy 203
Hypnotic, definition 225, 252
Hypoglycaemia, in insulin coma 271
Hypothyroidism 19, 279; screening 64
Hysterectomy 269; for abnormal smears 70

Ibuprofen (Brufen) 219
Id 198

IDDM (insulin dependent diabetes mellitus) 272
Idoxuridine (Herplex, Stoxil) 160, 241
Illness, mental 23
Imipramine (Tofranil) 228
Immune reactions 223; lymphocytes 283
Impetigo (school sores) causes, treatment, nephritis 123, 158, 161
Implosive therapy 202
Impotence, in treatment of blood pressure 246; behavioural therapy 202; in alcoholism 108
Inactivity, as factor in coronary heart disease 44
Incontinence, in dementia 279
Indigestion 131; confused with heart attack 142
Indocid (indomethacin) 219
Indomethacin (Indocid) 219
Infection, see Bladder; with corticosteroids 221; as complication of diabetes 273; in causation of stomach ulcer 131; mixed in otitis externa 151
Infectious diseases 163, 288
Infectious mononucleosis (glandular fever) 83, 122, 163, 288; rash with amoxycillin 122
Inflammation 167; response to steroids 218-24
Influenza 82, 136; influenza A 241
Inhalations, nasal 211; in asthma 211
Inoculations, trivac, divac, polio, morbilli, tetanus, diphtheria, hepatitis B 43, 55-6, 59, 61, 63-4
Inositol nicotinate (Hexopal) 249
Inotropic action, with digoxin 254
Insight, in psychotherapy 198
Insomnia, sleeplessness 277
Insulin 270f
Intal (sodium cromoglycate) 157
Intercourse, lubricants 177
Intertrigo, treatment 165
Intellectual impairment 279; in PKU 70
Intermittent claudication 115, 249
Internal examination 175
Intra-uterine device (IUD) 267; effect on periods 174, 180
Inversine 246
Iodine, food sources 93
Iritis 179
Iron deficiency 282; screening for 52, 54; anaemia 171,181
Iron, food sources 101; normal values 285; high in haemochromatosis 285
Irritable colon 80f; irritable bowel 80f, 134; food allergies 81
Ismelin (guanethidine) 246
Isogel, method of use 82; in constipation 260; in irritable bowel 81, 134
Isophane (NPH) insulin 274

Isoprenaline 154
Isoptin (verapamil) 247, 257
Isordil (isosorbide dinitrate) 248
Isosorbide dinitrate (Isordil) 248
Isoxsuprine hydrochloride (Duvalidan, Defencin) 249
Ispaghula plant 81
IUCD (see Intra-uterine device) 174

Jaundice 131
Jogging 44
Joint problems 169f; use of anti-inflammatory agents 213-4; pain in rheumatic fever 122; warm-up 105
Juvenile diabetes 272

Kanamycin 240
Kaolin 178
Keflex 238
Keratin 182-3
Ketoconazole (Nizoral) 176, 242
Ketones 271
Ketoprofen (Alrheumat, Orudis, Oruvail) 219
Ketotifen, in asthma 155
Kidney damage, with tetracyclines 239
Kidney, disorders 69; failure 255; in hypertension 245; use of Hydrallazine 246; in heart failure 255; in diabetes 273; as cause of back pain 127
Kinins 222
Knee jerks 127
Koplik's spots 163
Kubler-Ross, Elizabeth 173
Kwells (scopolamine) 178
KY-jelly 177
Kyphosis 127

Laboratory tests 282f
Labyrinthitis (vestibular neuronitis) 147
Lactulose (Duphalac) 260
Largactil (chlorpromazine) 227
Larodopa (levodopa) 233
Laroxyl (amitriptyline) 228
Lasix (frusemide) 240, 256
Laxatives, action 80, 135, 260
Lederfen (fenbrufen) 219
Legionnaire's disease 240
Leukaemia, use of steroids 221, 241
Levodopa (Larodopa) 233
Librium (chlordiazepoxide) 227
Lice, types, treatment 162
Life events 77; positions in transactional analysis 200
Lifting, dangers to back 125; approved method 126
Ligament disorders, use of anti-inflammatories 168
Lightheadedness (see Faint)
Lignocaine, in heart irregularities 257
Liquid paraffin 260

Lipids, normal values, hyperlipidaemias 285
Lithium carbonate (Camcolit), use in depression 195, 230
Liver, disorders 109; use of aspirin 218; contraceptives 261; role in clotting disorders 284; effect on bilirubin 284
Liver spots 166
Locoid (hydrocortisone 17-butyrate) 220
Lomotil (diphenoxylate) 178
Loniten (minoxidil) 247
Loperamide (Imodium) 178
Lorazepam (Ativan) 227
Lordosis 127
Loss of interest, as symptom of depression 195
Loss, reactions to 173
Lotion 212
Low density lipoprotein (LDL) 96
Ludiomil (maprotiline) 229
Lung cancer, and smoking 75, 115
Lymphadenitis, causes 134
Lymphatic tissue 222
Lymph nodes, in streptococcal infection 122; in rubella 163; in AIDS 278
Lymphocytes 222, 283; glandular fever 283
Lyndiol 263

Macrocytes, in pernicious anaemia 283
Madopar (benserazide) 233
Magnesium, food sources 93; with digoxin 255; carbonate as antacid 258, 260
Magnesium hydroxide 260
Magnesium sulphate (Epsom salts) 260
Malnutrition 88
Mammography 73
Manic-depression 195, 231
Manipulation 125
Maprotiline (Ludiomil) 229
Marihuana 252
Marital reconciliation, as cause of stress 77
Marvelon 264
Marzine (cyclizine) 177
Mast cells 222; in asthma 152, 155, 158, 222
Mastoiditis 150
Mature adult, qualities 113
Maxolon (metoclopramide), in migraine 139, 250; for nausea 177
Mazindol (Sanorex) 231
Meals on wheels 37
Mean corpuscular volume (MCV) 283
Measles (morbilli, rubeola) 56–7, 163, 288
Mebhydrolin (Fabahistin) 157
Mecamylamine (Inversine) 246
Meclizine (Antivert) 149

Medical checks (see Screening)
Medical emergency 17
Medical ethics 18
Medical students 38
Medicines 204f
Mefenamic acid (Ponstan) 219; in premenstrual tension 182
Melleril (thioridazine) 227
Meniere's disease, symptoms 148
Menopause 16, 180–1, 185–7, 261
Menorrhagia 181
Menstrual problems 179f
Menstruation, mechanism 180; the contraceptive pill 265–6
Meperidine 253
Mestranol 261f
Metabolic system 27
Metamucil, in constipation 260; in irritable bowel 82, 134
Metastases (secondaries) from breast 72
Metformin (Glucophage) 272
Methadone 253
Methylcellulose 260
Methyldopa (Aldomet) 246
Methysergide (Deseril) 139, 250
Metoclopramide (Maxolon), use in migraine 139; in nausea 177
Metronidazole (Flagyl), for trichomonas 176, 240
Mexiletine (Mexitil) 257
Mianserin (Tolvon) 229
Miconazole (Daktarin, Gyno-daktarin) 175, 242
Microcytes 283
Microgynon 264
Microlut 264
Microval 264
Mictral (nalidixic acid) 241
Midamor 256
Migraine 137–9; treatment 178, 250; with the contraceptive pill 262
Milestones, early childhood 4 weeks to 2 years 68–9
Milk, tryptophane 228; effect on sleep 228; in gastro-enteritis 178
Minerals, in diet 93
Minidiab 272
Minipress (prazosin) 247
Minocycline 239
Minoxidil (Loniten, Regaine) 247
Miscarriage, after conization 70
Mites, house dust, as cause of allergy 157, 222
Mittelschmerz 268
Moditen (fluphenazine) 227
Mogadon (nitazepam) 227
Moisturiser, in atopic eczema 164
Mole, danger signs, treatment 166
Monilia (candida albicans), thrush 242
Mono amine oxidase inhibitors (MAOIs) 195, 229; foods to be avoided 230; medicines to avoid 230, 233
Monocytes, normal range 283

'Morning after' pill 268
Morning stiffness, in rheumatoid arthritis 170
Morphine 252
Motor vehicle accidents 44f
Mouth, cancer 115; screening for 63; ulcers 124
Movements, unwanted 233; disorders in schizophrenia 197
Mucus 25, 81, 156; in asthma 152; in cough 128
Multiphasic screening 50
Multiple myeloma 126
Multiple sclerosis 77
Mumps 288; inoculation 57
Muscle, pain and spasm 126, 137; in headache 138; cramps 126; tension 191
Muscular dystrophy, screening for 61–2
Musculo-skeletal system 26
Mycardol 248
Myocardial infarction (heart attack) 254; as cause of heart failure 129
Mycoplasma 239
Mycostatin (Nystatin) 176, 242
Myopathy 108
Mysoline (primidone) 232

Nalcron (sodium cromoglycate) 157
Nalidixic acid (Negram, Mictral) 241
Napkin (diaper) rash 164
Naprosyn (naproxen) 218
Naproxen (Naprosyn) 218
Narcotics, definition 252
Nasal congestion, in coryza 135, 156
Nausea, with Antabuse 112; with analgesics 253; with vertigo 147; causes 177
Navidrex 256; Navidrex K 256
Neck problems, as cause of headache 138–9
Negram (nalidixic acid) 241
Neogynon 264
Neomycin 240
Neonaclex 256
Nephritis, sore throat 122–3
Nephrosis 273, 287; use of steroids 221; cholesterol in 285
Nervous system 26; autonomic 245–6; effects of diabetes 273
Neulactil (pericyazine) 227
Neurodermatitis 78
Neutrophils 283
Newborn child 67
Nicotine, chewing gum (Nicorette) 117
Nicotinyl alcohol (Ronicol) 249
NIDDM (non insulin dependent diabetes mellitus) 272
Nifedepine (Adalat) 247–8
Nipples 68
Nitrazepam (Mogadon) 227
Nitrobid 248
Nitrofurantoin (Furadantin) 240
Nitrostat 248

Nizoral (ketoconazole) 242
Nocturnal enuresis (bed wetting) 230; use of tricyclics 230; urine infections 184, 203, 230
Non specific urethritis (NSU) 174, 185
Non steroidal anti-inflammatory drugs (NSAIDs) 126, 170, 222; effect on stomach 218; osteoarthritis 170; for period pains 219
Nor-adrenalin (nor-epinephrine) 245
Nordette 264
Nordiol 264
Nor-epinephrine (see Nor-adrenalin)
Nor-ethisterone 263
Nor-ethynodiol 263
Norgestrel 264
Noriday 263
Norinyl 263
Nortriptyline (Allegron, Aventyl) 228
Nose bleeding 282
Nose drops, method of use 211
NPH (Isophane) insulin 274
NSAIDs (non steroidal anti-inflammatory drugs) 170, 218
Nuelin (aminophylline) 154
Numbness 31; in back problems 127
Nurses, role 36
Nutrients, essential 93
Nutrition, screening for defects 61, 63–4
Nystatin (Mycostatin, Nilstat) 176, 242

Obesity (see Overweight) 84f
Occupational disorders 35
Oedema 85; with cortisone 219; in heart failure 255; in urticaria 144
Oesophagus (gullet), spasm 142; cancer in smokers 116; regurgitation 142
Oestrogens 96, 180, 260; deficiency 186
Oil of evening primrose 182
Operant conditioning 203
Ophthalmoscope, in evaluation of headache 139
Opium, derivatives 252; as cause of vertigo 148
Orciprenaline (Alupent) 154
Organ transplants, rejection 223
Orgasm 26
Orinase (see tolbutamide) 272
Ornidazole 176
Orphenadrine hydrochloride (Disipal) 234
Orudis (ketoprofen) 219
Oruvail (ketoprofen) 219
Osmotic pressure 260
Osteoarthritis (osteoarthrosis) 86, 170
Osteoporosis 125, 186, 220; screening 63–5; loss of height 187; use of oestrogen 187

Otitis externa, causes 151
Otitis media 136, 149, 151, 157
Otrivine 136
Otosclerosis, and the pill 266
Ovaries 71; in breast cancer 72
Overbreathing (hyperventilation) 79–80
Over-the-counter (OTC) medicines 215
Overweight 86; dangers 86; amphetamines 86; relation to insulin needs 270; intertrigo 165
Ovostat 263
Ovral 264
Ovulen 263
Oxazepam (Serepax) 227
Oxygen, oxygen deficiency 53

Pacemakers, in heart 254, 257; artificial 257; metal detectors 257
Paget's disease 284
Pain 31; description 24f; in chest 141; in abdomen 130; on urination (dysuria) 183; with periods (see Dysmenorrhoea); from osteoporosis 187
Palpitations 80; with digoxin 255
Pancreas ('sweetbreads') 270; in smokers 116; effect of alcohol 108; amylase in 284
Pancreatitis, effect on amylase 284
Panic attacks, in anxiety 191
Papanicolaou smear (Pap smear) 70
Papular urticaria (hives) 143
Paracetamol 136; in migraine 250; in pain 218, 252
Paraffin, liquid 260
Parathyroid, deficiency, cataracts 208
Parenting, problems, screening 52, 54–7
Parkinson's disease 227, 233; levodopa 233; carbidopa 233
Parlodel (bromocriptine) 233
Passive smoking, symptoms 116
Pathology 282
Payment 16–17, 42
Peak flow meter 153
Penicillin 237; allergy 123, 206; rash 143, 145; action on streptococci 123, 159; need for 10 days' treatment in streptococcal throat 123
Penicillinase 237
Penicillium notatum 236
Penis 26; discharge 185
Pentaerythritol tetranitrate (Peritrate) 248
Pentazocine (Fortral, Talwin) 253
Peptic ulcer (see Stomach ulcer) 131
Peptide T, in AIDS 276
Perforation, in stomach ulcer 131; in diverticulitis 135; of ear drum 150
Percussion, in exam of chest 129
Perhexiline maleate (Pexid) 248
Periactin (cyproheptadine), effect on appetite 258

Peri-anal haematoma 167
Pericarditis 142
Pericyazine (Neulactil) 227
Periods 179f; heavy in anaemia 181
Peritonitis 134
Peritrate (pentaerythritol tetranitrate) 248
Pernicious anaemia 283
Perphenazine (Trilafon) 149, 227
Personality, type A, type B 47
Perspiration, in intertrigo 165
Pessary, applicator, in fungal infection, method of use 210
Pethidine (Demerol, Meperidine) for pain 252–3
Petit mal 232
Petrolagar 260
Pexid (perhexiline maleate) 248
Pharmacopoeia 204
Phenformin 272
Phenobarbitone 232
Phenolphthalein, as laxative 260
Phenothiazines 227; in schizophrenia 197; in nausea 258
Phentermine (Duromine) 231
Phenylalanine, in phenylketonuria 69–70
Phenylbutazone (Butazolidine) 219; action on the pill 266
Phenylketonuria (PKU), screening for 54, 69
Phenytoin (Dilantin) 232; over-development of gums 232; in heart irregularities 257; with the contraceptive pill 266
Phobias 202
Pholcodine 129
Phosphonoformate, in AIDS 276
Phosphorus, food sources 93
Physiotherapists (physical therapists) role 38; in rheumatoid arthritis 171
Piles (haemorrhoids), causes 166–7, 259
Pill, the contraceptive 261f
Pipanol (benzhexol hydrochloride) 234
Pipe smoking 115
Pirenzepine (Gastrozepine) 259
Piroxicam (Feldene) 219
Pituitary gland 180; in anorexia nervosa 88
Pizotifen (Sandomigran) 139
Placebo, origin 209
Plasma 282; plasma cells 222
Plasmalyte-O 178
PMT (see Pre-menstrual tension)
Platelets, in polycythaemia, in thrombocytopaenia, normal levels 283
Pleurisy 142
Pneumonia 116, 135; respiratory depressants 253; as cause of breathlessness 156
Podiatrist 274
Poliomyelitis 61, 160

Pollen, as cause of allergy 157, 223
Polyarteritis nodosa 223; use of steroids 221
Polycythaemia vera, producing excess red blood corpuscles 282
Ponderax (fenfluramine) 231
Ponstam (mefenamic acid) 182, 219
Positive reinforcement 112
Post herpetic neuralgia 160
Post menopausal bleeding 186
Post nasal discharge 124
Post nasal drip 135
Postural hypotension, causes 148
Posture, as cause of muscle pain 126; backache 126
Potassium, food sources 101; with digoxin 255; with diuretics 256; slow K 256; in diabetes 271; normal values 285
Practice nurse 36; as counsellor 190
Prazosin (Hypovase, Minipress) 247
Prednisolone 171
Pregnancy, screening for diabetes (see Screening); emotional problems 66; termination 66; as cause of stress 77; vaginal discharge 174; tetracyclines 239
Pre-menstrual tension (PMT) 181-2
Prematurity, in smoking 107
Prescription 16; abbreviations 212f
Prevention 15; primary, secondary 42, 43, 47
Primary care 32, 35
Primidone (Mysoline) 232
Pritiken diet 97
Probenecid (sulphinpyrazone) 172
Procainamide (Pronestyl) 257
Prochlorperazine (Stemetil) 177, 227
Progestagen 180, 262; oestrogen-like effect 262; action in migraine 139
Progestagen-only pill, breastfeeding 265
Progesterone 180
Promazine (Sparine) 227
Pronestyl (procainamide) 257
Prostaglandins 182, 261
Prostate gland, cancer 125; cause of urine infection 184; with tricyclics 229
Prostatitis 185
Prostitution, risks 52, 54
Protein, in diet 84; recommendations 88; cause of allergy 94
Protein in urine (proteinuria) 287
Prothiaden (Dothiepin) 228
Prothrombin time, normal values, clotting disorders 286
Protozoa, trichomonas vaginalis 240
Protriptyline (Concordin) 228
Pruritus ani 167; worms 167
Psoriasis 164f
Psychiatric history 28
Psychiatrist, role 190
Psychoanalysis 198
Psychologist, role 190
Psychosis, features 196

Psychosomatic disease 78
Psychotherapy, definition, theories 198f
Public health measures 43
Pulmadil (rimiterol hydrobromide) 154
Pulse, thready 31; rapid with low blood sugar 271; in feet 274
Pus 159

Q fever 239
Quinine, as cause of tinnitus 148

Radiation, of cervix 71
Ranitidine (Zantac) 133, 259
Rash, penicillin 123; allergic 143; non-allergic 158
Rastinon (see Tolbutamide) 272
Rational Emotive Therapy (RET) 199
Raynaud's syndrome 247, 249
Rauwolfia, derivatives, Reserpine, Serpasil 246
Reality therapy 201
Rebound, with nasal sprays 136; with steroids 221
Receptionist, role 37
Records 15, 22
Rectum, exam in appendicitis 133
Red blood corpuscles (RBCs), microcytes, macrocytes, mean corpuscular volume 282
Referral 18
Regaime 247
Registration, of patients 19
Regular (soluble) insulin 274
Regurgitation, of stomach contents 258
Rehabilitation 38
Relationships, interpersonal, doctor-patient 19; impaired in schizophrenia 197
Relaxation, techniques 192
Renal calculus (stone), as cause of pain 130
Renal colic 130
Renin 247
Renitec (enalapril) 247
Repetitive strain injury (RSI) 168; treatment 168
Reserpine 246
Respiratory depression 155
Restovar 263
Resuscitation, cardiopulmonary 289
Retinoic acid (Retina A) 182
Retina 147, 247
Retirement, as cause of stress 63
Retrovir, in AIDS 276
Rh status, screening 52f
Rheumatic fever 122, 237; heart valves 122; penicillin 123-4; breathlessness 155; use of steroids 221
Rheumatoid arthritis 170-1
Rheumox (azapropazone) 209
Rhythmodan (disopyramide) 257

Rimiterol hydrobromide (Pulmadil) 154
Ringworm, of fingernails 161; (see Fungal infection) 241
Rodent ulcer (see Basal cell carcinoma) 165-6
Rogers, Carl 199
Rohypnol (flunitrazepam) 227
Ronicol (nicotinyl alcohol) 249
Roseola infantum 163
RSI (repetitive strain injury) 168
Rubella (German measles) 288; screening 52, 57, 60, 62; complications 163
Rynacrom (sodium cromoglycate) 157

'Safe period' 268
Salbutamol (Ventolin) 154
Salicylates, aggravating allergy 95, 144-5
Saliva 246
Salmonella 239
Salt (sodium chloride) 101, 149, 256; in diabetes 271
Saluric 256
Sandomigran (pizotifen) 139
Sanorex (mazindol) 231
Scabies, symptoms, cause of impetigo 158; sites, treatment, scabs 161-2
Scapegoating, in alcoholism 111
Scarlet fever 288
Schizophrenia, diagnosis, treatment, impaired relationships, pre-occupation, anxiety, speech abnormalities, movement abnormalities, 196-8
Sciatica 127
Sclerosants 167
Scoliosis 127
Scopolamine (Hyoscine, Kwells) 178
Screening 49f; World Health Organisation criteria 50; multi-phasic 50; Canadian Task Force 51; antenatal 51
Seborrhoeic dermatitis, cause 164
Seborrhoeic wart ('senile' wart) 166
Secondaries (metastases), in breast cancer 72
Secondary care 35
Second opinion 22
Sedation, definition 252
Selenium sulphide (Selsun) 164
Self esteem 199, 201
Self-examination, of breast 73
Self-test, for alcoholism 109-10
Selsun (selenium sulphide) 164
Semicircular canals 147
Semilente insulin 270
'Senile' wart (seborrhoeic wart) 166
Senna 80; senna pods 80; senna tea 260; Senokot 260
Sensitivity (see Allergy)
Septrim (cotrimoxazole) 238
Septum, nasal, deviated 158

Serepax (oxazepam) 227
Serpasil 246
Serotonin 222
Serum 282
Sexual development, screening for 60–1
Sexual difficulties, as cause of stress 77
Sexual intercourse, increased desire with testosterone 262; vaginal secretions during 269; spread of AIDS by 277
Shingles (herpes zoster) 159, 241; in AIDS 278
Shock, use of steroids 221
Shock treatment (ECT), for depression 196
Shortness of breath 31; causes 152
Short sight, operative treatment 146
Shortwave diathermy 126
Sickle cell disease (thalassaemia), screening for 62
Side-effects, of medicines 205
Sigmoidoscopy 179
Silk, as vaginal lubricant 177
Silver nitrate, eye drops 54
Sinemet (carbidopa) 233
Sinequan (doxepin) 228
Sinusitis 136, 157; and tonsillitis and bronchitis 129
Skin 26, 143, 158; tests for allergy 94, 222;
Sleep, disturbance 66; problems in depression 195
Sleeping tablets 225f
Sleeplessness, see Insomnia 227
'Slipped disc' 124
Slow K 256
Smears, cervical 70–1
Smoke-free week 117
Smoking 43f; screening 61; lung cancer 115; and the contraceptive pill 261; risk factors 115; lung disease 156; passive 116; effect on heart 114; influence on unborn 117; strategies to stop 117; taxation 117; substitutes 117; 'Kick the habit' regime 118; hints for quitting 119; effect on longevity 117; as cause of ulcer 116, 131
Sneezing, in nasal allergy 157
Social worker 37; as counsellor 37
Sodium cromoglycate (Intal) 157,222; in asthma 154
Sodium, food sources 101; normal values 286; effects of steroids 286
Sodium, in heart 254; bicarbonate as antacid 258
Sodium valproate (Epilim) 232
Soframycin (framycetin) 240
Solar urticaria 146
Sore, non healing 48
Sore throat 122
Sparine (promazine) 227
Spasm, of blood vessels 138
'Spastic colon' 134

Specialist, dilution of experience 32
Speech, disorders in schizophrenia 197
'Speed' 87, 231
Speculum, in exam of vagina 175
Spermicide 267
Sphygmomanometer 71, 244
Spina bifida, screening 52
Spinal abnormalities, screening 52
Spinal collapse, with corticosteroids 220
Spironolactone 256; action on the contraceptive pill 266
Spondylolisthesis 127
Sputum (phlegm) 116; in bronchitis 116; significance if discoloured 128
Staphylococci, in impetigo 158; cause of food poisoning 177
Starvation 180
Stelazine (trifluoperazine) 227
Stemetil (prochlorperazine) 177, 227
Sterilisation 269
Steroids 171–2, 219; injection 221; in urticaria 144; in osteoporosis 187; other conditions 221
Stethoscope, in exam of chest 129
Stomach, emptying time 139, 206; irritation 177; acidity 258; steroids in 219; cause of nausea 177
Stomach ulcer 131; in smokers 116; with aspirin 219
Stoxil (idoxuridine) 241
Straining, in constipation 166
Streptococci, beta-haemolytic, in sore throat 122; rheumatic fever 122, 237; nephritis 123; in impetigo 158; in psoriasis 164
Streptomycin 240; effect on inner ear 148
Stress 45f; list of causative agents 78; on menstruation 180
Stroke (cerebro vascular accident) 247, 273
Sucralfate (Carafate) 259
Suggestion, power of 209
Suicide 31, 66; in depression 195; in trigeminal neuralgia 232
Sulfinpyrazone (Probenecid), interference by aspirin 172
Sulindac (Clinoril) 219
Sulphonamide 235
Sulphonylureas (see Tolbutamide)
Sun, herpes simplex 160; psoriasis 164; prevention of osteoporosis 187; sunscreen 166; sunburn 220
Super-ego 198
Suppositories 210; in migraine 250; in haemorrhoids 167
Surgam (tiaprofenic acid) 219
Surmontil (Trimipramine) 228
Swab, for organisms 124
Swimming, for asthmatics 155
Symmetrel (amantadine) 234
Symptoms 24, 226
Synovial membrane, in rheumatoid arthritis 171

Synphasic 263
Syphilis 279; screening 52, 54–5; as cause of psychosis 196
Systemic lupus erythematosus (SLE), use of steroids 221
Systole 243-4

Tablets, swallowing 210
Tagamet (cimetidine) 133, 259; use in herpes zoster 160
Talc 165
Tambocur (flecainide) 257
Tantrums 68
Tartrazine, in allergies 95, 144
Taste, effect of ice 210
Tea 228, 231; as cause of acidity 131
Team 36f; patient as team member 39
Teeth, effect of mixture 210; staining with tetracyclines 239
Tegretol 232; use in post herpetic neuralgia 160
Teldane (terfenadine) 157
Temazepam (Euhypnos) 227
Temgesic 253
Temperature, possible use in fighting infection 136; danger when very high 137; in appendicitis 133; otitis media 151
Tennis elbow, use of steroids 221
Tension headache 137–8
Tenuate (diethylpropion) 231
Tepid sponging 137
Terbutaline sulphate (Bricanyl) 154
Terfenadine (Teldane) 157, 223
Tertiary care 35
Testicles, in renal colic 130
Testosterone, and progestagens 261–2
Tetanus, inoculation 43
Tetracyclics, use in depression 195, 229
Tetracyclines 239; in acne 183; in bronchitis 239; for chlamydia 176
Thalassaemia (sickle cell disease), screening for 62
Theodur (see Theophylline) 154
Theograd (see Theophylline) 154
Theophylline 154
Therapeutic community 112
Thioridazine (Melleril) 227
Thirst, in diabetes 271
Throat, cancer of 115; infections 122f; streptococci 122
Thrombocytopaenic purpura, use of steroids 221; platelets in 211
Thrush 124; with the pill 262; (see also Fungal infections)
Thyroid, function, screening for disorders of 54, 63–4; disturbed with lithium 231; normal values 286; symptoms 286
Thyroid hormone, effect on menstruation 180; deficiency 285; excess causing osteoporosis 187
Thyrotoxic stare 286

Thyrotoxicosis, digoxin in 257
Tiaprofenic acid (Surgam) 219
Ticonazole (Gyno-trosyd) 176
Tinidazole 176
Tinnitus, in Meniere's disease 148
Tiredness, as symptom of depression 195; in AIDS 278
Tissue rejection 223
Tobacco 114; (see also Smoking)
Tobramycin 240
Tocainide (tonocard) 257
Tofranil (Imipramine) 228
Tolazamide (Tolinase) 272
Tolbutamide (Rastinon, Orinase) 272
Tolectin (tolmetin) 219
Tolerance 225; with morphine 253
Tolinase 272
Tolmetin (Tolectin) 219
Tolvon (Mianserin) 229
Tonic 141
Tonocard (tocainide) 257
Tonsillitis, and post nasal drip 124
Toxaemia of pregnancy 51
Toxoplasmosis, screening for 53
Tracheotomy 144
Trade name vs generic name 213
Trancopal (chlormezanone) 227
Tranquillisers 194; in migraine 251; as tonic 141
Transactional analysis 200
Transference, in psychotherapy, counter-transference 198-9
Transfusion, in AIDS 277
Transient ischaemic attack (TIA) 247
Treatment 221, 216
Tremor, in Parkinson's disease 233
Triazolam (Halcion) 227
Triamterene (Dytac, Dyrenium) 256
Trichomonas vaginalis, as cause of vaginal infection, odour, mode of transmission 175-6, 240
Tricyclics, use in depression 195, 207, 228; side-effects 228, 258; prostate problems 229; rapid heart beat 229
Trifluoperazine (Stelazine) 227
Trigeminal neuralgia, suicide 232
Trilafon (perphenazine) 149, 227
Trimethoprim 238
Trimipramine (Surmontil) 228
Trinitrate, glyceryl trinitrate, (Anginine, Trinitrin) 248
Trinitrin (glyceryl trinitrate) 248
Triphasil 264
Tri-potassium di-citrato bismuthate (De-nol), effect on bacteria, dark bowel motions 259
Tryptanol (amitryptiline) 228
Tryptophan 230
Tuberculosis, screening 60, 62; tuberculin testing 75; BCG inoculation 75; as cause of cough 129
Tuberculin 60, 62, 65
Twins, screening for 53
Type A personality, and heart disease 47
Type B personality 47
Typhoid 239

Ulcerative colitis 94; steroids 221
Ulcer, of stomach 131; gastric 131, 258; duodenal 131, 258
Ultrasonics 126
Umine (phentermine hydrochloride) 231
Unconsciousness 31
Urea, normal value 286
Ureter 130
Urethra 130
Urethritis 185
Uric acid, normal value 286; in gout 172
Urine 55; dysuria 183; infection 207, 273; tests 286-7
Urine infection 184; symptoms 25; follow-up examination 184
Urticaria 94; causes 143; 'giant urticaria' 144
Uterus (womb) 70; in overweight 86

Vagina, infection 175; acid/alkali balance 242; use of vinegar 242; dry with progestagens 262; examination 175
Vaginal discharge, causes, symptoms, prevention 174f, 240
Valium (diazepam) 106, 149, 227, 232
Valves, of heart in rheumatic fever 237
Varicella (chicken pox), symptoms 163, 288
Varicose veins 86, 166; in alcoholism 108
Vas deferens 269
Vasodilators, in heart failure 255; in arterial disorders 245f
Velosef 238
Ventolin (salbutamol) 154
Ventricles, fibrillation 256-7
Verapamil (Isoptin) 247, 257
Vertigo, definition, causes 147-9
Vestibular neuronitis (labyrinthitis) 147
Vinegar, use in vaginal infections 242
Viral infection 135, 235; white cell response 283
Virus 235; AIDS 276
Visiting the doctor 23f
Vision 31
Visual problems 146

Vitamin C 94, 241; action on the pill 266; action on tests for blood in bowel motion 76
Vitamin D 93; prevention of osteoporosis 187
Vitamins 93-4; deficiency in alcoholism 109
Vitamin K1, screening for deficiency 53
Vivactil (protriptyline) 228
Volmax (salbutamol) 154
Voltaren (diclofenac) 219
Vomiting 177; with Antabuse 112; with analgesics 253; with vertigo 147

Wart, genital 71
Warm-up 169, 105
'Waterbrash' 82, 132
Water retention 85, 254-5
Wax, in ears as cause of cough 130; cause of vertigo 148
Weight gain, with corticosteroids 219; with the pill 262
Weightlessness, a cause of osteoporosis 187
Weight loss, diet 87; in AIDS 278
Well baby, care 32
Weight, loss of weight 278; reduction 87
Wheeziness, as cause of cough 128; in asthma 153
White blood cells 283; types, normal values 283
Whole person care 79; in alcoholism 111
Whooping cough 288
Wind (flatus) 81
Withdrawal 106; of medicines 226
Womb (see Uterus)
Work surfaces 126
Worms 167; eosinophils in 283; in appendicitis 133

Xanthopsia, with digoxin 255
X-rays, radiation hazards 51; breast cancer 73; barium meal 131
Xylocard 257

Yeasts 239
Yoghurt 239, 242

Zadine (azatadine maleate) 157
Zantac (ranitidine) 133, 259
Zarontin (ethosuximide) 232
Zasten (ketotifen) 155
Zidovudine (Retrovir) 276
Zovirax (acyclovir) 160, 241
Zyloprim (allopurinol) 172